Visit our website

to find out about other books from Churchi
and our sister companies in Harcourt Healtl

Register free at
www.harcourt-international.com

and you will get

- **the latest information on new books, journals and electronic products in your chosen subject areas**

- **the choice of e-mail or post alerts or both, when there are any new books in your chosen areas**

- **news of special offers and promotions**

- **information about products from all Harcourt Health Sciences' companies including Baillière Tindall, Churchill Livingstone, Mosby and W. B. Saunders**

You will also find an easily searchable catalogue, online ordering, information on our extensive list of journals...and much more!

Visit the Harcourt Health Sciences' website today!

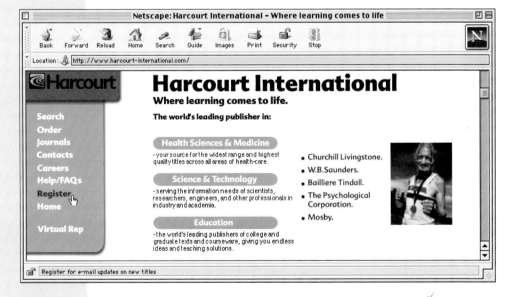

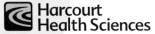

ESSENTIALS OF PATHOLOGY FOR DENTISTRY

Commissioning editor: Michael Parkinson
Project development manager: Barbara Simmons
Project manager: Nancy Arnott
Designer: Erik Bigland

ESSENTIALS OF PATHOLOGY FOR DENTISTRY

R F T McMahon BSc MD FRCPath
Senior Lecturer in Pathology, University of Manchester;
Honorary Consultant Pathologist, Manchester Royal Infirmary, Manchester

P Sloan BDS PhD FRCPath FDS RCS (Eng)
Professor of Experimental Oral Pathology, University of Manchester;
Honorary Consultant Oral Pathologist, Turner Dental School, Manchester

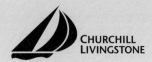

CHURCHILL
LIVINGSTONE

EDINBURGH LONDON NEW YORK PHILADELPHIA ST LOUIS SYDNEY TORONTO 2000

CHURCHILL LIVINGSTONE
An imprint of Harcourt Publishers Limited

© Harcourt Publishers Limited 2000

 is a registered trade mark of Harcourt Publishers Limited

First published 2000

ISBN 0443 057060

British Library of Cataloguing in Publication Data
A catalogue record for this book is available from the British
Library.

Library of Congress Cataloging in Publication Data
A catalog record for this book is available from the Library of
Congress.

Medical knowledge is constantly changing. As information
becomes available, changes in treatment, procedures, equipment
and the use of drugs become necessary. The author and publisher
have, as far as it is possible, taken care to ensure that the
information given in the text is accurate and up-to-date. However,
readers are strongly advised to confirm that the information,
especially with regard to drug usage, complies with current
legislation and standards of practice.

The
publisher's
policy is to use
**paper manufactured
from sustainable forests**

Printed in China

Preface

The curriculum in dental schools is in the process of evolution at present, within which the contribution of pathology is as vital as ever. However, such change inevitably presents an opportunity for re-evaluation of the ways in which we present traditional discipline-based subjects within an increasingly integrated course.

One of the newer methods of education being introduced in many undergraduate curricula is the Problem-Based Learning (PBL) approach which depends heavily on adult learning principles. Underpinning the PBL system is a sound knowledge base and the aim of this book is to provide the essential aspects of a traditional pathology undergraduate course within a PBL framework for students of dentistry and professions allied to dentistry.

This book is designed to cover the major aspects of general pathology which are essential for the understanding of disease processes, particularly with regard to inflammation and wound healing, neoplasia and vascular pathology. They have been supplemented by additional chapters on the genetic basis of disease, the principles of immunopathology and an introduction to microbiology. In addition, those aspects of systemic pathology of relevance to dental practice in its broadest sense, both general dental practice and hospital-based oral and maxillo-facial medicine and surgery, have been included. There is no intention in this book to provide the detailed aspects of oral pathology which are covered well elsewhere, although by the end of a course in general and systemic pathology as outlined in this textbook, students should be fully prepared for progression to an oral pathology course.

Each chapter contains a summary of the main pathological principles and specifically those of dental relevance. In the systemic pathology section, illustrative cases (or scenarios) are presented, in which clinical cases are used to accentuate various pathological principles by the insertion of directed questions at appropriate points. Later, suggested discussion points are provided. Student groups using the book would be expected to generate their own hypotheses and develop strategies for understanding the principles incorporated in the case. In addition, the cases described are designed to stimulate consideration of the pathological basis of disease alone, albeit within a clinical context, rather than a broader overview of the patient. Nonetheless this approach allows students to gain a deeper understanding of pathological processes within a patient based clinical environment. This book is based on the changes introduced into the Manchester dental undergraduate curriculum, where a wholly PBL approach is employed in year 1 and where a mixed PBL-traditional system is used in year 2, where the bulk of pathology learning takes place. This book can be used in either type of course but it is planned to be of particular benefit in curricula where some form of PBL will take place.

Manchester 2000   RFTM
                                                        PS

Acknowledgements

Contributors

This book could not have been produced without the help and encouragement of a large number of people.

We particularly wish to thank our wives and daughters for the time taken away from them in the preparation of this book.

We are immensely grateful to our illustrator Ray Evans for converting our ill-formed doodles into works of art. We would also like to thank our secretary, Irene Bohanna, for making sure that things got sent in a suitable format and our photographer, Jane Crosby, for her help with the photomicrographs.

We thank in particular our additional contributors for delivering (on time!) such excellent material on microbiology (Sujatha Panikker), on immunopathology (Tony Freemont) and, at very short notice, on genetics (Nalin Thakker).

Also, thanks are due to the surgeons Reg Kingston at Trafford General Hospital and Bob Pearson at Manchester Royal Infirmary.

Finally, we would like to thank the people at Churchill Livingstone who made this book happen: Mike Parkinson for suggesting the idea and Barbara Simmons for her tremendous patience and good humour.

N. Thakker BDS MSc PhD MRCPath
Senior Lecturer in Medical Genetics and Oral Pathology, University of Manchester, Honorary Consultant Oral Pathologist, Turner Dental School

A.J. Freemont BSc MD FRCP FRCPath
Professor of Osteoarticular Pathology, University of Manchester, Honorary Consultant Pathologist, Manchester Royal Infirmary

S. Panikker MB BS MSc DTM&H
Lecturer in Bacteriology and Virology, University of Manchester

Contents

BASIC PATHOLOGY

1 Cellular processes in pathology

CELLS IN DEVELOPMENT AND TISSUE MAINTENANCE

Morphogenesis

This is the process of embryological development by which tissues and organs develop their structural shape and form. It is a highly complex process and involves a series of genetically controlled events. Interactions between epithelium, mesenchyme, extracellular matrix and growth factors occur. Coordinated growth and differentiation of cells takes place and unwanted cells are eliminated by apoptosis (individual cell death).

Differentiation

This is the process in which cells develop a specialized morphology or function. It occurs in embryonic and adult life. Cells pass through several stages of differentiation and the process is due to selective expression of particular sets of genes. Fully differentiated cells may assume distinctive appearances, e.g. the acinar cell in a salivary gland possesses particular cytoplasmic membranes and organelles for its function, or a distinctive biochemistry, e.g. an endocrine cell producing a particular hormone.

Growth

This is the process of increase in size, generally applied in pathology to cells, tissues, organs, whole organisms and populations. Growth can be achieved by increase in cell number by mitosis, increase in cell size or by accretion of extracellular matrix. Combined patterns frequently occur during development and healing processes. Remodelling,

or tissue turnover, is also an important process in morphogenesis and tissue maintenance. Extracellular matrix remodelling is important in bone and soft tissues. Cell turnover occurs in many, but not all, tissues.

SUMMARY BOX
MORPHOGENESIS, DIFFERENTIATION AND GROWTH

- Morphogenesis: process of embryonic development determining shape and form of organ and individuals.
- Differentiation: process of cellular development leading to specialized morphology or function.
- Growth: increase in size; can be applied to cells, tissues, organs, organisms and populations.

Turnover of cells

Growth and tissue maintenance in adult life depends upon a balance between cell proliferation and cell death. In adult tissues, cells tend to lose their capacity to divide rapidly. Cells fall into three categories in relation to their regenerative capacity:

- *Labile cells* continue to divide rapidly and constantly throughout adult life. They have a short life span and are quickly replaced. Examples of labile cells include the epithelial cells of the oral cavity (which renew in around 5 days), gut, exocrine glands, urinary bladder and other linings. Labile cells are particularly susceptible to injury by radiation and cytotoxic drugs which target dividing cells. Dry mouth due to salivary gland damage and oral ulceration are common unwanted effects of these agents.
- *Stable cells* normally divide infrequently but cell loss

2

or injury stimulates rapid mitosis for regeneration. Examples of stable cells include those in bone, fibrous tissue, liver and kidney.

- *Permanent cells* cannot divide normally in adult life and therefore they are not replaced when lost or injured. Examples of permanent cells include cardiac muscle, skeletal muscle and neurons.

SUMMARY BOX
TURNOVER OF CELLS

- Growth depends on a balance of cell proliferation and death.
- Regeneration is the process of replacement of injured or dead cells.
- Cells may be labile, stable or permanent.
- Cell cycle is modified by growth factors and cyclins.
- Cell replacement occurs from the stem cell pool.
- Cell turnover is regulated by inhibitors and inducers of cell cycle (entry and activity) and apoptosis.

Cell cycle (Fig. 1.1)

The cell cycle comprises a short stage of cell division termed the M phase (mitosis) and a long intervening interphase which comprises S phase (synthesis of DNA), G_1 phase (gap between M and S phase) and G_2 phase (gap between S and M phase). Cells normally only enter S phase if they are committed to mitosis; non-dividing cells are in a resting phase termed G_0.

The DNA content of the cell doubles during S phase; each chromosome contains four DNA strands (DNA duplex) from towards the end of S phase to the end of metaphase in mitosis. After this point the 92 chromosomes formed are shared between the two daughter cells.

Quiescent cells are stimulated to enter the cell cycle by the actions of growth factors such as epidermal growth factor (EGF), insulin-like growth factors (IGF 1 and 2) and platelet-derived growth factor (PDGF). Cells may leave the cycle at G_1 by entering the resting G_0 phase or escape permanently by undergoing terminal differentiation. The G_1 phase may last for hours or days but the S, G_2 and M phases are fairly constant in duration.

Modulation of the cell cycle is achieved by cyclin proteins which phosphorylate various proteins involved in the cell cycle mechanism. Cyclin-dependent kinases can inhibit the action of cell cycle inhibitors such as the product of the retinoblastoma gene (pRb).

Injured or lost cells are replaced from the stem cell pool which acts as a reservoir of determined, but not differentiated, cells with the potential to renew the tissue population. When a stem cell undergoes mitosis, one daughter cell proceeds along a pathway of differentiation and the other retains stem cell characteristics. Stem cells are generally a small population within any given tissue and they often occupy a particular niche, e.g. the stem cells in the oral mucosa reside in the basal layer adjacent to basement membrane. Mutations in stem cells can be propagated whereas those occurring in terminally differentiating cells cannot.

The control of cell proliferation and its relation to wound healing and growth disorders is discussed in Chapter 6.

Apoptosis

Individual cell death, also known as programmed cell death or apoptosis, is a process of cell death quite distinct from necrosis. It is an energy-dependent process and has a role in embryonic development and control of tissue and organ size, e.g. in atrophy. Defective or unwanted cells can be deleted by apoptosis (Fig. 1.2). Factors which influence apoptosis include intracellular and extracellular factors.

- Apoptosis inducers include loss of attachment to matrix, growth factor reduction, glucocorticoids, viruses, free radicals, ionizing radiation, cytotoxic drugs and immune-mediated cytolysis.
- Apoptosis inhibitors include growth factors, attachment to extracellular matrix, sex steroids and certain viral proteins.

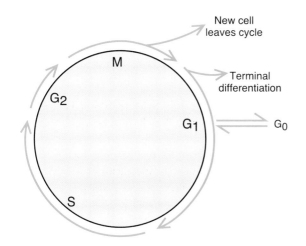

Fig. 1.1 Cell cycle. Schematic representation of cell cycle (see text for details).

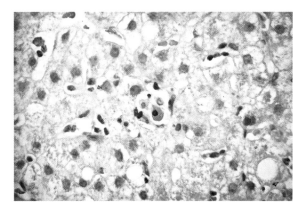

Fig. 1.2 **Apoptosis.** Section of liver from a patient with hepatitis C virus infection demonstrating an apoptotic body within the hepatic lobule. Note the eosinophilic cytoplasm and pyknotic nucleus.

Inducers or withdrawal of inhibitors activate a distinctive chain of events culminating in cell shrinkage and destruction. These events are mediated by endogenous proteases and endonucleases which cause fragmentation of DNA, degradation of cytoskeleton and loss of mitochondrial function. The cells shrink, develop an eosinophilic cytoplasm and eventually the cell membrane breaks down. Remnants may then be phagocytosed or break down into free apoptotic bodies. Unlike necrosis, where lytic enzymes liberated from the dead cells stimulate inflammation, apoptosis does not induce an inflammatory reaction.

Apoptosis is a fundamental process in many diseases, and alteration of apoptotic rate is thought to be important in a variety of conditions.

- Increased apoptosis contributes to the loss of cells in neurodegenerative disease and conditions where there is a low peripheral blood white cell count, such as the reduction in CD4 lymphocytes in AIDS. Viral proteins in HIV may activate CD4 and destroy uninfected cells. Apoptosis is also thought to play a role in cell loss after exposure to ionizing radiation.
- Reduced apoptosis leads to cell accumulation. Failure of inhibition of apoptosis may follow loss of p53 protein (which switches defective cells to apoptosis before mitosis) or increased expression of *bcl*-2 protein (which inhibits apoptosis). Defective cell accumulation is important in multistage carcinogenesis. It has also been suggested that apoptosis inhibition may contribute to autoimmune disease by failure to destroy cells directed against self antigens.

CELL INJURY

Causes

Various chemical, physical and biological agents are associated with cell injury. A number of common mechanisms operate and widely differing injurious stimuli may utilize similar pathways.

- Chemical agents include drugs, poisons, caustic chemicals and toxic gases. Drugs such as aspirin may cause local cell death and hence ulceration when held inappropriately in the mouth. Poisons act in a dose-dependent way and tend to exert their effects in a systemic fashion. Some are highly toxic metabolic inhibitors, some affect specific tissues such as nerve, or lung in the case of inhaled gases. Caustic agents, because of their marked acidity or alkalinity, cause local cell death rapidly. They also coagulate protein and corrode the tissue.
- Physical causes of cell injury include heat, cold, electrical charge, ionizing and ultraviolet radiation and mechanical trauma. Thermal and electrical trauma disrupt cells and denature proteins, leading to cell injury and death. In addition, secondary effects may occur owing to elimination of local blood supply. Ionizing radiation and ultraviolet radiation damage DNA, though free radicals generated can affect cell cytoplasm and membrane. Mechanical trauma also directly disrupts cells and can cause secondary effects by ischaemia through interference with blood supply.
- Infection causes cell injury by a variety of mechanisms. Often there is a metabolic product or secreted toxin which acts directly on the cells, e.g. bacterial products released from dental plaque can cause chronic inflammation of the gingivae. Intracellular infections may directly disrupt cellular processes. More often, damage is mediated by the inflammatory or immune response to the infectious agent.
- Immunological reactions to infection, autoimmunity and hypersensitivity reactions damage cells by a variety of mechanisms.

Mechanisms

- Blockage of specific metabolic pathways may occur as a result of the action of toxins and poisons. Respiration of the cell can be arrested, for example by cyanide which binds to cytochrome oxidase. Disruption of protein synthesis also compromises cell vitality and some antibiotics such as streptomycin and chloramphenicol can be toxic to cells in this way.

- Deprivation of essential metabolites is an important mechanism leading to cell injury. Glucose is an essential source of energy, and inadequate utilization of glucose in diabetes mellitus may damage CNS neurons, which have a high requirement for glucose. Oxygen is equally essential to cellular respiration, although anaerobic glycolysis can maintain viability for a short period. Shortage of oxygen resulting from reduced blood flow is termed ischaemia. Lack of blood flow leading to ischaemic necrosis is referred to as infarction. Sensitivity of cells to reduced oxygen is variable; neurons in the CNS can survive for a few minutes only. When the blood supply to the ischaemic area is restored, reperfusion injury may occur. This is thought to be due to the generation of free radicals. The injured cells are subsequently removed by apoptosis.
- Free radicals are highly reactive atoms or groups of atoms which are generated in tissues by ionizing radiation or oxidation–reduction reactions. Free radicals damage the polyunsaturated fatty acids which are essential to the integrity of the cell membrane. Oxygen toxicity, tissue damage in inflammation and the actions of some poisons are mediated by free radical damage to cell membranes. Antioxidant drugs are used to minimize such cell injury.
- Loss of membrane integrity also occurs when there is damage to ion pumps, leading to osmotic disruption of the cell. Agents which deplete ATP can cause lysis in this way. Damage to intramembrane channels, membrane lipids and cross-linking of membrane proteins all have serious consequences for the cell. The cytotoxic actions of activated complement and perforin are mediated by cell membrane damage.
- DNA damage is an important feature of ionizing radiation, chemotherapy and free radical generation. In rapidly dividing cells, injury or death may be immediate. Where cells survive, mutation may occur and can be passed on to the daughter cells.
- Trauma due to mechanical action, heating, freezing and laser application can disrupt cells causing leakage of cytoplasmic contents. Osmotic imbalance can also disrupt cells, for example in accidental injection of non-isotonic fluids.

Fatty and hydropic change

Fatty change is due to accumulation of lipid droplets in the cytoplasm. Alcohol and diabetes mellitus are common

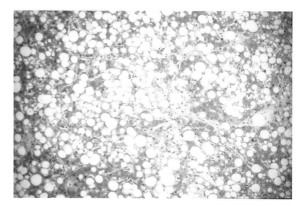

Fig. 1.3 Fatty change. Histological section of liver showing well-developed fatty change as a consequence of alcohol excess. Most of the hepatocytes are filled by a single droplet of fat.

causes of fatty change in the liver (Fig. 1.3). Damage to the cell is caused by disordered ribosomal function and uncoupling of lipid from protein metabolism. Mild fatty change is reversible but if the stimulus persists, then severe irreversible fatty change may develop.

Hydropic change is caused by fluid accumulation, and the cytoplasm of affected cells appears pale and swollen. It is the result of metabolic disturbance due to a variety of stimuli. Early change produces cloudy swelling and with further damage the cytoplasm becomes vacuolated. Hydropic change is generally reversible, but if the causative agent persists, then cell death may follow.

SUMMARY BOX
CELL INJURY

- Causes: trauma, chemical, physical, infection, immunological.
- Mechanisms: metabolic pathway blocks, deficiency of essential metabolites, free radicals, failure of membrane integrity, DNA damage and trauma.
- Reversible cell injury includes fatty and hydropic degeneration.

Amyloidosis

This is a condition where there is deposition of an abnormal extracellular fibrillar protein called amyloid. Physically, amyloid has a characteristic appearance of rigid straight fibrils in β-pleated sheets, producing hyaline pink staining on haematoxylin and eosin preparations. In Congo red stains, it has an orange-red appearance with a typical apple-green birefringence under cross-polarized light. Despite a typical physical manifestation, chemically the protein may be derived from a number of precursor amino acids and proteins. The two commonest are AL protein, light chains from immunoglobulins, especially in patients with multiple myeloma, and AA protein in patients with chronic inflammatory conditions, such as tuberculosis, bronchiectasis and rheumatoid disease, and some neoplasms, such as Hodgkin's disease. Some patients with inherited conditions, endocrine neoplasms and Alzheimer's disease and on haemodialysis may develop less common forms of amyloidosis. The protein may be deposited systemically in a variety of organs, especially the kidneys producing the nephrotic syndrome, spleen, liver and heart, or locally in response, for example, to pancreatic or thyroid tumours.

Fig. 1.4 Fat necrosis. Histological section of fatty tissue in which there is extensive inflammatory cell infiltration to the right of the section in response to necrotic fat.

Necrosis

Death of cells and tissue is referred to as necrosis. Many injurious stimuli, including ischaemia, trauma and metabolic upset, cause necrosis. Typically, necrotic cells undergo autolysis and leak enzymes into the surrounding tissues. Often this provokes an inflammatory response. Necrotic tissue may be removed by phagocytosis or be walled off. It should be noted that necrosis is a process distinct from apoptosis. Differing patterns of necrosis are recognized at the gross and microscopic level. The nature of the injurious stimulus and type of tissue involved determine the pattern of necrosis seen.

- *Coagulative necrosis* is the most frequently encountered type of necrosis and it may occur in any tissue. Protein coagulation occurs and cells retain faint outlines. At the outset, tissue texture will be normal or stiff. In certain circumstances, haemorrhage into the necrotic area will occur. With time, the area of coagulative necrosis will soften as a result of the action of enzymes released from polymorphs and macrophages. At this stage the necrotic tissue may disrupt, with severe effects in some organs.

  Microscopically, areas of coagulative necrosis show retention of their outline structure with loss of nuclear staining. Unfolding of protein causes the tissue to take up eosin dye strongly. Inflammatory cells are frequently seen, with polymorphs infiltrating in the early stages, and later the cells associated with organization and repair.
- *Colliquative necrosis* is seen in the brain and is the result of liquefaction of necrotic neural tissue, which lacks a substantial supporting extracellular matrix. A glial (CNS macrophage) reaction occurs around the area of liquefaction, walling it off and eventually forming a cyst. Vital, but injured, neuronal tissue surrounding the area may then resume function and this accounts for the recovery which sometimes follows strokes.
- *Caseous necrosis* is so called because of its cheese-like consistency. It is a characteristic but not pathognomonic feature of tuberculosis infection. Microscopically, it is structureless and it consists of eosinophilic amorphous material often containing fragmented cell nuclei. In tuberculosis, it is mainly formed from dead macrophages and tissue fluid in granulomas.
- *Fat necrosis* results from trauma to adipocytes which release their lipid content. This provokes an intense inflammatory reaction, and subsequent organization of the area leads to formation of a nodule (Fig. 1.4). Release of pancreatic lipase may provoke fat necrosis in acute pancreatitis.

Gangrene is putrefaction of necrotic tissue which may spread to involve adjacent vital tissue. It is most often associated with bacteria such as the clostridia. Breakdown of haemoglobin stains the gangrenous tissue black. Gangrene may complicate necrosis, particularly in the bowel where clostridia are common. Alternatively, infection by bacteria such as clostridia and bacteroides may result in putrefaction necrosis as a primary process in infected wounds.

CELL SENESCENCE AND AGEING

Multiple pathologies are common in the elderly and it is widely accepted that ageing involves an interaction of genetically determined cellular events and environment. Human cells are capable of around 50 divisions in culture (Hayflick limit), after which they undergo senescence and die. There are two principal theories of ageing:

- *Clonal senescence theory* suggests that there is an intrinsic genetic mechanism which determines life span. Evidence for this comes from cell culture experiments which suggest the presence of specific ageing genes on chromosome 1. Also, natural models of genetically determined premature ageing (progerias) in humans, such as Werner's syndrome and Down syndrome, provide evidence for the existence of ageing genes.

  Telomeric shortening has been proposed as one mechanism which may limit the cell's life span. Telomeres are located at the tips of each chromosome and are not fully copied prior to mitosis. At each cell division the telomeres are shortened until further replication is impossible. Only germ and embryonic cells show telomeric replication by the enzyme, telomerase.

- *Replication senescence theory* suggests that 'wear and tear' leads to accumulation of sublethal cellular damage. Toxic by-products of metabolism, protein cross-linking, DNA mutation, loss of DNA repair mechanisms and peroxidation of cell membranes have all been proposed as possible cumulative defects. The replication senescence theory suggests that 'wear and tear' eventually leads to failure of critical tissues, e.g. neurons and cardiac muscles cells, which lack regenerative ability.

Environmental and genetic factors appear to play a role in cell ageing. The clonal and replicative senescence theories are not mutually exclusive.

SUMMARY BOX
CELL AGEING AND DEATH

- Necrosis: death of tissue following irreversible injury; often involves areas of tissue.
- Apoptosis: individual (programmed) cell death; may be part of embryonic development, physiological or pathological cell turnover.
- Clonal senescence theory of ageing proposes an intrinsic genetic mechanism.
- Replicative senescence theory suggests 'wear and tear' causes accumulation of cellular damage.

2 Genetic basis of disease

INTRODUCTION

This chapter deals with three principal points:

- the different consequences of genetic aberrations in the germ cells (sperm and ova) and somatic cells (all other cells)
- what sort of aberrations occur in our genetic material (genotype)
- how these genetic changes result in identifiable biological traits (phenotype).

Readers should already be familiar with the structure and function of chromosomes, the structure of DNA, meiosis, mitosis and protein synthesis. The aim of this chapter is to provide an overview of the mechanisms in molecular pathogenesis with reference to relevant examples. Details of clinical conditions are not provided. Instead the reader is referred either to the On-line Inheritance in Man (OMIM; http://www3.ncbi.nlm.nih.gov/Omim), which is a catalogue of all known inherited conditions.

Diseases can be either environmental or genetic in origin or, more commonly, due to an interaction between the two. Ignoring any diseases that can be considered purely environmental in origin, the genetic influence in disease can occur at several levels. At one end of the spectrum we have conditions that are considered to have a purely genetic aetiology. These include the classical familial conditions such as haemophilia that are due to defects in single genes. These conditions, also known as single gene – or Mendelian – disorders, are relatively rare. At the other end of the spectrum, are the relatively common multifactorial conditions such as cardiovascular disease, diabetes, non-syndromic cleft lip and palate, etc. that are due to the interaction of environment with a gene or, more likely, multiple genes. In between these extremes we can have conditions that are polygenic, i.e. involve many genes, each contributing to a greater or lesser extent to the final phenotype. Also, in some ways, environmental factors play a part in what we consider as purely genetic conditions. For example, in phenylketonuria, an autosomal recessive condition caused by deficiency of phenylalanine hydroxylase, there is failure of conversion of phenylalanine to tyrosine. As a result of this there is accumulation of phenylalanine in the tissues, which leads to mental retardation in early childhood. By restricting dietary phenylalanine (complete avoidance of phenylalanine is not possible because it is an essential amino acid) from a very early age, mental retardation can be avoided.

Finally, when considering the genetic basis of disease, we must remember that DNA is not only found in the nucleus of a cell but is also present in the mitochondria, and mutations of this DNA are also associated with certain familial diseases.

Changes in the genetic material arise either through errors that occur during replication or because of exposure to some environmental genotoxic agent. These errors are normally detected by the cell's DNA repair system and corrected. However some errors persist because the cell is either not capable of repairing certain types of changes or just fails to correct them correctly or at all. It is important to appreciate that errors/accidents can occur anywhere in the 600 million bases of the DNA arranged in the 46 long molecules. This contains 80,000 genes but these only make up 3% of the total sequence.

The different consequences of genetic aberration in germ cells and somatic cells

Germ cells

The genetic constitution of any individual is the sum of the genetic material of the sperm and ova from which that individual is derived. Thus, any genetic change in a germ cell is also present in all cells (i.e. constitutively) in the individual derived from that germ cell. Also, once a genetic change is present constitutively in any individual, it is then possible for it to be passed on to the next generation through that individual's germ cells (see below).

Somatic cells

When there is a change in genetic material of a somatic cell, the change is only passed to the daughter cells resulting from mitotic division of the cell. All other cells in the body are normal. However, the extent of tissues affected will depend on when the change occurs.

If, for example, change occurs after development, only a limited number of cells will carry the genetic change and the disease will not be passed on through the germ cells to any offspring. This is what happens in sporadic (non-familial) cancers (see Ch. 6).

If there is a change in genetic material of one of the cells in the early post-conception cell divisions, then a much larger proportion of cells in the body (all derived from that one cell) will also carry the same change. Such an individual is in effect a somatic mosaic, i.e. has two types of cells each with slightly different genetic constitution. If some of the germ cells are derived from the cell with the genetic change, then the individual also has germ line mosaicism and is at risk of passing the condition to his or her offspring. Germ line mosaicism can also occur without accompanying somatic mosaicism if mutation has occurred in one of the precursor cells of the gamete during development.

Meiosis

To understand the nature of the chromosomal changes and also inheritance of disease, the reader needs to have a very clear understanding of the process of meiosis. Essentially, it is cell division that is used to generate haploid gametes from diploid precursor cells. Thus, unlike mitosis (Fig. 2.1A), where each daughter cell is identical to the parent cell, the daughter cells in meiosis (gametes) have half the number of chromosomes of the parent cell (Fig. 2.1B). It occurs over two phases.

The key features of the first phase (meiosis I) are:

1. The DNA duplicates in the diploid precursor cell, giving a cell with twice the diploid content with each chromosome consisting of two sister chromatids.

2. Homologous (the maternal and paternal copy) chromosomes align as a pair (synapsis) during this process; exchange (cross-over or recombination) of material takes place between the homologous chromosomes. The result is that each chromosome consists of a patchwork of paternal and maternal genetic material. This is important for increasing genetic diversity.

3. There is an independent segregation of the maternal and paternal chromosomes to each of the daughter cells, i.e. each cell randomly receives either the maternal or the paternal copy of every chromosome. Thus, a cell may have paternal copies of chromosome 1, maternal copies of chromosomes 2 and 3 and so on.

4. The daughter cells consist of 23 chromosomes but have diploid DNA content because each chromosome consists of two sister chromatids.

The essential features of the second phase (meiosis II) are:

1. There is no further DNA duplication.

2. There is a symmetrical distribution of the genetic material, one of the two sister chromatids that make up each chromosome going to each of the two daughter cells.

3. Each daughter cell has 23 chromosomes and a haploid DNA content.

On fertilization, two haploid gametes fuse to form a diploid conceptus which has:

- two copies of every autosomal chromosome (or autosome; chromosomes 1 to 22)
- if female, two copies of the X chromosome
- if male, a copy each of the X and Y chromosomes.

So, each normal individual has two copies of every autosomal gene. Females, in addition, have two copies of genes on the X chromosome and males have one set each of X and Y chromosome genes.

HOW DO CHANGES IN THE GENETIC MATERIAL CAUSE DISEASE?

We can consider this question in two parts: (1) what sort of changes occur in the genetic material and (2) what are their consequences?

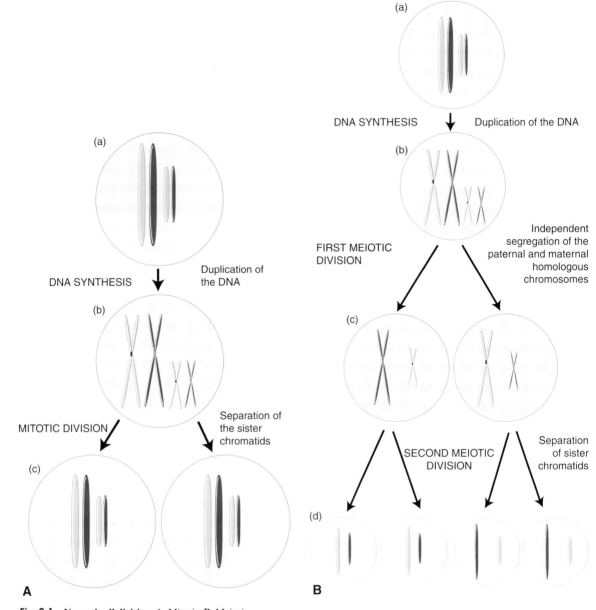

Fig. 2.1 **Normal cell division. A.** Mitosis. **B.** Meiosis.

Genetic aberrations can be:

- gross: occurring at the chromosomal level, resulting in abnormalities of numbers or structure of chromosomes, or
- subtle: occurring at the molecular level, resulting in alterations in the DNA sequence.

Chromosomal changes

Chromosomal abnormalities are relatively common. They are estimated to be present in approximately 7.5% of conceptions. However, it is likely that a majority of the fetuses with such abnormalities undergo spontaneous abortion as such abnormalities are seen in only 0.5% of newborns. Consistent with this is the observation that 50% of early spontaneously aborted fetuses and 5% of late spontaneously aborted fetuses or stillborn babies have chromosomal abnormalities.

Abnormalities of chromosomes can be structural or numerical.

Numerical abnormalities of chromosomes

- Normal germ cells (sperm and ova) have a haploid chromosomal constitution, i.e. 23 chromosomes (often referred to as N). Any exact multiples of N are referred to as euploid. A normal somatic cell (i.e. all cells other than germ cells) has diploid or 2N chromosomes.
- Polyploidy is a state in which cells have chromosomes in multiples of N greater than 2N, e.g. a triploid cell has 69 chromosomes (3N).
- Aneuploidy is a state in which there is a variation in the number of chromosomes that is not in multiples of N. For example, an extra copy of a particular chromosome is referred to as trisomy of that chromosome (e.g. trisomy 21, Down syndrome), and loss of a copy of a chromosome is referred to as monosomy of that chromosome. All complete monosomies of autosomal chromosomes are lethal, although partial monosomies may be observed in unbalanced translocations (see below). The only complete monosomy that is not lethal is that of the X chromosome and this presents as Turner syndrome.

Polyploidy. Triploidy is the commonest form of polyploidy and usually results in a miscarriage of the fetus. Triploidy arises by:

- fertilization of an egg by two spermatozoa (dispermy), or
- failure of maturation of the egg or sperm resulting in a diploid gamete.

Tetraploidy arises from failure of completion of the first zygotic mitotic division and is incompatible with life.

Aneuploidy. This can result from:

- nondisjunction – failure of chromosomes or sister chromatids to separate at anaphase in cell division
- anaphase lag – delayed movement of chromosomes after separation at anaphase.

The end result of either nondisjunction or anaphase lag during meiosis or mitosis is one daughter cell with an extra copy (disomic) and the other daughter cell lacking a copy of the affected chromosome (nullisomic) (see Figs 2.2, 2.3 and 2.4).

Consequences of meiotic nondisjunction involving an autosome. Fertilization of a disomic gamete results in a trisomic zygote, whilst fertilization of a nullisomic gamete results in a monosomic zygote (Figs 2.3 and 2.4). Zygotes monosomic for autosomes are non-viable. The commonest trisomy observed is that of chromosome 21 (Down syndrome) and this, in most cases, arises from nondisjunction in the first division of meiosis in oogenesis in the mother.

Consequences of meiotic nondisjunction involving sex chromosomes. This depends on whether the nondisjunction occurs in oogenesis or spermatogenesis and

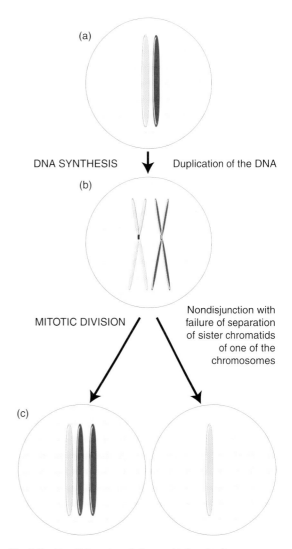

Fig. 2.2 **Nondisjunction of chromatids in mitosis.**

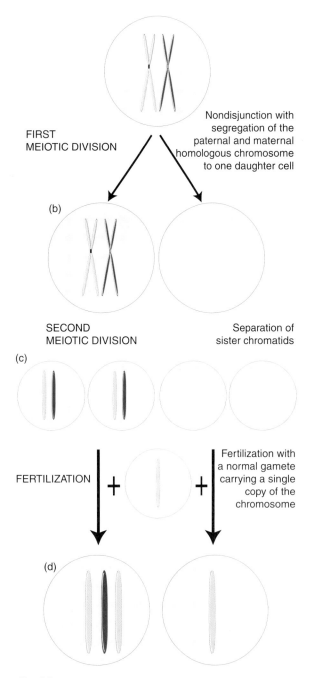

Fig. 2.3 Nondisjunction of chromosomes in the first meiotic division.

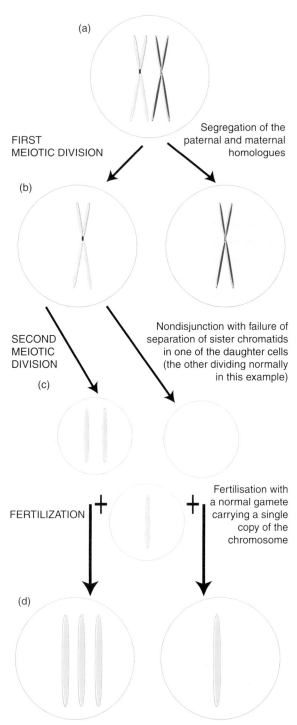

Fig. 2.4 Nondisjunction of chromatids in the second meiotic division.

also on the stage of meiosis in which it occurs. The end result is abnormalities of numbers of sex chromosomes, some of which are associated with distinct phenotypes characterized by sexual immaturity in females (Turner syndrome) or males (Klinefelter syndrome).

Nondisjunction in either stage of meiosis in oogenesis can result in gametes that have two copies of the X chromosome (disomic) or no copies of the X chromosome (nullisomic). Fertilization of the disomic ovum with an X chromosome-bearing sperm can result in a zygote with trisomy of X, whilst fertilization with a Y chromosome-bearing sperm will result in a zygote having XXY genotype (Klinefelter syndrome). Fertilization of the nullisomic gamete with an X chromosome-bearing-sperm can result in a zygote with monosomy of the X chromosome (Turner syndrome), whilst fertilization with a Y chromosome-bearing sperm will result in a zygote having monosomy of the Y chromosome (YO genotype) which is lethal to the embryo.

Nondisjunction in either stage of meiosis in spermatogenesis can result in gametes that have two copies of the X or the Y chromosome (disomic) or no copies of the X or the Y chromosome (nullisomic). Fertilization of a normal ovum by a sperm disomic or nullisomic for the X chromosome will result in XXX or XO genotypes respectively. Fertilization of a normal ovum by a sperm disomic or nullisomic for the Y chromosome will result in XYY or XO genotypes respectively.

Nondisjunction or chromosome lag in mitosis can also give rise to trisomic and monosomic cells (Fig. 2.2). The trisomic cell will give rise to trisomic daughter cells by further mitotic division, whilst the monosomic cell will not persist. All other cells proceed normally with their divisions giving rise to disomic daughter cells. Thus the individual in whom this occurs will be a mosaic consisting of two genetically different types of cells (disomic and trisomic). This is only likely to be significant in terms of phenotypic changes if it occurs in the mitotic division of one of the cells in the early embryo so that a substantial proportion of cells in the individual are trisomic.

Structural abnormalities of chromosomes

These result from chromosome breakage and usually involve one or two chromosomes. The chromosome breakage can be spontaneous. However, the rate of breakage can be markedly increased by exposure to mutagenic agents such as ionizing radiation and certain chemicals. The rate is also increased in certain inherited conditions with defects of DNA replication and repair, e.g. Bloom's syndrome.

Several types of structural abnormalities are observed. Those involving a single chromosome include:

- deletions – loss of a part of a chromosome
- inversions – inversion of a segment of a chromosome

which may (pericentric inversion) or may not (paracentric inversion) involve the centromere

- duplications – duplication of a chromosomal segment in tandem or in inverse configuration with the original sequence
- isochromosome – duplication of one arm of the chromosome coupled with loss of the other arm so that the chromosome consists of two identical arms.

Chromosomal structural aberrations involving more than one chromosome include the following:

- insertions – breakage of material from one chromosome and insertion into another chromosome
- translocations – exchange of material between two chromosomes.

Translocations are of two major types (Fig. 2.5A and B):

- reciprocal translocation – reciprocal exchange of material between two chromosomes
- Robertsonian translocations – these only involve acrocentric chromosomes (chromosomes with very small short arms: chromosomes 13, 14, 15, 21, 22).

The exchange of material usually does not involve loss of significant material. Individuals with such balanced translocations do not have any phenotypic effects unless, rarely, the translocation actually disrupts a gene or genes (see examples above). However, such individuals are at increased risk of having unbalanced gametes because of altered pairing in meiosis (Fig. 2.5). Fertilization of an unbalanced gamete results in a conceptus with an unbalanced chromosomal constitution (Fig. 2.5).

Consequences of chromosomal abnormalities

The phenotype in individuals with chromosomal abnormalities depends on the extent of the abnormality, i.e. whether it involves a single gene, a small group of genes or large regions of chromosomes with many genes.

Structural aberrations could disrupt a single gene leading to loss of its product (e.g. neurofibromatosis type I gene), translocate it to a region of active chromatin domain so that it is inappropriately expressed (e.g. *myc* in Burkitt's lymphoma) or create a chimaeric gene that expresses an altered protein (e.g. ABL in chronic myeloid leukaemia).

Where there is deletion of a small group of genes, the resulting phenotype can be attributed to the lack of product of several genes and is referred to as contiguous gene syndrome.

Chromosomal abnormalities involving large regions (e.g. large deletions) or whole chromosomes (missing or

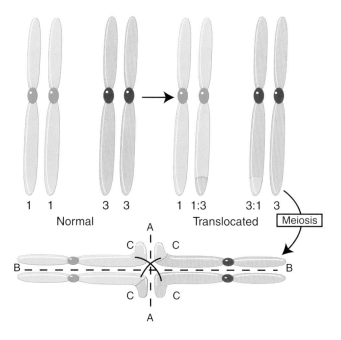

Segregation can occur along planes A or B, or alternative pairing may occur as indicated by C.
Gametes resulting from this are:

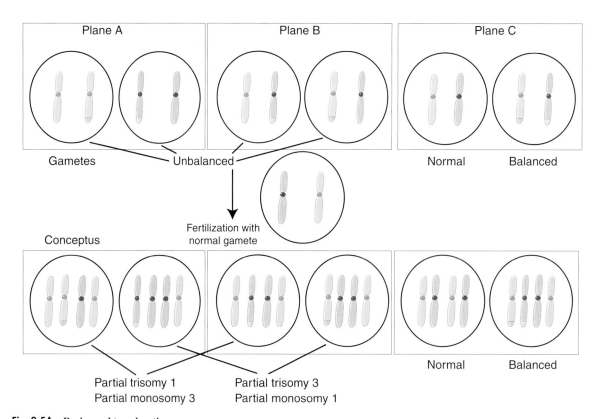

Fig. 2.5A Reciprocal translocation.

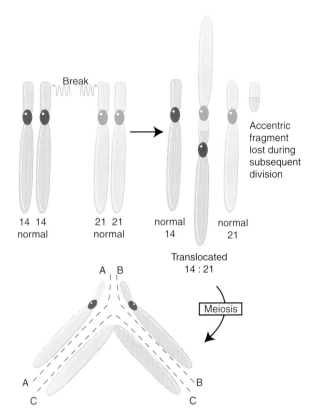

Segregation can occur in planes A, B or C generating gametes with different genetic constitution

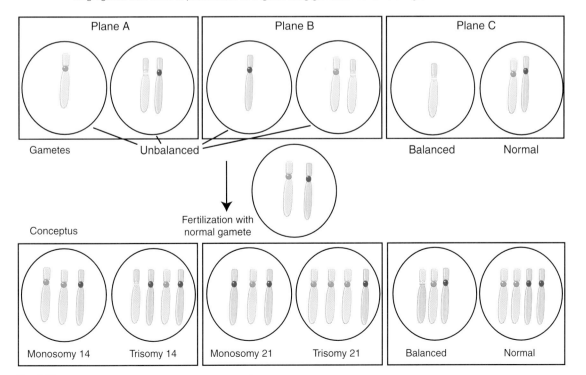

Fig. 2.5B Consequences of Robertsonian translocation.

extra chromosomes) generally result in severe birth defects, the general features of which often include mental and growth retardation together with more specific abnormalities. The main phenotypic changes that occur because of an extra copy of a chromosome or a lack of one chromosome are largely due to dosage imbalance of only a few genes of those chromosomes. For most genes, having an extra copy of the gene which results in 50% increase in its product is unlikely to be significant. Similarly, for most genes, a lack of one copy of the gene and consequent 50% reduction in protein is also unlikely to be significant.

SUMMARY BOX
CHROMOSOMAL ABNORMALITIES

- Chromosomal abnormalities are common, often resulting in spontaneous abortion.
- They may be numerical or structural.
- Numerical abnormalities may be polyploid (multiples of N = 23), resulting from dispermy or failure of maturation, or aneuploid, resulting from nondisjunction or anaphase lag.
- The major effects of numerical abnormalities may be caused by dosage imbalances in a few identifiable genes.
- Structural abnormalities result from chromosome breakage and include deletions, inversions, duplications, isochromosome, insertions and translocations.
- The consequences of structural abnormalities depend on the extent of abnormality.

Molecular changes

Molecular changes can abolish or modify normal gene function by:

- structural changes or mutations, or
- non-structural changes such as methylation.

Mutations

These may involve a single nucleotide (point mutations) or larger segments of the DNA. The sequence can be altered in a variety of ways (Fig. 2.6):

- Silent point mutation – change of a single nucleotide which does not result in change of the amino acid coded by a codon.
- Missense mutation – change of a single nucleotide which does result in change of the amino acid specified by a codon. The missense change can be conservative or non-conservative, i.e. replacement by an amino acid which is chemically similar or dissimilar respectively.

- Nonsense mutation – change of a single nucleotide which results in a change of codon specifying an amino acid to a termination codon.
- Insertion/deletion – insertion or deletion of one or more nucleotides in the normal sequence. If insertion or deletion involves nucleotides in multiples of three, then the reading frame is maintained and results in the addition or removal of amino acids in the final protein sequence.
- Frameshift mutation – insertion or deletion of nucleotides not in multiples of three resulting in shift in the reading frame. Translation of this sequence results in an altered amino acid sequence beyond the mutation; also, depending on the position of a stop codon in the altered sequence, the protein may be longer or shorter than the normal protein.
- Splice mutation – changes in the sequence at the intron–exon border or in the introns, leading to aberrant splicing and resulting in altered exons or exon skipping (Fig. 2.7).
- Expansion of trinucleotide repeat sequences – expansion of tandem nucleotide repeats within or outside the coding sequence is observed in a number of hereditary neurological conditions. This can result in an altered protein (e.g. in Huntington's disease) or in inhibition of transcription of the gene (e.g. fragile X) respectively.

Methylation

Structural changes in the sequence are not the only way to abolish gene function. Another way in which gene transcription can be switched off is by methylation of nucleotide bases, particularly cytosine. Many genes often have in their promoter regions a sequence that is rich in the dinucleotides cytosine (C) and guanine (G) linked together by cytosine 3′ and guanine 5′ phosphodiester bonds. These sequences are known as CpG islands. Methylation of CpG islands associated with a particular gene results in repression of the transcription of that gene and, under normal circumstances, provides a way for regulating the expression of genes.

However, this mechanism of switching off the expression of a gene is also often observed in pathological conditions. For example in cancer, tumour suppressor genes (see Ch. 6) such as those coding for cyclin-dependent kinase inhibitor 2A (CDKN2A or p16INK4a) and retinoblastoma (Rb) are often inactivated by methylation of CpG islands in their promoter regions.

In some cases, mutations or chromosomal abnormalities involving genes with unusual methylation patterns

Normal DNA sequence:	TTT	TCA	CCC	ACC	AAT	GTG	AAG
Normal amino acid sequence:	F	S	P	T	N	V	K

(F: phenylalanine, S: serine, P: proline, T: threonine, N: asparagine, V: valine, K: lysine)

SILENT POINT MUTATION

Altered DNA sequence:	TTT	TCG	CCC	ACC	AAT	GTG	AAG
Amino acid sequence	F	S	P	T	N	V	K

Change in one nucleotide (A to G) but no change in amino acid coded for by the altered codon

MISSENSE MUTATION

Altered DNA sequence:	TTT	CCA	CCC	ACC	AAT	GTG	AAG
Altered amino acid sequence:	F	P	P	T	N	V	K

Change in the amino acid coded for by the altered codon (serine to proline)

NONSENSE MUTATION

Altered DNA sequence:	TTT	TGA	CCC	ACC	AAT	GTG	AAG
Altered amino acid sequence:	F	X	P	T	N	V	K

Codon (TCA) for an amino acid (serine, S) altered to a stop codon (TGA) leading to premature truncation (X) of the protein

IN-FRAME INSERTION OF NUCLEOTIDES

Altered DNA sequence:	TTT	TCA	CGA	CCC	ACC	AAT	GTG	AAG
Altered amino acid sequence	F	S	R	P	T	N	V	K

Insertion of nucleotides (CGA) in a multiple of three resulting in maintenance of the reading frame and insertion of one extra amino acid (arginine, R) in the protein

DELETION OF NUCLEOTIDES IN MULTIPLES OF THREE (IN-FRAME)

Altered DNA sequence:	TTT	CCC	ACC	AAT	GTG	AAG
Altered amino acid sequence:	F	P	T	N	V	K

Deletion of nucleotides (TCA) in a multiple of three resulting in maintenance of the reading frame and deletion of one amino acid (serine, S) in the protein

FRAMESHIFT DELETION MUTATION

Altered DNA sequence:	TTT	TCC	CCA	CCA	ATG	TGA	AG
Altered amino acid sequence:	F	S	P	P	N	X	

Deletion of a single nucleotide (A) causing a frameshift resulting in alteration of the amino acid sequence downstream from the mutation and introduction of a premature stop codon (TGA)

FRAMESHIFT INSERTION MUTATION

Altered DNA sequence:	TTT	TTC	ACC	CAC	CAA	TGT	GAA	G
Altered amino acid sequence:	F	F	T	H	G	C	G	

Fig. 2.6 Mutations. Silent point, missense, nonsense, in-frame insertion, in-frame deletion, frameshift deletion and frameshift insertion mutations.

can cause disease. For most genes, both alleles (paternal and maternal) are expressed. However, for some genes, only one allele is expressed (monoallelic expression). This occurs by methylation and transcriptional silencing of one copy of the gene. For example, genes on one of a pair of X chromosomes in females are transcriptionally silenced by methylation in the process of Lyonization so that males (with their single X chromosome) and females have the same dosage of products of chromosome X genes. Monoallelic expression is also observed in other situations. In some cells, only the paternal allele or the maternal allele of certain genes is expressed; this process is known as genomic imprinting. Disease can result if, by chance, the gene that is normally expressed in a cell suffers an inactivating mutation or if there is uniparental disomy. This occurs where, instead of receiving one of a pair of homologous chromosomes from the father and the other from the mother, an individual receives both from the same parent. An interesting example of such a mechanism causing disease is deletion of an imprinted region

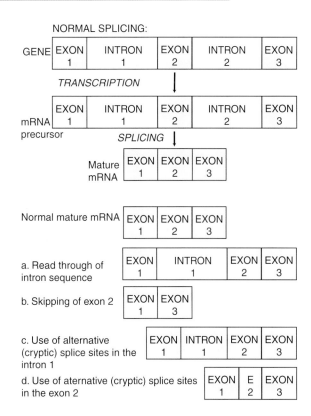

Fig. 2.7   Normal transcription and mRNA splicing. Mutations altering the splice sites at exon–intron borders may cause various errors in splicing which result in (a) inclusion of an intron ('read through') or (b) exclusion of an exon ('exon skipping') in the mature mRNA. Such mutations can also result in the use of alternative (cryptic) sites in either an intron (c) or an exon (d), leading to inclusion of some of the intronic sequence or exclusion of some of the exonic sequences in the mature mRNA. Mutations not affecting splice sites but creating new splice sites could also have the same effect.

on chromosome 15q12. Within this domain there are genes which show opposite patterns of imprinting, i.e. some are only expressed if derived from the mother and others are only expressed if derived from the father. Deletion on the chromosome inherited from the father or uniparental disomy where both chromosomes 15 are from the mother results in the Prader–Willi syndrome which is characterized in infancy by hypotonia, moderate mental retardation, hypogenitalism (in boys) and, later in childhood, additionally by obesity. In contrast, deletion in this region of the maternally derived chromosome 15 or uniparental disomy where both chromosomes 15 are derived from the father results in the Angelman syndrome which is characterized by mental and motor retardation, jerky movements, absence of speech and paroxysmal laughter.

Consequences of molecular changes in the genome

The genetic material is the 'blueprint' for synthesis of proteins. Very simply, the consequences of mutations depend on three factors:

- the effect of the genetic change on protein synthesis or function – this is dependent on the nature, type and site of mutation
- the function of the protein that the gene encodes
- whether the genetic changes occur in a somatic cell or a germ cell.

The effect of the genetic change on protein synthesis or function

The changes in the genetic material may lead to:

- No changes in protein synthesis or structure because the genetic change occurs in a non-essential region of the gene such as the introns (and does not affect splicing), is a silent mutation (see above), or is a conservative change in the protein that does not have any effect on the protein synthesis or function.
- A quantitative change with failure or excessive/ inappropriate synthesis of protein. This occurs in a variety of ways. The genetic change could delete the whole gene or disrupt it substantially, prevent transcription by altering the promoter site and/or by other means such as trinucleotide expansion, affect splicing and generate unstable transcripts or transcripts that are altered substantially (gain or lose sequence), or truncate the protein or alter the sequence in a manner that makes it highly unstable.
- A qualitative change with synthesis of protein that is non-functional or of abnormal function. This results from mutations in the coding sequence such as missense changes, or in frame insertions or deletions that allow the synthesis of an altered protein.

The difference between quantitative and qualitative changes in some sense is artificial. It is easy to understand that changes such as deletion of a whole gene would lead to a deficiency of the product, i.e. quantitative change. It is also easy to understand that, if there is a missense change which alters the sequence and also the function of the protein, there is a purely qualitative change. However, sometimes qualitative changes in the protein result in an unstable protein which is rapidly degraded, thus causing a quantitative deficiency of the protein. Also with qualitative changes, production of a non-functional protein results in a quantitative deficiency of the normal protein. This is well illustrated by considering the haemoglobinopathies (see Ch. 8). In thalassaemias, there is a deficiency of the globin chains of haemoglobin, i.e. a quantitative defect. Thus, α-thalassaemia results from deletion of one or more α-globin genes resulting in deficiency of the α-chains. In the other haemoglobinopathies, the problem is that of an abnormal haemoglobin, i.e. a qualitative defect. For example, in sickle cell anaemia, there is a substitution of a single amino acid in the β-globin chain which results in an abnormal haemoglobin; this makes the red blood cells undergo distortion with subsequent reduction in their life span and also gives them a tendency to occlude capillaries. However, some forms of thalassaemias arise because of a qualitative change in globin chains. For example, in β-thalassaemia, mutations result in unstable proteins which are rapidly degraded to cause a deficiency of β-chains.

Thus, in terms of understanding the likely effect of a mutation on the phenotype, it is better to think in terms of what the mutation does to the function of the protein. We can expect phenotypic changes to occur when genetic alterations result in:

- loss of function of a protein, i.e. failure of synthesis of a protein or synthesis of a non-functional protein, or
- gain of function of a protein, i.e. inappropriate synthesis of a protein or synthesis of a protein of abnormal function.

Loss of function mutations

In general, loss of function mutations are recessive, i.e. both alleles of the gene need to be inactivated for this phenotype to occur. This is because, for most proteins, loss of 50% of the product is not critical. This is well illustrated by the fact that most inherited conditions involving metabolic enzymes (the so-called 'inborn errors of metabolism') are recessive, e.g. albinism.

In some cases, with loss of function mutations, 50% of the gene product is inadequate, and can lead to a dominant phenotype, e.g. hereditary angio-oedema, which is characterized by recurrent episodes of submucosal and subcutaneous oedema involving the respiratory and gastrointestinal tracts and including the oral cavity and lips.

Gain of function mutations

Most gain of function mutations are dominant, i.e. only one of the two copies of a gene needs to be affected.

However, some dominant mutations result in proteins that are not only non-functional but also interact with the product of the normal gene and prevent it from functioning. This is referred to as a dominant negative effect and is particularly observed with proteins that are oligomers (consisting of two or more subunits). The mutant protein that forms a subunit of an oligomeric protein can disrupt either the oligomerization or the function of the oligomer.

An example of this is observed with some mutations of the p53 tumour suppressor gene which normally functions as a tetramer. Mutations of one allele can produce polypeptide chains which disrupt the tetramer formed with the normal polypeptides produced by the normal allele. Another example of dominant negative effect is seen with mutations of collagen which is also a multimeric protein. These can result in various forms of osteogenesis imperfecta which are characterized by bone fragility and also sometimes with defects of dentine formation (dentinogenesis imperfecta). Collagen fibrils are made up of procollagen units, each of which consists of three polypeptide chains (two encoded by one gene and the other encoded by another gene) wound in a triple helix. Mutations of one allele of the genes encoding type I collagen polypeptides, which result in production of altered polypeptide chains, disrupt formation of the triple helix with normal chains produced by the normal alleles, leading to production of very little normal collagen despite the fact that only one allele is mutated. In fact, what might be considered as more severe mutations of these collagen genes (i.e. those which completely abolish synthesis of protein), actually lead to milder disease because in these cases, the normal polypeptides produced by the unaffected alleles are able to form the triple helix molecules, albeit at 50% of normal quantity.

In some genes, both gain of function mutations and loss of function mutations are observed and result in widely different phenotypes. For example, constitutional loss of function mutations in the RET oncogene, which codes for a transmembrane tyrosine kinase receptor, results in Hirschsprung's disease which is characterized pathologically by absence of enteric ganglia along variable lengths of the intestine, whereas constitutional gain of function mutations in RET result in multiple endocrine neoplasia syndrome 2A (MEN2A) or MEN2B or familial medullary thyroid carcinoma; these syndromes are characterized by neoplasia or thyroid carcinoma with or without other tumours.

In general, mutations resulting in loss of function of the protein are likely to be varied. This is because a variety of changes (e.g. deletions, nonsense mutations, etc.) could have the same end result of loss of function of the protein. In contrast, mutations resulting in gain of function have to be more specific to result in a defined change in function of the protein. This is very well exemplified by mutations of oncogenes in cancer which result in gain of function (see Ch. 6). As mentioned above, gain of function mutations of the RET oncogene can lead to MEN2A and familial thyroid carcinoma. These mutations are nearly all missense changes specifically in one of five cysteine residues of the extracellular domain of the RET protein which constitutively activate RET tyrosinase kinase mimicking the effect of ligand binding to RET.

Changes in the function of protein

So far we have considered how changes in the genetic sequence affect protein synthesis or function and how this in turn may affect the phenotype. Obviously, the possible clinical consequences of any mutation or other genetic change also depend on the nature and function of the protein itself and, also, when and where it is required.

In simplest terms, some proteins have a more critical role than others and defects of such proteins are likely to lead to more serious clinical phenotypes. In general, disorders of haemoglobin, collagen or cell proliferation regulators have more serious consequences (haemoglobinopathies, connective tissues disease and cancer respectively) than mutations of keratin 4 and 13 which are observed in an autosomal dominant condition called white spongy naevus merely leading to benign hyperkeratosis of the oral, vaginal, rectal and nasal mucosa. However, this does not mean that all mutations of keratin genes are likely to be relatively harmless. Mutations of keratin 5 and 14 genes, for example, cause a skin-blistering disorder (epidermolysis bullosa simplex; see Ch. 15).

It may also be expected that proteins which are expressed in many tissues would have more widespread effects than those with more localized expression. However, expression patterns are not a reliable indicator of which tissues are likely to be affected. The retinoblastoma gene is widely expressed in all tissues and is one of the most important regulators of the cell cycle. It might be expected that constitutional mutations of this gene would predispose to tumours of a wide variety of tissues. However, in reality only tumours of the retina (retinoblastoma) or bone (osteosarcoma) are observed.

Another factor that needs to be considered in understanding the consequences of genetic changes is when the protein is required. In α-thalassaemia, deficiency of α-globin will affect a fetus because fetal haemoglobin is made up of α- and γ-globin chains. However, mutations affecting the β-globin chain which cause β-thalassaemia, will not have any effect until after birth when adult haemoglobin, consisting of two α and two β chains, becomes the predominant haemoglobin (see Ch. 8).

SUMMARY BOX
MOLECULAR ABNORMALITIES

- Molecular changes include structural changes such as mutations, and non-structural changes such as methylation.
- Mutations may involve a single nucleotide or larger DNA segments, and include silent point, missense, nonsense, insertion/deletion, frameshift and splice mutations and expansion of trinucleotide repeat sequences.
- Consequences depend on the effect on protein synthesis/function, the function of the protein encoded by the gene, and whether the changes occur in a germ cell or a somatic cell.
- There may be no effect on protein expression, quantitative change (e.g. failure, excessive or inappropriate expression) or qualitative change (synthesis of abnormal or non-functioning protein).
- Mutations may lead either to loss of function of a protein (generally recessive) or gain of function (generally dominant).

HOW ARE DISEASES INHERITED?

Single gene (Mendelian) inheritance

It is very easy to understand how single gene disorders are passed on through generations if we understand how chromosomes segregate in meiosis (see Fig. 2.1, pp. 9, 10).

All individuals, because of independent segregation of chromosomes, pass either a paternal or a maternal copy of any chromosome to their gametes and hence to the offspring resulting from fertilization of the gamete. Thus, individuals with a mutant copy of the gene on one of a pair of homologous autosomes have a one in two chance of passing the normal copy of the gene or the mutant copy of the gene to their offspring. If individuals have two mutant copies of any gene (one on each of a pair of homologous autosomes), then all their gametes will carry a mutant copy of the gene. For genes on the X chromosome, a man always passes his single copy of the X chromosome (and any mutant genes on it) to his daughter(s), who are thus obligate carriers of any mutant gene on the father's X chromosome. Thus, there is never any male-to-male transmission of X-linked conditions (sons receive the Y chromosome from the father). For a woman, the situation is exactly as for autosomes since she has two copies of the X chromosome.

Autosomal dominant inheritance

A condition will show an autosomal dominant mode of inheritance if it is caused by disruption of a single gene on an autosome and the phenotype is expressed in a heterozygote state.

The chief features of this mode of inheritance are shown below and in Figure 2.8A.

SUMMARY BOX
AUTOSOMAL DOMINANT INHERITANCE

- Both males and females are affected.
- Both males and females transmit the condition.
- There is a vertical pattern of transmission with affected individuals in every generation.
- Any child of a heterozygous parent has a 50% chance of inheriting the condition.
- Affected homozygotes are rarely observed for most rare autosomal dominant conditions.

There are several conditions which complicate this basic pattern.

Non-penetrance or reduced penetrance. Penetrance refers to manifestation of the phenotype in someone who carries a mutant copy of the gene. A fully penetrant condition is one where all people who carry the mutant gene manifest the phenotype associated with the condition. If a condition has reduced penetrance, then some people who carry the gene will not manifest the condition. Thus in a pedigree, the condition may occasionally skip a generation as shown in Figure 2.8B. This may pose problems in counselling because individuals who have not manifested the condition cannot be given reassurance based on the clinical findings alone that they have definitely not inherited the condition and that they have no risk of passing the condition to their offspring.

Variable expressivity. In some autosomal conditions, affected individuals, even within the same families and carrying the same mutation, manifest different features or have different degrees of severity of the condition. Such conditions are said to have variable expressivity. Sometimes affected individuals may show very minor changes and may not be diagnosed as being affected. In such situations, the risk estimations of passing the

condition to their offspring will be wrong. Another problem with genetic counselling in conditions with variable expression is that it is difficult to provide accurate information about the severity of the phenotype for any individual.

Variable expression and reduced penetrance are essentially part of the same spectrum and both are probably due to the influence of other genes or the environment in the development of some or all of the phenotypic changes.

Age-dependent onset. Certain familial conditions do not present early in life. Examples of this include Huntington's disease which is characterized by progressive loss of mental function accompanied by abnormal movements, and some inherited cancer syndromes such as hereditary non-polyposis colorectal cancer (HNPCC). In Huntington's disease, the onset is usually after age 35 and individuals who have inherited the disease gene can develop the condition at any age up to about 70. Thus, you may observe the situation shown in Figure 2.8C which may be misleading in interpreting pedigrees and in risk estimation.

Homozygous affected individuals in autosomal dominant conditions. In most rare autosomal dominant conditions, individuals homozygous for the mutant allele are rare because there is little chance of both parents being heterozygotes. However, in some relatively common conditions such as familial hypercholesterolaemia, mating between heterozygotes does occur, resulting in affected homozygote offspring. In autosomal dominant conditions where homozygotes are seen, they generally tend to be more severely affected than heterozygotes, often with the condition proving lethal in early life (e.g. in Marfan's syndrome). However, in Huntington's disease, there does not appear to be any difference in the severity or phenotype between homozygotes and heterozygotes.

Autosomal recessive inheritance

A condition will show an autosomal recessive mode of inheritance if it is caused by disruption of a single gene on an autosome and the phenotype is expressed in a homozygous state for the mutant allele. These conditions are usually observed in the offspring of clinically unaffected parents heterozygous for the mutant allele (carriers). These conditions are also more likely to arise in situations where the parents are related to each other (consanguineous mating) and share some genes. This increases the probability that both the parents carry the same mutation from a common ancestor.

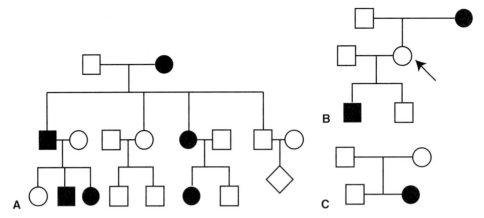

Fig. 2.8 Autosomal dominant inheritance. A. Autosomal dominant pedigree. **B.** Pedigree pattern in an autosomal dominant condition with reduced penetrance. Although the individual marked with an arrow is not manifesting the phenotype, she must carry the mutant gene responsible for the condition since she has an affected child and an affected parent. **C.** The affected individual in this pedigree could represent a new mutation. Alternatively, one of the parents is a heterozygote but has not yet manifested the condition (age-dependent onset). In the case of the former, the probability of the unaffected sibling having inherited the mutant gene is very small, whereas in the latter situation the probability is 50%.

The chief features of this mode of inheritance are shown below and in Figure 2.9.

SUMMARY BOX
AUTOSOMAL RECESSIVE INHERITANCE

- Both males and females are affected.
- Parents are usually unaffected heterozygotes for the mutant allele.
- There is an increased incidence of parental consanguinity.
- There is a horizontal pattern of transmission with affected individuals usually in a single generation.
- Any child of heterozygote parents has a 25% chance of inheriting the condition.
- Any child of heterozygote parents has a 50% chance of being a carrier.

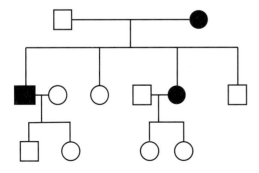

Fig. 2.9 Autosomal recessive pedigree.

X-linked recessive inheritance

A condition will show an X-linked recessive mode of inheritance if it is caused by disruption of a single gene on the X chromosome and phenotype is expressed mainly in males because they have a single X chromosome (i.e. they are hemizygous for the X chromosome) and in females who are homozygous for the mutant allele.

The chief features of this mode of inheritance are shown below and in Figure 2.10.

SUMMARY BOX
X-LINKED RECESSIVE INHERITANCE

- Generally only males are affected.
- Parents are usually unaffected with the mother heterozygous (a carrier) for the mutant allele.
- Females may be affected if they have an affected father and a carrier mother or rarely as a result of non-random X inactivation.
- Any son of a heterozygote mother has a 50% chance of inheriting the condition.
- Any daughter of a heterozygote mother and an unaffected father has a 50% chance of being a carrier.
- All daughters of an affected father are obligate carriers of the mutant allele.
- Male-to-male transmission does not occur.

X-linked dominant inheritance

A condition will show an X-linked dominant mode of inheritance if it is caused by disruption of a single gene

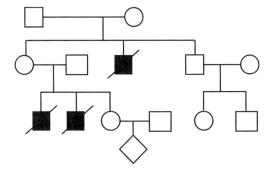

Fig. 2.10 X-linked recessive pedigree.

on the X chromosome and the phenotype is expressed in males and also in females homozygous for the mutant allele.

The chief features of this mode of inheritance are shown below.

SUMMARY BOX
X-LINKED DOMINANT INHERITANCE

- Both sexes are affected but more females than males.
- Males are generally more severely affected than females who show a variable expression of the phenotype because of Lyonization.
- Any child of a heterozygote mother and an unaffected father has a 50% chance of inheriting the condition.
- All daughters of an affected father inherit the condition.
- Male-to-male transmission does not occur.

Mitochondrial inheritance

Mitochondrial inheritance is entirely maternal since mitochondria are cytoplasmic organelles and the cytoplasm of a fertilized ovum is derived from the ovum itself, the sperm having very little cytoplasm. Thus, mitochondrial diseases are only transmitted by females but can affect both males and females.

Mutations in mitochondrial DNA occur more commonly than in nuclear DNA, the mutation rate being almost 20-fold higher. This could be due to the generation of oxygen radicals coupled with the limited DNA repair capacity in the mitochondria.

Two key features of mitochondrial diseases are the wide variability in the phenotype even within the same families and the tissue specificity. This is likely to be due to several factors:

- A cell has many mitochondria and on cell division

there is not an equal segregation to the daughter cells. Thus, the proportion of mitochondria carrying a particular mutation in their DNA can vary. In some mitochondrial diseases, all mitochondria in all cells carry the causative mutation in their DNA (homoplasmy). In other cases, a variable fraction of the total number of mitochondria in any particular cell carry the mutation in their DNA (heteroplasmy).

- Certain tissues such as cardiac muscle, skeletal muscle and the central nervous system are highly dependent on oxidative phosphorylation (normal function of mitochondria) and are more likely to be affected by mutations in mitochondrial DNA. Thus, myopathy and encephalopathy are often observed in many mitochondrial diseases.

- Mitochondria accumulate mutations in their DNA with age and this is accompanied by a decrease in their oxidative phosphorylation capacity. Thus, within individuals, there is an evolution of mitochondrial mutations with age.

Overall, the phenotype in mitochondrial diseases is dependent on the proportion of the mitochondria with mutations in their DNA in a critical tissue. This in turn is dependent on the degree of heteroplasmy and the continuing evolution of mutations in individuals with age.

SUMMARY BOX
MITOCHONDRIAL INHERITANCE

- Mitochondrial inheritance is maternally derived.
- Mitochondrial DNA mutations are more common than in nuclear DNA.
- There may be a wide variability in phenotype even within families and tissues.
- This may be related to non-equal segregation in daughter cells, increased sensitivity of tissues to oxidative phosphorylation, and increasing age.

Non-Mendelian inheritance

Few diseases are purely genetic or purely environmental in origin; most are likely to involve interaction between the two and can be included under the broad umbrella of multifactorial conditions. The genetic influence in such diseases may be determined by a few (oligogenic) or many (polygenic) genes with each gene contributing to a lesser or greater extent to the final phenotype. It is important to realize that unlike in single gene disorders, in multifactorial conditions the genetic factors do not directly cause the disease but are responsible for predisposition to a disease in the presence of suitable environmental triggers. Thus individuals may not necessarily develop the condition. Also, unlike the single gene disorders, predisposition may be determined by normal variants (alleles) of the genes that are not pathogenic in isolation.

The role of genetic factors in the common diseases is suggested by:

- Studies showing a higher risk of certain diseases in relatives of affected individuals compared to the general population that is proportional to the degree of relatedness. This is well illustrated by non-syndromic cleft palate and schizophrenia. Of course similar relationships may be observed because of a shared environment.

- Twin studies. If a disease is purely genetic, then monozygotic twins (who have all their genes in common) should show 100% concordance (have the same phenotype, i.e. both affected or both not affected), whilst dizygotic twins and siblings (who share 50% of their genes) show 50% concordance. In contrast, if a disease is purely environmental, then there should be no difference in concordance between monozygotic twins, dizygotic twins and siblings. Furthermore, this should be considerably less then 100%, although it may still be relatively high because of shared environment. Finally, if a disease has a part genetic and part environmental (multifactorial) aetiology, then monozygotic twins will show a higher concordance than dizygotic twins and siblings, but this will be less than 100%.

- Adopted twins studies. Because twins also share their environment, it may be difficult to completely exclude the role of environmental influences in conventional twin studies. Studies of twins who have been separated at birth avoid this problem and provide an even more powerful method of detecting genetic influence in any disease.

Threshold model of multifactorial inheritance

It is easy to appreciate the role of a number of genes in determining continuous variable characters such as height, weight or blood pressure, with each allele of the genes contributing to a variable degree to the final phenotype. Alleles of such genes will show a normal distribution in the general population. So, for example, with a character such as height, a minority of the people have a combination of alleles that leads to unusually short or long stature whilst a majority of people have combinations of alleles that lead to height between these two extremes (Fig. 2.11).

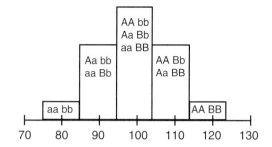

Fig. 2.11 Distribution of a hypothetical character with a mean value of 100 in a population where the character is determined by the additive codominant effect of two loci, A and B.

It has been proposed that even for a dichotomous or discontinuous character such as disease (you can either have the disease or not have the disease) it is possible to think of an underlying continuous normally distributed genetic liability in the general population which predisposes to the disease. As for continuous characters such as height, the liability is determined by a combination of alleles of a number of relevant genes. However, unlike continuous characters, disease occurs only when a certain liability threshold is exceeded by an individual having a certain combination of alleles of a number of relevant genes (see Fig. 2.12).

- Because affected individuals share a greater proportion of their genes with their relatives than with the general population, the distribution of genes and thus the genetic liability in their family members is shifted to the right (Fig. 2.12). The result of this is that the proportion of individuals in the family that exceed the threshold will be higher than in the general population, i.e. relatives of affected individuals have a greater predisposition than the general population to having the disease.

- Furthermore, this shift is proportional to the degree of relatedness. Thus, first-degree relatives because they share more genes with the affected individual have a greater shift to the right then second-degree relatives and so on. Thus, the closer the relationship, the greater the predisposition.

- The greater an individual's liability, the greater the likely shift to the right in distribution of the liability in his family. Genetic liability is a reflection of the number of relevant alleles of particular genes an individual has; thus, the greater the liability, the greater the number of relevant alleles of these genes in the individual. His relatives who have genes in common with him are thus also more likely to have a greater number of relevant alleles of these genes.

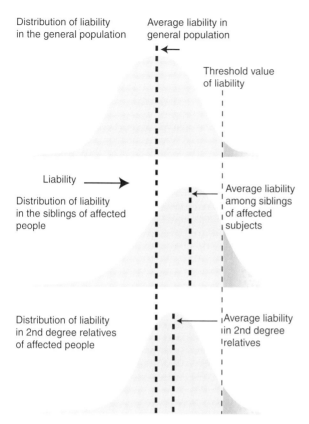

Distribution of liability
in the general population

Average liability in
general population

Threshold value
of liability

Liability ⟶

Distribution of liability
in the siblings of affected
people

Average liability
among siblings
of affected
subjects

Distribution of liability
in 2nd degree relatives
of affected people

Average liability
in 2nd degree
relatives

Fig. 2.12 **Distribution of genetically determined liability among relatives in a multifactorial threshold model.**

Unlike in Mendelian conditions, we cannot estimate risks in multifactorial conditions from our knowledge of their mode of inheritance. We know that individuals whose genetic liability exceeds the threshold level will have predisposition to a particular disease. However, whether or not they develop the disease may depend on exactly how much over the threshold their genetic liability is and also on environmental factors. Since we do not know these, the only reasonable way we can estimate risks for any individual is from empirical data from studies of incidence of the condition in the general population, risks within families of affected individuals and so on.

Also, from the threshold model of multifactorial inheritance, we can deduce that the risk for an individual increases:

- With the number of affected individuals in his or her family. If there is more then one affected individual within a family, i.e. more than one person over the threshold, then it is likely that genetic liability in this family is shifted more to the right of the normal popu-

lation compared to a family with just a single affected individual. This is well demonstrated by considering recurrence risks of cleft lip (with or without cleft palate). The risk for an individual with one affected sibling is about 4% whilst the risk for an individual with two first-degree relatives is 10%.

- With the severity of the condition in the affected individuals in his or her family. Assuming that severity reflects the underlying genetic liability, the greater the severity of the disease the more any affected individual's liability exceeds the threshold. Thus the distribution of liability in her family is likely to be to the right of a less severely affected individual. Again using cleft lip as an example, the recurrence risk for a sibling of a child with just cleft lip is about 2.5% whilst the risk for a sibling of a child with cleft lip and palate is in the order of 6%.

- If the affected individual(s) in the family are of the usually less commonly affected sex. Some diseases are more common in one sex. This suggests that for the less commonly affected sex, the threshold is higher than it is for the more commonly affected sex. Thus, for members of the less commonly affected sex to have the condition, they must have a greater genetic liability than members of the more commonly affected sex. A good example is that of congenital pyloric stenosis. This is five times more common in boys than in girls, suggesting that the threshold in girls is higher. Relatives of affected females have higher recurrence risks than those of affected males, e.g. children of affected mothers have greater recurrence risks than children of affected fathers.

Whilst this model provides a good framework for understanding multifactorial conditions with a genetic basis, it must be stressed that it may not apply to all non-Mendelian conditions.

SUMMARY BOX
NON-MENDELIAN INHERITANCE

- Diseases are rarely either purely genetic or purely environmental.
- Most diseases are multifactorial, where the genetic influence may be by a few (oligogenic) or many (polygenic) genes.
- In multifactorial conditions, genetic factors lead to a predisposition to disease in the presence of environmental triggers, as shown by increased risk in relatives of affected individuals and from twin studies.
- The threshold model of multifactorial inheritance for discontinuous characters suggests that disease occurs only when a certain liability threshold is exceeded.

3 Inflammation

Inflammation is the response of living tissue to injury. The possible injurious stimuli are many but the inflammatory response in the first instance is rather stereotyped and follows the same pattern regardless of the cause.

The cardinal features were described nearly 2000 years ago by Celsus and still apply.

- *Rubor:* the redness noted in acute inflammation is a consequence of increased vascularity to an area of tissue damage.
- *Calor:* the heat generated in inflammation is a result of a combination of increased blood flow and the release of inflammatory mediators, especially cytokines.
- *Dolor:* inflammation is often accompanied by pain caused by the stretching of pain receptors and nerves by the inflammatory exudate and by the release of inflammatory mediators.
- *Tumor:* the swelling in inflammation occurs because there is exudation of fluid including proteins and cells into an area of tissue damage.

Later, another feature was added to the four described by Celsus which represented a combination of the effects of those already mentioned, i.e. loss of function (*functio laesa*, to maintain the Latin theme).

The inflammatory stimuli include physical agents such as heat, cold and radiation, chemical agents such as acids and alkalis, microbiological agents such as bacteria, viruses, fungi and protozoa, and immunologically mediated damage through antigen–antibody complexes.

The functions of the inflammatory response are to provide an exudate which brings proteins, fluids and cells to an area of damage to act as a local defence mechanism, to destroy and/or eliminate the injurious agent, and to break down the damaged tissue and remove the debris. The exudate is derived from local vessels in the area of the tissue damage and contains fluids including salts; proteins including immunoglobulins; the end-product of the coagulation system – fibrin; and cells including polymorphs in the early stages and lymphocytes, plasma cells and mononuclear cells at a later stage.

SUMMARY BOX
INFLAMMATION

- Response of living tissue to injury, characterized by heat (calor), redness (rubor), pain (dolor), swelling (tumor) and loss of function.
- Stimuli include physical agents (heat and cold), chemical agents (acid), microbiological injury (bacteria, viruses and fungi), and immunologically mediated damage.
- It is a defence mechanism, providing an exudate (proteins, fluids) and cells, which destroys or localizes an injurious stimulus, breaks down the damaged tissue and removes the debris.
- It is classified according to the timescale involved into acute and chronic inflammation, which also have characteristic differences in the cells involved.

Inflammation may be categorized as acute or chronic but these are rather arbitrary classifications. In general, acute inflammation is short-lived for minutes, hours or days and is characterized by neutrophil polymorphonuclear cell infiltration, while chronic inflammation is longer-lasting for days, weeks, months or years and contains mononuclear cells such as lymphocytes, plasma cells and macrophages.

ACUTE INFLAMMATION (Fig. 3.1)

This can be conveniently divided into three phases:

* The initial vascular phase, where there is vasodilatation with increased blood flow to the area of tissue damage. This results in sluggish blood flow, increased local hydrostatic pressure and increased permeability of the vessel walls, which may be exacerbated by the release of inflammatory mediators (see below).
* The formation of a cell-free, protein-rich exudate (oedema fluid) which functions as a diluent and buffer for the injurious stimulus (Fig. 3.1B). It provides nutrients for inflammatory cells and allows the diffusion of inflammatory mediators. Important proteins present include fibrin converted from fibrinogen following activation of the coagulation cascade, immunoglobulins which act as opsonins for phagocytosis, and components of the complement and kinin systems which are potent chemical mediators.
* The cellular phase of the inflammatory response is mediated by various chemical messengers which activate the endothelium to permit adherence of polymorphonuclear leukocytes (PMNs), and activate the PMNs to increase their capacity for phagocytosis, bacterial killing and the production of further inflammatory mediators. PMNs then move to the area of tissue damage by the process of chemotaxis (Fig. 3.1C).

Phagocytosis

This is the process by which PMNs engulf invading organisms. PMNs attach to microorganisms by membrane receptors, particularly the Fc component of immunoglobulins. The process may also be activated by various fragments of the complement cascade and by some bacterial polysaccharides. When the microorganism has been bound, it is surrounded by pseudopodia, projections of the PMN which are formed by the sequential assembly and disassembly of actin filaments. The pseudopodia fuse to form an endocytotic vesicle, which then becomes a phagosome, which fuses with lysosomes. The lysosomes contain a variety of enzymes designed for bacterial killing, including myeloperoxidase and other substances capable of generating oxygen-derived free radicals. This leads to destruction of the invading microorganism which is then cleared up by the macrophage system. Foreign material ingested and destroyed in this way may be further packaged into residual bodies prior to macrophage clearance.

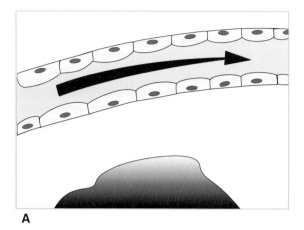

A

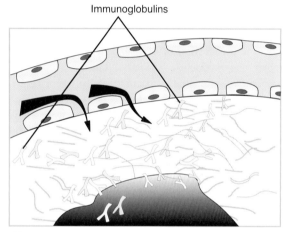

Immunoglobulins

B

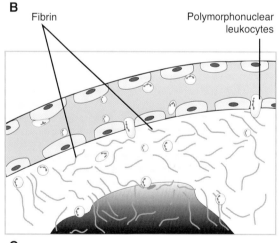

Fibrin

Polymorphonuclear leukocytes

C

Fig. 3.1 **Acute inflammation. A.** Normal blood vessel with intact endothelial layer. **B.** Exudative phase of inflammatory response: separation of endothelial cells and movement of plasma proteins including immunoglobulins and fibrin to site of injurious stimulus. **C.** Cellular phase of inflammation: polymorphs adhere to endothelium, move through gaps (diapedesis), and migrate to site of injury (by chemotaxis).

Types of inflammation

The naming of the type of inflammation is determined by the predominant part of the inflammatory process involved. Where abundant exudation of low-protein, relatively acellular fluids and salts occurs, this is serous inflammation, such as in the pleural and peritoneal cavities.

When there is pronounced activation of the coagulation system with conversion of fibrinogen to fibrin, the form of inflammation which results is fibrinous. This occurs particularly in body cavities such as the pericardium after myocardial infarction, in uraemic pericarditis and less commonly nowadays, as part of acute rheumatic fever (Fig. 3.2A).

When tissue damage has been extensive, the end product of the inflammatory process is known as pus, which is a collection of dead and dying PMNs, tissue debris and products of bacterial killing. Purulent or suppurative inflammation occurs usually when there is infection with a pyogenic (pus-forming) organism such as *Staphylococcus aureus* and where there is extensive tissue destruction (Fig. 3.2B). This often results in the formation of an abscess, which is a localized mass of necrotic tissue. In the acute phase, this is surrounded by an acute inflammatory infiltrate which will continue to expand as long as the organism responsible continues to proliferate. Later, the central necrotic area becomes surrounded by granulation tissue (see p. 31), eventually leading to the development of scar tissue. Nevertheless, the central area may contain organisms still capable of reproduction for prolonged periods.

Tissue damage

Although the main purpose of the inflammatory reaction is a protective one, by its nature the possibility of damage to tissue or organs exists. The hypersensitivity reactions are so called because they represent an immunological response to what may be a trivial injurious stimulus with an exaggerated overactivation of the inflammatory response. They are dealt with later in the section on immunopathology. Where the formation of the cell-free protein-rich inflammatory exudate occurs in an enclosed space such as in the epiglottis in young children infected with *Haemophilus influenzae* type B, the end result potentially is the complete occlusion of the airway with respiratory failure and sudden death. When there is extensive suppurative inflammation within the lining of the brain (meninges) caused by organisms such as *Haemophilus influenzae* type B, *Neisseria meningitidis* (meningococcus) or *Streptococcus pneumoniae* (pneumococcus), meningitis occurs with the development of raised intracranial pressure because of the limited space available for the brain to expand. Thus, the acute inflammatory process may be harmful to the tissues or organs in which it occurs.

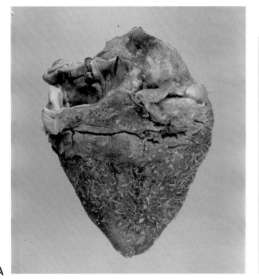
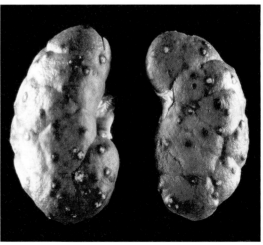

A **B**

Fig. 3.2 Types of inflammation. A. Fibrinous inflammation of pericardium in a patient with acute rheumatic fever. **B.** Pyogenic inflammation of kidneys in a patient with pyaemic abscesses from staphylococcal septicaemia.

Inflammatory mediators

The mediators of acute inflammation may be either cellular or derived from circulating plasma.

Cellular mediators

The cellular mediators in turn may either be preformed and stored in cells such as mast cells, basophils and platelets (e.g. histamine) or be derived from active synthesis within a variety of cells. A major group of mediators is derived from the effect of phospholipase A_2 on the long-chain fatty acids of cell membranes, leading to the formation of arachidonic acid (Fig. 3.3). Two further pathways of metabolism of arachidonic acid exist, via cyclooxygenase to thromboxanes and prostaglandins and via lipoxygenase to leukotrienes. The chemicals thus formed have a complex role to play in the initiation, continuation and cessation of acute inflammation and many of its major effects. Other substances such as platelet-activating factor (PAF), cytokines (intercellular messengers such as interleukin-1 (IL-1), IL-8 and tumour necrosis factor-alpha (TNF-α)), and nitric oxide (NO) also have roles to play, particularly in relation to endothelial and vascular reactivity and to platelet interactions with endothelium.

Plasma-derived mediators

These include the cascade systems such as coagulation (clotting), complement, kinins and fibrinolysis. These systems again have a complex series of interactions which in normal situations maintain an equilibrium between tissue defence and inflammation. When the stimuli to activation of these systems are sufficiently powerful and long-lasting, then inflammation as a pathological process ensues. It is likely that in the majority of cases of trivial injury, the process is self-limiting with no or minimal tissue injury.

A number of commonly used drugs have effects on the inflammatory process by reducing the availability of chemical mediators: corticosteroids are used to damp down the inflammatory reaction by their inhibition of phospholipase A_2, thus preventing the formation of arachidonic acid; and non-steroidal anti-inflammatory drugs such as ibuprofen and aspirin inhibit the cyclo-oxygenase pathway, thus preventing the synthesis of prostaglandins and thromboxanes.

Sequelae

The possible sequelae of acute inflammation are:

1. resolution, which is the restoration to complete structural and functional normality of a tissue after inflammation
2. suppuration where there is extensive tissue damage with the formation of pus, usually by the effect of pyogenic organisms, which inevitably leads to
3. healing by regeneration/repair which is the process by which damaged tissue is replaced by either similar tissue (regeneration) or scar tissue (repair), or
4. chronic inflammation where there is continuing inflammation at the same time as attempts at healing.

SUMMARY BOX
ACUTE INFLAMMATION

- Initial response of tissue to injury.
- Vascular phase: blood flow increased at site of damage, accompanied by increased vascular permeability.
- Exudative phase: formation of cell-free protein-rich exudate in the tissues.
- Cellular phase: tissue infiltration by neutrophil polymorphs.
- The inflammatory response is facilitated by cellular mediators (prostaglandins, leukotrienes, cytokines) and by plasma components (coagulation factors, complement, kinins).
- Some forms of acute inflammation are characterized by prominence of one phase: haemorrhagic, serous, fibrinous or purulent.
- Outcome: resolution (restoration to normal), suppuration (pus formation), healing (by regeneration and repair) or chronic inflammation.

ORGANIZATION AND REPAIR

Where there has been extensive tissue damage as a result of inflammation, the tissue must be replaced. How this occurs is determined by the extent of tissue damage, whether the supporting stroma (connective tissue framework) of the tissue is damaged, the nature of the tissue damaged (whether stable, labile or permanent) and the general condition of the patient's health.

Regeneration is the process which occurs when tissue is replaced by similar tissue, which indicates that the tissue damaged in the inflammatory process is either labile (renewing, i.e. constantly in the cell cycle) or stable

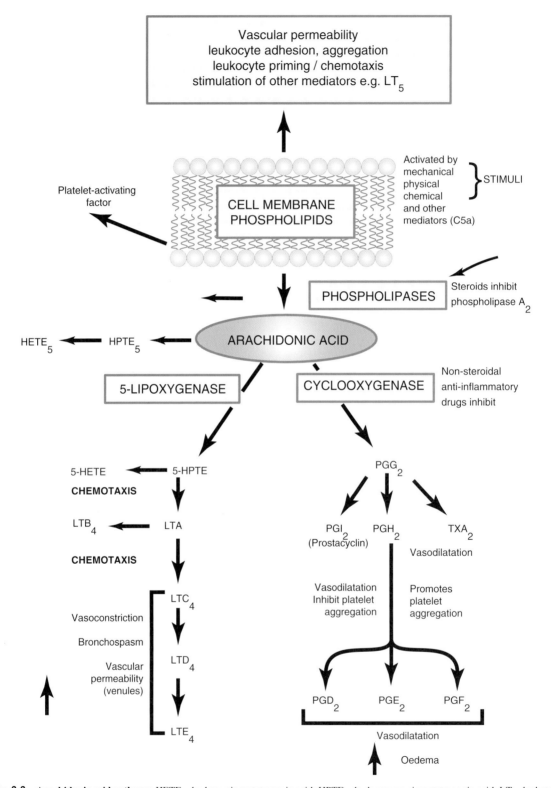

Fig. 3.3 Arachidonic acid pathway. HETE = hydroxyeicosatetraenoic acid; HPTE = hydroperoxyeicosatetraenoic acid; LT = leukotriene; PG = prostaglandin; TX = thromboxane. (See text for details.)

(conditionally renewing, i.e. capable of entering the cell cycle), and thus capable of self-replication, and that the supporting stroma of the tissue is preserved (see Ch. 1).

Repair is the process whereby damaged tissue is replaced by collagenous scar tissue. This indicates either that the damaged tissue is incapable of self-replication (i.e. composed of static/permanent cells, outside the cell cycle) or that the connective tissue framework is damaged irrevocably.

Granulation tissue

The main contributor to the healing process is the formation of granulation tissue. This is a dynamic process in which there is ingrowth of new capillaries into an area of tissue necrosis where there is demolition of the inflammatory exudate by macrophages. In the early stages of healing, granulation tissue is extremely vascular. As the healing process continues, the relative proportion of vascular tissue to fibroblastic tissue producing collagen decreases. Over a period of days to weeks or months, there is a change in the proportion of vessels, fibroblasts and mature collagenous scar tissue, so that eventually only collagen remains.

The process of healing varies according to the tissue involved and well-defined sequences have been described for healing in, for example, skin wounds and bone fractures.

Healing of skin wounds

Because of the accessibility of the skin to detailed studies, much information on this form of wound healing is available. It includes epithelial regeneration and repair of connective tissue with the development of scar tissue. When the edges of a skin wound are in close apposition, e.g. a sutured surgical incision, healing occurs by first intention leading to primary union. Where there is a large tissue defect with the wound edges widely separated, healing occurs by second intention leading to secondary union. In the latter form of healing, the amount of granulation tissue, fibrosis and scarring is greater than in the former; however, the differences in the two types is quantitative rather than qualitative.

Healing by first intention (primary union)

Initially, after the skin incision, there is some death of cells with haemorrhage into the incised area. This leads to blood clot formation and the generation of fibrin and

the release of fibronectin; this combination of substances provides a provisionally stable wound. Dehydration of the clot on the surface leads to scab formation. An inflammatory reaction ensues in the first 1–2 days, and this is followed by demolition by polymorphs and macrophages in the subsequent 2–3 days.

Epithelial regeneration occurs in a sequence of cell migration, proliferation and remodelling. Cell migration begins after 18–24 hours, possibly as a result of a release from contact inhibition. There is then proliferation of epithelial cells from the edge of the wound with increased numbers of mitotic cells after 24–36 hours. These cells migrate over viable tissue only and, as the cells migrate, they release factors, such as collagenase and plasminogen activators, which allow their ingress into the damaged area. As they regenerate the epithelium, cells also produce their own new basement membrane. Proliferation continues for several days, during which the thickness of the epithelium is restored to normal.

Repair develops initially by neovascularization (angiogenesis), i.e. by the ingrowth of new capillaries from vessels at the edge of the skin incision. This requires local degradation of the parent capillary basement membrane and changes in the extracellular matrix (ECM) mediated by factors such as collagenase and stromelysin produced by endothelial cells. This process may be modified by metalloproteinases and tissue inhibitors of metalloproteinases (TIMPs). The new blood vessels produced lack basement membrane in the early stages and, thus, there is leakiness of vessels with extensive oedema. Lymphatics also infiltrate the damaged tissues. The second major component of granulation tissue is fibroblasts, which migrate into the damaged area and undergo increased synthetic activity to produce components of the ECM including glycosaminoglycans, proteoglycans, fibronectin and collagens, particularly types I and III. Significant collagen deposition is first noticed at 3–4 days and initially collagen type III predominates. With remodelling by collagenases from macrophages and fibroblasts, type I eventually becomes the main type present. The stability of the collagen formed is enhanced by cross-linking both within and between collagen fibrils.

Healing by second intention (secondary union) (Fig. 3.4)

This is a slower process than primary union. It is characterized by a more intense inflammatory reaction with greater granulation tissue production, which potentially may lead to deforming scars. A particular problem is

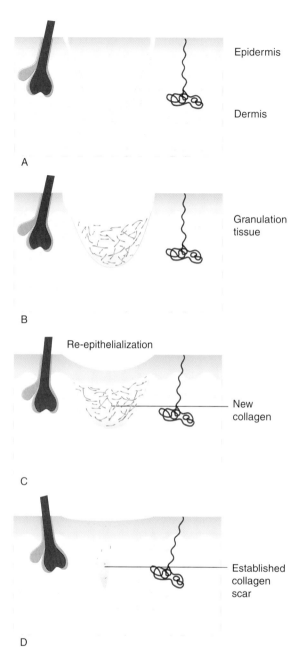

A

Epidermis

Dermis

B

Granulation tissue

Re-epithelialization

C

New collagen

D

Established collagen scar

Fig. 3.4   Wound healing in skin by secondary intention.
A. Injury to skin involving epidermis, dermis and adnexal structures, with edges widely separated. **B.** Loss of epidermis with underlying inflammatory response and ingrowth of granulation tissue, comprising capillaries and myofibroblasts (2–10 days). **C.** Re-epithelialization of epidermis and deposition of new collagen in dermis (10 days +). **D.** Replacement of dermal structures by established collagenous scar (weeks to months).

wound contraction which arises as a result of myofibro-blastic contraction of contractile filaments, rather than shortening of collagen fibres. This may cause important clinical problems of obstruction in healing of peptic ulcers and puckering of skin, especially in burns. Epidermal migration continues as previously described but may be supplemented by proliferation of epithelium from hair follicles and other skin adnexal structures. The scar tissue formed runs parallel to the skin surface and generally lacks dermal papillae, rete ridges and adnexae.

Factors which may influence wound healing

Local

- *Blood supply:* patients with arterial disease or impairment of venous drainage tend to heal less well than those with normal vasculature.
- *Infection:* the presence of infection delays wound healing and therefore there is a need for wound debridement for complete healing to occur. This may occur by the infiltration of polymorphs and macrophages, or larger wounds may require surgical cleansing.
- *Early movement:* this is a particular cause of delay in bone fracture healing (see later).
- *Foreign material:* the presence of suture material, dead tissue and other debris may prevent healing.
- *Ionizing radiation:* tissues which have recently been irradiated heal less well than normal and this can be a problem in surgery on patients who have been given radiotherapy as a method of reducing tumour bulk.

Systemic

- *Metabolic factors:* the process of healing requires the production of new proteins and thus patients who are deficient in protein generally or in sulphydryl-containing amino acids, such as methionine, particularly do not heal as quickly as normal. Vitamin C (ascorbic acid) is important in the cross-linking of collagen fibres and zinc is a cofactor in DNA and RNA polymerases, so patients lacking these factors heal slowly. Diabetics generally do not heal as well as the non-diabetic population, nor do other patient groups who are more prone to infection.
- *Corticosteroids:* it has been shown in experimental animals that these drugs impair the healing response, probably by impairing the inflammatory response in the early phase of healing.

- *Cytotoxic drugs:* these drugs interfere with macromolecular synthesis and may have inhibitory effects on proliferating cells.

Complications of wound healing

- *Wound dehiscence:* in the early stages of the healing response, the tensile strength of the newly formed collagen is weak and there is a possibility of the wound breaking down. This is particularly a problem in patients with deficiencies of vitamin C and proteins.
- *Hypertrophic scars/keloid:* these occur when there is excessive production of scar tissue, with thick hyalinized collagen bundles in whorls, especially on the face, neck, anterior chest and shoulder. Hypertrophic scars tend to recede with time whereas keloids, in which racial or familial factors play a part, tend to persist.
- *Contracture/cicatrization:* when myofibroblasts are a major component of granulation tissue, there is a possibility of severe deformity. This is seen in healing of skin wounds as a result of burns, and in the gastrointestinal tract in peptic ulcer disease or Crohn's disease.
- *Neoplasia:* increased turnover of proliferating tissues may lead to the development of neoplasia at the site of healing, e.g. squamous carcinoma arising at the edge of chronic venous ulcers in the lower limbs (Marjolin's ulcer).

Control mechanisms

- The *chalone hypothesis* has long been suggested as an explanation for the loss of contact inhibition which occurs early in the healing phase of epithelial regeneration. Chalones are thought to be diffusible, tissue-specific, chemical agents released by epithelial cells, which inhibit cellular proliferation. This hypothesis has never been proven.
- A variety of growth factors are known to be involved in the control of healing. They are released by injured cells, platelets, macrophages and lymphocytes and act in a paracrine fashion on adjacent tissues. They are necessary for angiogenesis, mitogenesis of fibroblasts, chemotaxis and motility of active cells, fibrogenesis and remodelling of extracellular matrix.
- Platelet-derived growth factor (PDGF): this is a chemoattractant for smooth muscle cells and fibroblasts, a mitogen for mesenchymal cells and is involved in the synthesis and remodelling of ECM.
- Transforming growth factor beta (TGF-β): this is a mitogen for mesenchymal cells and an inhibitor of epithelial cell proliferation.

- Fibroblast growth factors (basic bFGF and acidic aFGF): these are involved in neovascularization of tissues, with aFGF requiring the presence of heparin for its action.
- Cytokines: the secretory products of lymphocytes and macrophages such as interleukin-1 (IL-1) and tumour necrosis factor-alpha (TNF-α) increase the number and facilitate the activation of fibroblasts.
- Epidermal growth factor: this is responsible for cellular proliferation and increases angiogenesis.

SUMMARY BOX
ORGANIZATION AND REPAIR

- Factors in attempts to replace damaged tissue include the extent of damage, the underlying connective tissue framework and the nature of the damaged tissue.
- Regeneration refers to replacement by similar tissue.
- Repair refers to replacement by scar tissue.
- Organization is the process by which damaged tissue is replaced by scar tissue and involves the development of granulation tissue; an example is healing of a skin wound (either primary or secondary).
- Factors which delay wound healing include local problems (blood supply, infection, early movement, foreign material and ionizing radiation) and general factors (nutrition, diabetes mellitus, and drugs).
- Complications of wound healing in skin include wound dehiscence, hypertrophic scars, contracture and cicatrization, and the development of neoplasia.

CHRONIC INFLAMMATION

This is the process in which there is continuing inflammation at the same time as attempts at healing. This may occur when there is an ineffective acute inflammatory response resulting in persistence of the injurious stimulus or may arise de novo.

The chronic inflammatory process is characterized by the presence of mononuclear cells such as lymphocytes, plasma cells and monocyte-derived macrophages. There is usually an active inflammatory component (neutrophil polymorphs) associated with the chronic inflammatory cells and features of healing such as granulation tissue, epithelial regeneration and collagen deposition may also be seen. The combination of inflammation with healing leads to the alternative succinct description of chronic inflammation as 'frustrated healing'.

The single most characteristic cell of chronic inflammation is the macrophage. This is a cell derived from monocytes, released from bone marrow, and converted by the action of interferon-γ to macrophages. When activated, the cells change morphology and come to resemble squamous epithelial cells and thus are termed 'epithelioid'. Occasionally, macrophages may fuse their cytoplasm to form multinucleated giant cells (MNGC) which are known by a number of names including Touton giant cells (often incorporating fat and with a circumferential ring of nuclei), foreign body-type giant cells (a haphazard arrangement of nuclei within fused cytoplasm and possibly surrounding foreign material) and Langhans'-type giant cells (where nuclei are arranged in a peripheral horseshoe pattern). The change in cell morphology is associated with a change in cell function, whereby macrophages transform from purely phagocytic cells to cells capable of secreting a variety of active agents such as platelet-activating factor, arachidonic acid derivatives, oxygen metabolites, proteases and other proteolytic enzymes, cytokines such as interleukin-1 and tumour necrosis factor-α, and growth factors including platelet-derived growth factor (PDGF), epidermal growth factor (EGF) and basic fibroblast growth factor (bFGF).

Chronic inflammation may be classified as either non-specific, where only general features of inflammation are apparent, or specific, where a recognizable pattern of inflammation may be seen allowing a confident attempt at the aetiology of the condition. The latter form of chronic inflammation is often associated with the presence of granulomas.

SUMMARY BOX
CHRONIC INFLAMMATION

- Continuing inflammation at the same time as attempts at healing.
- Mononuclear cells predominate including lymphocytes, plasma cells and particularly macrophages.
- Chronic inflammation may follow acute inflammation or may arise de novo.
- Histological features may be non-specific (general features of inflammation only) or specific (where typical features may be present, e.g. tuberculosis, syphilis).
- Granulomas are aggregates of macrophages which may be accompanied by multinucleated giant cells, including Touton type incorporating fat, foreign body type and Langhans' type commonly seen in TB, sarcoidosis and Crohn's disease.

Granulomatous inflammation

A granuloma is a discrete collection of macrophages and the terminology may be qualified on the basis of the cell type predominating or on the stimulus causing the inflammation.

- In general with regard to microbiological agents, the stimulus to the inflammatory process is of low pathogenicity but capable of generating an intense immunological response. Characteristically, this is a type IV hypersensitivity reaction where there is a delayed T cell-mediated immune response to, for example, mycobacteria. Tuberculosis and leprosy are examples of this form of inflammation.
- Granulomatous inflammation may occur as a result of exposure to inanimate foreign material, which may be either exogenous such as silica or endogenous such as uric acid, fat or keratin.
- Fungal infection may also lead to granulomatous inflammation. Examples include the response to infection with *Aspergillus*.

In some cases, it is not possible to identify a specific aetiological agent. The best-known examples of this are sarcoidosis, affecting lymph nodes and lung mainly (see p. 131), and Crohn's disease, a disease of any part of the gastrointestinal tract from mouth to anus (see p. 154).

Tuberculosis

When the body encounters *Mycobacterium tuberculosis* for the first time, there is little or no acute inflammatory response, since the polymorph enzymes have limited impact on the mycobacterial cell wall. The organism is recognized by T lymphocytes and there is then recruitment of macrophages to the site of infection. The macrophages become epithelioid in nature, they fuse to form Langhans'-type giant cells and with the effect of macrophage-derived proteolytic enzymes there is central caseation necrosis (Fig. 3.5). The organism may be identified in tissue sections by the use of the Ziehl–Neelsen stain. This combination of features is characteristic of a tubercle, which may also be described as caseating epithelioid granulomatous inflammation. The response to the organism is determined by a number of factors including the loading, infective dose; the host response which is often impaired at the extremes of life in neonates and the elderly, respectively, in malnourished patients and in patients on corticosteroids; the development of resistance to the organism which is becoming more of a problem in the USA; and the use of specific antituberculous therapy. Immunity against tuberculosis can be induced artificially by the use of bacille Calmette–Guérin (BCG). See Chapter 9 on respiratory disease for more details of tuberculosis.

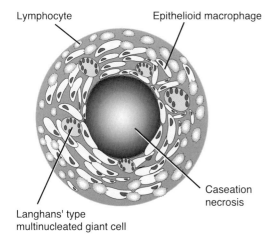

Lymphocyte   Epithelioid macrophage

Caseation
necrosis

Langhans' type
multinucleated giant cell

Fig. 3.5   Chronic inflammation: granuloma. A granuloma is a
localized collection of macrophages. In this example of
tuberculosis, there is central caseation necrosis with surrounding
macrophages and lymphocytes. Langhans'-type giant cells are
multinucleated giant cells formed from fusion of macrophages.

SUMMARY BOX
GRANULOMATOUS INFLAMMATION
(TUBERCULOSIS)

- Specific form of chronic inflammation, in which there is T
  cell-mediated recruitment of macrophages at the site of
  exposure to the organism *Mycobacterium tuberculosis*.

- Macrophages are epithelioid in type and aggregate to
  form a granuloma.

- The granuloma is often accompanied by multinucleated
  Langhans'-type giant cells and central caseation necrosis,
  characteristic of destruction of mycobacterial cell walls.

4 Basic principles of immunology

INTRODUCTION

Immunology is the study of the immune system. The immune system is that part of the body's defence system mediated by lymphocytes. It imparts specific protection against pathogenic microorganisms and other antigens.

ANTIGENS

Antigens and the concept of 'self' and 'foreign'

With the exception of identical twins, the structure of many complex circulating and cell surface-bound molecules within our bodies shows distinct differences between individuals. Our own molecules are described as 'self' and the different variants found in others as 'foreign'. Many foreign molecules are also derived from non-human organisms – animals, plants and microbes. Foreign molecules are described as antigens and can stimulate an immune response.

Antigens are therefore personal to the individual. They are defined as large, organic molecules, usually protein but sometimes polysaccharide, nucleic acid or lipid, which in chemical structure are different from the molecules found normally in the individual's body, and that can stimulate the immune system to attack them and attempt to eliminate them. Such molecules may be soluble or insoluble free molecules or they may be part of the surface of a cell, notably a cellular pathogen, such as a bacterium.

Although an antigen is generally a single molecule, it is made up of a number of parts, and it is these different parts that determine how the immune system reacts with the antigen. Some parts of the antigen determine the extent of the immune reaction, others the specificity. Those parts of the antigen that react directly with the immune system are described as epitopes or antigenic determinants; the rest of the antigen is called a carrier. Extracted epitopes can stimulate the immune system by themselves. Some molecules that are too small to do this might still become epitopes but only if they bind to larger molecules. These small molecules are known as haptens and can be defined as molecules that, whilst not themselves antigenic, can function as antigens should they become attached to a large carrier molecule. Some such molecules are well recognized by everyone because they are common causes of unwanted immunological reactions (see below). They include some drug allergies such as those caused by penicillin.

Antigen entry to the body and tissue retention

The route by which an antigen enters the body influences the immune events. Whether the antigen enters through the skin, the respiratory tract or some other route modifies the recipient's response, just as does the amount of antigen. For instance, many antigens entering the gastrointestinal tract are destroyed or changed by digestion so that antigenic reactivity is lost or specifically altered. Nevertheless, some protein antigens can be absorbed unchanged from the intestine. This is best exemplified by those antigens, such as egg albumen, which can enter the body unchanged from the bowel and induce an allergic response (see below).

Antigens are more likely to provoke an immune

response if they are retained locally in tissues, an effect that can be brought about experimentally by substances, such as certain oils, which are described as 'adjuvants'.

SUMMARY BOX
ANTIGENS

- An individual's own molecules are recognized as 'self' and different molecules are recognized as 'foreign'.
- Some parts of antigens determine the extent of the immune response and others the specificity.
- Antigens may enter the body at a variety of sites, especially skin, respiratory tract and gastrointestinal tract.

THE IMMUNE RESPONSE

The nature of the immune response

The immune response is a defence mechanism mediated by lymphocytes and stimulated by antigens. Normally it is capable of recognizing and destroying every antigen that gains access to the body, whether the antigen is free within the extracellular environment of the body's tissues or part of the surface of a foreign cell.

There are two forms of immune system responses to antigens – humoral (chemical) and cellular (mediated by specific cells). In humoral immunity, protection is afforded by the formation of chemicals called antibodies. In cellular immunity, protection is mediated by cells called cytotoxic lymphocytes.

The most remarkable aspect of the immune response is that the recognition and destruction of each antigen is absolutely specific, in that it is targeted at that antigen alone. Bearing in mind the huge number of antigens with which we come into contact during our lives, from food, from infection, and generally from contact with our environment, it is difficult to comprehend either how or why such a defence system has evolved. As our understanding of the immune system has increased, it is apparent that the main reason why the immune system (as opposed to our non-specific defence system) has evolved is to allow us a 'memory' for infections so that should we survive an attack by a pathogen any future attacks are more easily and rapidly repelled and the effects are lessened. It is also becoming apparent that the method by which such a paradoxically diverse and yet specific defence system is possible is because of two related families of genes. These genes code for two molecules that lie at the heart of the control of the immune response (the T cell recep-

tor, which is the molecule on the T cell membrane that recognizes antigen; and immunoglobulins, which are the molecules used by B cells both for recognizing antigen and mediating humoral immunity – see below). These genes have evolved in mammalian cells with the potential for such huge degrees of subtle rearrangements, allelic deletion and alternative splicing that they are capable of producing the tremendous variations in the structure of their protein products essential for specific recognition and response to all antigens.

The immune response has evolved as a complex defence system. Like so many complex systems it has the potential for malfunctioning. When this happens the immune responses may cause damage to the tissues of their own (host) body. This adverse response is described as hypersensitivity (see below). Occasionally it is not the response that malfunctions but the recognition process and 'self' antigens are thought by the body to be 'foreign'. When this happens the body attacks its own tissues causing autoimmune disease.

In this chapter the mechanisms underlying and the complexities involved in the normal and abnormal immune response will be described and discussed. By necessity such a description must be broad based and incomplete. For more detail, specialized books should be consulted.

SUMMARY BOX
IMMUNE RESPONSE

- A defence mechanism mediated by lymphocytes stimulated by antigens.
- Humoral response is through chemicals (antibodies) and cellular response is through specific cells.
- Specific antibodies recognize single specific antigens.
- Initially T cells recognize antigens, then B cells produce antibodies.
- A rapid response is mounted on subsequent exposure to antigens through memory T and B cells.
- Potential malfunctions include hypersensitivity (overactivity in response to trivial stimulus) and autoimmunity (self-antigens being recognized as foreign).

Lymphocytes

Lymphocytes are the type of white blood cells responsible for all specific immune reactions. They have three functions. They may (a) be actively involved in destroying the antigen, (b) direct other cells to help in eliminating antigens and (c) act as a 'memory' for the antigen so that if encountered on a second or subsequent occasion a more rapid and powerful response can be evoked. This last is the principle exploited in immunization.

Lymphocytes that undertake or regulate immune events are said to be 'effector cells' whereas those responsible for retaining information about past antigenic challenge are described as 'memory cells'.

Lymphocytes are small cells with relatively large, round nuclei, little cytoplasm and few organelles. They are found in large numbers in the bloodstream, the specialized lymphoid organs (spleen, lymph nodes, mucosa-associated lymphoid tissues, and thymus) and in low numbers in other organs. The peripheral blood normally contains approximately 250 000 lymphocytes per decilitre so that these cells constitute about one-third of the circulating leukocyte population. From the bloodstream, lymphocytes enter into tissues which they patrol looking for antigens. After spending a variable length of time in the tissue they leave, using the same route as tissue fluid, i.e. via the lymphatics. They are the only constant cells to be found in lymph, hence their name. Subsequently they return to the bloodstream through the connections between the lymphatics and the venous side of the haemic circulation. Thus they are continually recirculating through the body. Periodically they arrive in special lymphoid organs such as the lymph nodes, spleen and mucosa-associated lymphoid tissues (tissues looking like lymph node but an integral part of the wall of those tubes in contact with the outside, e.g. the bowel, bronchi, etc.). Here the lymphocytes come into contact with other lymphoid cells, specialized antigen-presenting cells (see later) and other immune system cells. These organs are the site of lymphocyte replication in the adult and where many immune reactions take place.

There are two classes of lymphocyte: B lymphocytes (B cells) and T lymphocytes (T cells). The cells in each class look the same but they can be distinguished by their reactions to antigen and by the presence of unique molecules found only on the surfaces of specific lymphocyte cell types (see 'Cluster determinants (CD)' below).

- B cells recognize antigen, using molecules called immunoglobulins bound to their cell membranes and are responsible for the production of secreted immunoglobulins (antibodies) that bind to antigens and lead to humoral immunity.
- T cells recognize antigen by means of receptor molecules (the T cell receptor) located in the plasma membrane of the cell. T cells are the essential elements of cell-mediated immunity.

Although in adults most lymphocyte replication occurs within lymphoid tissues, the specific pool of lymphocyte stem cells is within the bone marrow. During early life, undifferentiated lymphocytes from the bone marrow recirculate through the thymus, or through a different, and to date still unidentified, part of the body, analogous to the bursa of Fabricius in other animals, where they mature, respectively, into T and B lymphocytes (Fig. 4.1). These cells are still not capable of inducing an immune response. For this they must encounter antigen, but any antigen will suffice. Once the lymphocyte has been challenged with antigen a remarkable change occurs in the

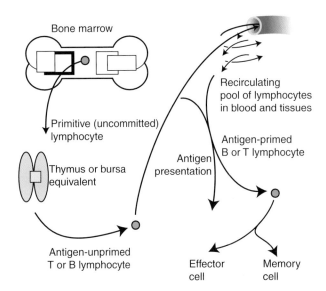

Fig. 4.1 Diagrammatic representation of the differentiation pathways of lymphocytes.

cell that causes it to participate in the immune response, but now the cell, and its progeny, will only respond to one specific antigen. Effectively lymphocytes pass through three stages: immature cells just formed within the bone marrow; maturation to a cell that is differentiated towards a B or T lymphocyte; and, finally, a specific antigen-primed cell that can only recognize and respond to a single antigen.

The thymus involutes during adolescence meaning that no further lymphocytes can differentiate into T cells, and the same may apply to B cells. It follows that after involution of the thymus, the precursor pool in the bone marrow can no longer be used to replenish the body's lymphocyte population. To compensate, lymphocytes have developed a system whereby they can proliferate within lymphoid organs, notably lymph nodes and the spleen.

T cells

The effector cells of the T cell lineage are of two varieties: cytotoxic and regulatory.

- Cytotoxic cells (including CD8+ T cells) directly destroy foreign target cells that they recognize by virtue of antigens expressed on their surfaces.
- Regulatory T cells are of two main types: CD4+ (helper (T_H) cells) and CD8+ (suppressor (T_S) cells), that promote or inhibit immune reactions respectively.

T cells constitute 70% of peripheral blood lymphocytes and circulate continually from the blood to the tissue and then to the lymph. Circulating T cells tour the body, within the blood and almost every tissue, continuously monitoring it for foreign antigen. The T lymphocyte cannot detect antigen directly. For this it requires a cell capable of presenting it with antigen in a suitable form. This necessitates the presenting cell expressing, on its surface, a molecule called a major histocompatibility complex antigen (MHC), either class I (for cytotoxic cells) or type II (for regulatory cells (see 'Antigen-presenting cells' below)) coupled with the specific antigen peptide. The MHC can be considered to be like a docking site. The way in which the T cell recognizes antigen and its 'docking site' on the antigen-presenting cell is via a

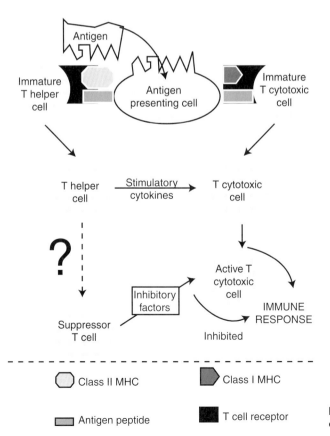

Fig. 4.2   Interactions between T effector cells.

molecule on its cell membrane known as the T cell receptor. Specificity of the T cell response is conferred through changes in the structure and conformation of this molecule, induced by the presence of properly presented, specific antigen. Once they recognize presented antigen, a signal is generated via intracellular second messenger pathways that profoundly modifies T lymphocyte behaviour. Activated cells may become regulatory or cytotoxic effector cells or memory cells (Fig. 4.2).

Regulatory cells either stimulate or inhibit the immune response. CD4+ T helper (T_H) cells can either stimulate activation of further T cells or cooperate with B lymphocytes to induce immunoglobulin formation, whereas CD8+ T suppressor (T_S) cells suppress these and other functions of the immune response.

Cytotoxic T cells, once activated, enter the tissues and circulation and, when they encounter cells bearing the antigen on the surface, destroy those cells. This process necessitates binding to the target cell via the T cell receptor (TCR).

Memory cells preserve, permanently or semipermanently, a memory of the antigen.

B cells (Fig. 4.3)

Like T lymphocytes, after antigen recognition, B lymphocytes transform. The non-antigen-primed B lymphocyte expresses immunoglobulin (M) molecules on its cell surface. These can bind to free antigen. Rarely, this is sufficient to initiate transformation by itself. More commonly

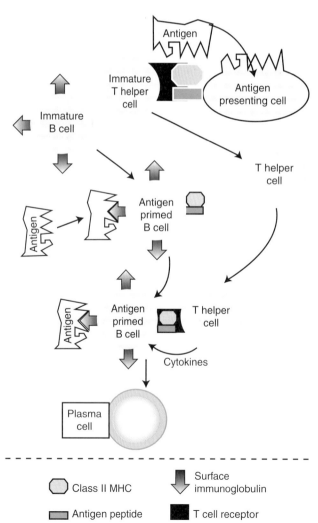

Fig. 4.3 Interactions between T helper cell and B lymphocytes.

the antigen-primed B lymphocyte has to bind to a T helper cell when direct contact and cytokine release (see 'Cytokines' below) lead to transformation to the B lymphocyte effector or memory cell. The effector B lymphocytes are plasma cells and they manufacture antibodies for secretion into the body fluids. Morphologically, plasma cells are 15–20 µm in diameter, round or ovoid. They have eccentric nuclei which display peripheral clumps of nuclear chromatin, giving an appearance described as being like a cartwheel. Because they are highly biosynthetic the cytoplasm of these cells contains many ribosomes and much rough endoplasmic reticulum, which gives them a basophilic (blue-purple) coloration in haematoxylin and eosin-stained tissue sections.

The primary function of the plasma cell is the production of secreted immunoglobulins or antibodies (the terms are synonymous).

Immunoglobulins (antibodies)

Antibodies are secreted by mature plasma cells. They are glycoproteins and are present in the plasma and most extracellular fluids. Diversity and heterogeneity are central to antigenic recognition, and immunoglobulin structure reflects this requirement.

Each immunoglobulin (Ig) molecule consists of a functional unit made up of four polypeptide chains, two long (or heavy) and two short (or light) chains arranged in a shape reminiscent of a fork.

There are five different types of heavy chain molecule each with a molecular weight of approximately 60 000, called α, δ, ε, γ and µ and two different types of light chain κ and λ with a molecular weight of 22 000. Each functional unit contains two identical heavy chains and two light chains either of which could be κ or λ. The functional units may exist singly or as groups of two or five linked by 'joining' or 'J' chains. Differences in molecular size and composition within the heavy chains allow five classes to be recognized (Table 4.1), each class being known by the English equivalent of its Greek heavy chain letter (A, D, E, G, M). They have distinctive properties and functions.

If immunoglobulin molecules undergo enzyme digestion in vitro they break up, not into four chains, but into two fragments. The first is formed of a pair of antigen-binding (fragment antigen-binding (Fab)) sites while the second has a less variable structure and, because it can easily be crystallized, is termed Fc (Fig. 4.4).

Within each of the five classes of immunoglobulin, an enormous number of detailed variations in molecular structure is possible. These variations are confined to the variable end of the Ig molecule, which is also the Fab segment, and are coded for by large numbers of specific genes responsible for the construction of the Ig molecules. By building diversity into the chemical structure of the Ig molecule it is possible to give it specificity, in terms of antigen recognition.

The five classes of Ig also have other characteristic and

TABLE 4.1
A DESCRIPTION OF THE VARIOUS TYPES OF IMMUNOGLOBULIN

Class	No. of functional units	Features
IgA	2	20% of immunoglobulin in the blood. Found in all body secretions including saliva. Consists of two molecules joined by a J chain. Secreted IgA is bound to another molecule called 'secretory fragment' which stops its breakdown by natural digestive enzymes. It binds to organisms, particularly bacteria, in the lumen of the hollow viscera and prevents their entry into the body
IgD	1	About 1% of all immunoglobulin. Found on inactive cells. Important recognition of lymphocyte-specific antigens
IgE	1	This is mostly bound to mast cells. It is involved in allergy and parasite responses
IgG	1	75% of immunoglobulin in the blood and tissue fluid. Crosses the placenta, and gives passive immunity to the fetus
IgM	5	10% of immunoglobulin. This is the immunoglobulin expressed on the surface of B lymphocytes that acts as the primary protein antigen recognition molecule. It is also secreted as a pentamer. Because of its size it is usually found in the circulation and rarely escapes into tissue fluid. It does not cross the placenta

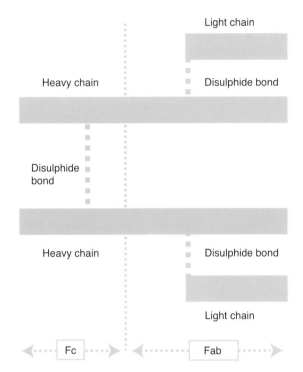

Fig. 4.4 **The basic structure of an immunoglobulin molecule.**

- White blood cells are actively involved in destroying antigens, directing other cells to help in eliminating antigens and acting as memory for the antigens.

- They are found in the bloodstream and specific lymphoid organs (spleen, lymph nodes, thymus and mucosa-associated lymphoid tissue), and are in constant recirculation.

- Two main classes (T cells and B cells) are distinguished by cell surface markers, known as cluster determinants (CD).

- T lymphocytes develop from bone marrow stem cells and mature on exposure to antigen through the thymus; they may be cytotoxic or regulatory (helper or suppressor).

- T cells recognize antigen and antigen-presenting cells via the T cell receptor.

- B lymphocytes develop from the human equivalent of the bursa of Fabricius (B cells) and transform after antigen recognition.

- Primed B cells link with T helper cells to lead to the formation of plasma cells (effector B cells) which produce specific antibodies (immunoglobulins).

constant structural and biological properties. These are a function of the easily crystallizable, constant (Fc) part of the molecule.

The mechanism by which immunoglobulins function in the immune system are described below in the section entitled 'Infection and immunity'.

NK cells

There is a group of cytotoxic cells that is not strictly of the T cell lineage. These are natural killer (NK) cells. They possess receptors that bind to antibody molecules attached to cell surfaces. They work in a different way from other cytotoxic T cells which react to specific cell surface-bound antigens. NK cells recognize and bind to any antibodies that have already bound to specific cell membrane antigens. This type of reaction, known as antibody-dependent cell-mediated cytotoxicity (ADCC), causes non-specific destruction of a target cell, whose surface antigens have already been the subject of attack by specific antibodies.

Other cells and the immune system

The immune response as part of chronic inflammation. Activation of the immune system is one of the mechanisms that gives rise to the state of chronic inflammation, which has already been discussed (see Ch. 3). Thus, the chronic inflammatory phenomena of fibrosis and vascular proliferation are seen as part of a typical immune reaction. Lymphocytes produce cytokines, which can activate many other cells, including fibroblasts, endothelial cells, etc., recruiting them into specific defence, but in a non-specific fashion.

Two cells, however, stand out from the others as being fundamental to the immune system in a way that the others are not. These cells are the antigen-presenting cells and tissue macrophages.

Antigen-presenting cells and macrophages. In terms of the immune system both antigen-presenting cells and macrophages are important because they present antigen to T lymphocytes. Antigen-presenting cells are specifically differentiated for this purpose. They are found in the epidermis and lymphoid tissues and scattered throughout other tissues. They endocytose the antigen, change and concentrate it on their cell surfaces and then interact with T lymphocytes.

Their interaction is mediated by 'docking' molecules encoded by a group of genes on chromosome 6 called the major histocompatibility complex (MHC). These molecules, called MHC antigens, are intricately variable cell membrane glycoproteins which, in man, are known as human leukocyte-associated antigens (HLA antigens). These molecules play a central role in immune recognition.

The two major groups of gene products are called the class I and class II antigens:

- Class I antigens are found on all nucleated cells and are encoded by parts of three different sets of MHC genes known as A, B and C.
- Class II antigens, sometimes called Ia (immune associated) antigens are encoded by genes in the D region of the MHC. The D region itself has three parts known as DP, DQ and DR. These antigens are expressed on antigen-presenting cells, macrophages and B lymphocytes and are involved in presentation of antigen to regulatory T cells.

The MHC genes are highly polymorphic, meaning that at any one site (A, B, C or D) there are huge numbers of possible gene permutations. Common molecules are recognized and numbered, e.g. A4, B25, DR3, etc.

Not all antigen comes into contact with the relatively rare antigen-presenting cells. In other sites the macrophage performs this role, although they are only about 5% as efficient as the specialized antigen-presenting cells.

The macrophage also acts directly as an immune system cell and can be turned into an effector cell (either a cell that synthesizes cytokines and other active molecules or one capable of phagocytosis) by lymphocytes stimulated by specific antigens.

HLA in disease. The expression of certain HLA subtypes is associated with an increased risk of certain diseases. Thus those individuals with HLA-B27 are 90 times more likely to develop the spine disease, ankylosing spondylitis, and being HLA-DR4-positive increases the risk of developing rheumatoid arthritis fourfold.

Cluster determinants (CD)

T cells, B cells and many other cells are recognized by the use of specific, artificially synthesized, immunoglobulins called monoclonal antibodies, which identify the presence of cell surface antigens that are found only on cells of a single type. By international agreement, these antigenic markers are categorized by number in a 'cluster of determinants' (CD). Thus, CD45 is an antigen common to all leukocytes, CD20 is an antigen common to all B cells, CD3 identifies all T cells, while macrophage markers

include CD14, CD25 and CD68. Helper T cells are usually CD4; cytotoxic and suppresser T cells are CD8. Often different types or functional groups of lymphocytes are recognized by this nomenclature.

Interactions between cells in the immune response

Summary of the role of B and T cells in the immune response

The mechanism by which lymphocytes recognize antigens and undergo transformation is very complex. It can be summarized, however, as follows.

A T lymphocyte, following presentation with antigen in conjunction with a class II MHC molecule by an antigen-presenting cell becomes transformed into a T helper cell. This involves a complex series of intracellular events that lead to the production of novel molecules. One group are the T cell receptor molecules, modified specifically for the presented antigen. Others, known as cytokines, are released into the extracellular fluid and cause changes in adjacent cells by binding to receptor molecules expressed by those cells.

Many of the cells in the vicinity of activated T cells are B or T lymphocytes. These cells are transformed, by direct binding or through cytokines, to become (a) effector cells (plasma cells for B cells and cytotoxic cells for T cells) which mediate the immune response, or (b) memory cells. The life span of different populations of memory cells is very variable, and whilst some exist for a long time, imparting almost life-long immunity, others exist for a much shorter time with correspondingly shorter immunity.

Cytokines

Cytokines can be thought of as locally acting hormones. They are a huge family of molecules that are produced by one cell and act on the same or other cells. To work, it is essential that the cell to which the cytokine is directed (the target cell) can bind the cytokine. This is done by the expression of cell surface molecules known as cytokine receptors. Cytokines can work in three ways:

- Some are produced by a cell that also expresses the receptor. The cell autostimulates itself, a process called an autocrine effect.
- Frequently, receptors are found on cells in the immediate vicinity of the cell synthesizing the cytokine. Stimulation through this route is known as paracrine.

- Occasionally, the cytokines are not broken down in the tissue of origin and escape into the circulation where they can be taken anywhere in the body to cells expressing receptors. Because this resembles the way in which a hormone works it is known as an endocrine effect.

The production of cytokines and their receptors is very complexly controlled by the chemical and physical tissue environment.

It is of more than academic interest to understand cytokines as many modern approaches to disease management are directed at interfering with the synthesis or action of cytokines or their receptors.

The site of the immune response

This sequence of contact with, and response to, antigens can occur either in the tissues or within the specialized lymphoid organs. It follows that some cells, notably B lymphocytes, whose effector cells do not require to be close to the antigen to work (because they destroy antigen by the production of soluble antibodies that can be taken to the antigen by the circulation and/or tissue fluid) can be activated away from the site of antigen entry, allowing a response to be initiated in a more controlled environment and permitting dissemination of the immune response throughout the body, should the antigen, or more usually antigen-bearing cells (such as bacteria), escape the confines of their tissue of entry.

SUMMARY BOX
OTHER IMMUNE CELLS

- Antigen-presenting cells contain major histocompatibility complex antigen (MHC) on their surface: type I for cytotoxic cells and type II for regulatory cells. MHC binds to specific T cell receptors.
- Regulatory cells either stimulate (CD4+, T helper) or inhibit (CD8+, T suppressor) interactions with other T cells or with B cells for immunoglobulin synthesis.
- Antigen-presenting cells are specifically differentiated for this purpose and are found particularly in the skin (Langerhans' cells) and lymphoid tissues.
- Macrophages are present throughout the body and can function as less specialized antigen-presenting cells, capable of producing cytokines or of phagocytosis.
- Cytokines are substances which act on the same (autocrine effect) or target cells, locally (paracrine) or more distally (endocrine), through specific cytokine receptors.

INFECTION AND IMMUNITY

General aspects of immunity to infectious organisms

Immunity to infectious organisms comes from innate or acquired immunological responsiveness to foreign antigens, either on or induced in host cells by microbial organisms. The resistance may be general, a state that includes all those heritable, nutritional and metabolic factors that raise the quality and quantity of resistance, or it can be local. Immunity may be natural or it may be acquired, actively (by induction of host immunity) or passively (through being given antibodies against the microbial antigens).

Active immunity is conferred in two ways; by recovery from infection with microorganisms; or by inoculation. In the latter, antigen or whole dead or inactive organisms are injected into the host. Antigen reaches lymphoid tissues and is endocytosed and processed by antigen-presenting cells. It stimulates an immune response which eliminates the antigen but leaves a long-lasting memory. Sometimes more than one dose of antigen (a booster) is required to achieve optimal levels of immunity.

Passive immunity is conferred in utero by the transplacental transfer of maternal IgG, but not by the much larger IgM antibody molecules which do not pass the placental barrier. After birth it can also be conferred by ingestion of breast milk. In later life, passive immunity is given by the parenteral injection of sera containing preformed antibodies, such as those in convalescent serum (i.e. serum of someone recovering from the infection). Nowadays, passive immunity is largely confined to prophylactic treatment against infections such as hepatitis A and B. Where possible, it is preferred also to boost active immunity by the further injection of the appropriate antigen, for example hepatitis B virus vaccine.

Paradoxically, a hazard of the passive administration of crude serum containing antibody is the development of an immune reaction in response to the presence of foreign serum proteins. This danger is now largely avoided by the use of purified human gamma-globulin or antibodies produced through the techniques of molecular genetics.

Cell-mediated immunity

Cell-mediated immunity is a necessary defence mechanism in dealing with intracellular microorganisms, particularly viruses, mycobacteria, chlamydia and some protozoa that, by virtue of their intracellular location, are little affected by antibodies. Their destruction is a property of T lymphocytes. The intracellular organisms cause changes in the host cells that are manifest as expression of antigens on the surface of the infected cell. These are recognized by T lymphocytes. The host cell and its included infection are then destroyed. The characteristics of T cell-mediated responses are typified by the response of the sensitized or immunized individual to *Myco-bacterium tuberculosis* which is described elsewhere in this book (see Chs 3 and 9).

Although antiviral responses are predominately cell mediated, small amounts of circulating antiviral antibody form when the virus is extracellular, during transfer from cell to cell or on arrival in the host. These antibodies are able to neutralize virus at sites of entry or bind to virus in the stage of primary viraemia. The active stimulation of antiviral antibody formation to provide protection against viruses such as polio virus, using orally administered attenuated strains, or the passive administration of pre-formed antimeasles virus gamma-globulin, are examples of effective antivirus prophylaxis attributable to humoral antibody. The presence of antiviral antibody in rising titres can be a useful diagnostic aid in suspected viral disease.

Humoral immunity

Humoral immunity to organisms is best illustrated by reference to bacterial infection. Humoral immunity protects against many bacteria, including *Streptococcus pneumoniae* and *Haemophilus influenzae*, and against bacterial exotoxins, such as those of the clostridia and *Corynebacterium diphtheriae*. However, humoral immunity is relatively ineffective in responding to organisms such as mycobacteria which live within macrophages.

Humoral immunity affords protection against bacterial infection in a variety of ways. Before these can be understood it is necessary to examine a remarkable group of plasma proteins collectively known as complement.

SUMMARY BOX
INFECTION AND IMMUNITY

- Active immunity is acquired by recovery from infection with microorganisms or by vaccination.
- Passive immunity is acquired from the mother or by injection of immune serum.
- Cell-mediated immunity protects against intracellular organisms.
- Humoral immunity is active against bacteria and involves the complement system.

Complement

Complement is a series of proenzymes produced by the liver and secreted into the blood. Rather like the clotting system, complement is activated on the basis of a cascade in which the initial stimulus produces a few molecules of the first enzyme, but this then rapidly leads to a stepwise amplification in the numbers of effector enzyme molecules. The key molecule in this cascade is complement factor 3, or C3. This is converted into its active components, C3a and C3b, by two different mechanisms. The first, or 'classic pathway', is initiated by antigen–antibody complexes and leads through complement components 1, 4 and 2 to the production of C3 convertase, the enzyme which changes C3 to C3a and C3b. C3 convertase production can also be stimulated through the second, or 'alternative pathway', activated by endotoxins, complex polysaccharides and aggregated globulins. C3b has three major effects:

1. It feeds back into the alternative pathway and inhibits the production of C3 convertase (a negative feedback).
2. It activates the fifth component of complement (C5) to form C5a and C5b.
3. It is a powerful opsonin in its own right (see below).

C3a increases vascular permeability as does C5a; the latter is also highly chemoattractive to most leukocytes. C5b initiates the action of a further four enzymes (C6, 7, 8 and 9) within the cascade to form a large complex, which is a powerful enzyme able to perforate the cellular membrane of bacteria. This bypasses the sodium pump; sodium and water enter the cell, which swells and 'explodes'.

SUMMARY BOX
COMPLEMENT

- A complex series of proenzymes activated in a cascade mechanism.
- The central step is activation of C3 into its active components (C3a and C3b).
- Activated products of complement function through opsonization, induction of vascular permeability, and chemotaxis for leukocytes.
- Complement is particularly important in bacterial infections.

There are three mechanisms by which humoral immunity affords protection against bacterial infection, two are mediated wholly or in part by complement.

- *By the direct action of complement.* C7, C8 and C9 together exert selective effects on the bacterial cell wall, which are particularly important for the destruction of Gram-negative bacteria. Antibody binds to the bacterial wall, complement is fixed, and the cascade activated, finally leading to permeabilization of the organism's wall and thus destruction of the microorganism itself.
- *By opsonization.* Opsonization is mediated by opsonins, which prepare bacteria for phagocytosis. Commonly, opsonins are complement (C3b and C5b) and IgG antibodies against the antigens of bacterial capsules or cell walls. They are particularly effective against extracellular pyogenic microorganisms, especially those that are encapsulated, such as *Streptococcus pneumoniae*. Neutrophil granulocytes and macrophages identify the complement products or the free Fc part of the opsonizing antibodies, which are attached to antigens on the surface of the bacterium. Some bacteria possess mechanisms to counter opsonization. For instance, the opsonization of *Staphylococcus aureus* can be prevented by the production of a membrane molecule by the bacterium, called protein A, that blocks the free end of the antibody molecule.
- *By the neutralization of bacterial exotoxin.* Bacteria may mediate their damaging effects by secreting protein-based poisons. These are recognized as foreign and neutralized by immunoglobulins.

DISEASES OF THE IMMUNE SYSTEM

Immunodeficiency

Immunodeficiency is a state of diminished immune reactivity. It may be a primary (congenital or heritable) defect, or a secondary result of disease, drugs, infection, irradiation and other causes. The patient with immunodeficiency is said to be immunocompromised.

Primary immunodeficiency

Primary immunodeficiency is classified, first, according to whether T cells, B cells, or both, are defective or absent, and, second, according to the phase of T cell or B cell development and function that is affected.

There are many categories of more or less severe primary immunodeficiency disease. They are rare conditions of which some examples are given below.

- *A complete lack of B cells.* An absence of B cells, and thus of antibody synthesis, is encountered. The most common form of this disorder is known as Bruton-type agammaglobulinaemia. Children affected with this disorder are highly susceptible to bacterial infection but have a normal degree of T cell-mediated immunity to viral, fungal and mycobacterial disease.
- *A complete lack of T cells.* An absence of T cells, and thus of cell-mediated immune responses, is encountered in the DiGeorge syndrome in which the thymus does not form. Individuals with this rare syndrome have normal humoral immune responses to pyogenic bacterial infections but display little resistance to viral infections, such as measles and chickenpox, and to mycobacterial infection. In these individuals the local injection of attenuated *Mycobacterium tuberculosis* in BCG vaccine is followed by progressive local and even systemic infection.
- *Combined immunodeficiency.* In severe forms of combined immunodeficiency, both B cell and T cell formation is defective and there is a lack of both humoral and cell-mediated immune responses. Consequently, an extreme defect of resistance to all forms of infection prevails. Children with this condition usually die of infections.

Secondary immunodeficiency

Disease of the lymphoreticular tissues may lead to secondary immunodeficiency. These diseases are usually either infections or neoplasms.

Malignant tumours of the reticuloendothelial system can cause secondary immunodeficiency. Thus, although the cells of myeloma (a malignant proliferation of plasma cells) usually secrete large quantities of immunoglobulin, it is always abnormal and the presence of malignant plasma cells suppresses normal cell function leading to an overall B cell deficiency resulting in a defect of humoral immunity. Hodgkin's lymphoma is associated with a deficiency of T cells and lowered resistance to viral, mycobacterial and fungal infections.

Infections such as with human immunodeficiency virus (HIV) can also lead to secondary immunodeficiency, often by stimulating T suppressor cells.

Immunosuppression

The immune system can also be inhibited by the deliberate use of certain drugs. Suppression of the T cell immune reaction against a graft (transplant) is required to permit prolonged survival of the transplanted organ or tissue. Immunosuppressive drugs are also used to treat autoimmune disorders such as rheumatoid arthritis. The major hazard of prolonged immunosuppression is the emergence of an unexpectedly high incidence of infections, often by organisms that are not usually pathogenic such as certain fungi. Such organisms are described as opportunistic. Many opportunistic infections manifest themselves in the mouth.

Immune suppression and immunodeficiency can also predispose to cancers, such as leukaemia, lymphoma and malignant melanoma. Sometimes these cancers are caused by oncogenic infective agents such as Epstein–Barr virus (EBV), latent within the B cells of normal adults. Cytotoxic T cells normally regulate the transformation of EBV-infected cells, and suppression or lack of T cell activity allows infected B cells to behave without this constraint.

SUMMARY BOX
IMMUNODEFICIENCY

- Primary immunodeficiency may be (a) primarily B cell deficient (affected individuals prone to bacterial infections), (b) primarily T cell deficient (affected individuals display little resistance to viral and mycobacterial infections), or (c) combined immunodeficiency where individuals are prone to all forms of infections and die relatively young.
- Secondary immunodeficiency is caused by diseases of the lymphoreticular system including neoplasms such as myeloma and lymphomas, and infections such as human immunodeficiency virus (HIV) causing acquired immunodeficiency syndrome (AIDS).
- Immunosuppression is caused by the use of certain drugs such as corticosteroids and cytotoxic antineoplastic agents.
- Patients on such treatments are prone to infection with low-virulence organisms, so-called opportunistic infections.

HYPERSENSITIVITY

Hypersensitivity is a group of conditions in which undesirable tissue damage follows the development of a state of humoral or cell-mediated immunity. Hypersensitivity is particularly likely when large amounts of foreign antigen persist while antibody formation is occurring. Individuals sensitized by first exposure to foreign antigen develop a beneficial primary immune state. Later exposure to the same antigen boosts this immunity. Hypersensitivity represents an unwanted alteration of this secondary reaction.

There are four types of hypersensitivity: types I, II and III hypersensitivity are 'immediate' and expressed by reactions between antigen and the humoral arm of the immune system; type IV hypersensitivity is 'delayed' and is mediated by T lymphocyte surface receptors.

Type I hypersensitivity

Certain individuals exposed to some foreign antigens are prone to form IgE antibodies (Fig. 4.5). The Fc parts of IgE molecules have an affinity for, and adhere to, the surface of mast cells. When there is further contact with the original sensitizing antigen, the antigen binds to free, Fab parts of the IgE molecules. This initiates a sequence of cell surface and intracellular events that causes the mast cells to degranulate and release histamine, heparin, the leukotrienes and other factors into the nearby tissues or circulation. This causes changes in vascular tone and permeability and alterations in other smooth muscle beds, notably in the bronchi where bronchospasm ensues.

Type I hypersensitivity is called anaphylaxis. The responses of type I hypersensitivity may be generalized or localized, depending on how antigen reaches the tissues.

Local anaphylaxis

Local anaphylactic reactions in man are commonplace. They include hay fever, extrinsic asthma and urticarial (the production of focal swellings within skin (wheals) and lining tissues) responses to foods.

Generalized anaphylaxis

Generalized anaphylaxis in man is rare but life-threatening. The injection of certain molecules including some drugs, such as penicillin, leads to widespread mast cell degranulation with circulatory collapse and generalized oedema (most dangerously in the larynx). This is a life-threatening condition requiring immediate treatment. It is therefore important to have antihistamines, adrenaline and steroids (the drugs used to treat generalized anaphylaxis) to hand when giving patients drugs.

Type II hypersensitivity – cytotoxic

Cytotoxic hypersensitivity is directed against cells by antibody molecules bound to cell surfaces. It may be mediated either by complement activation or by killer cells. One result is cell lysis – hence the name. Cytotoxic

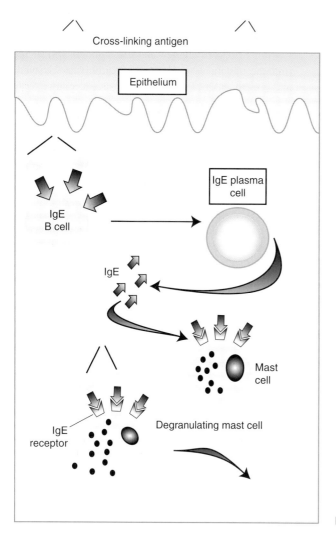

Cross-linking antigen

Epithelium

IgE plasma cell

IgE B cell

IgE

Mast cell

IgE receptor

Degranulating mast cell

Fig. 4.5 IgE-mediated anaphylaxis.

hypersensitivity is exemplified by the haemolytic reactions accompanying the transfusion of incompatible blood and by some drug reactions.

Type III hypersensitivity – immune complex mediated

Free, soluble antigen and antibody, present in the circulation in appropriate (optimal) proportions, can combine to form immune complexes, the presence of which can be shown by laboratory tests. Soluble immune complexes lodge in or pass through blood vessel walls, fix complement, and initiate inflammatory, tissue-damaging reactions. Polymorphs are attracted by chemotaxis. In turn, these cells release enzymes such as elastase and neutral

collagenase. Platelets aggregate and thrombus formation is encouraged.

- *Systemic immune complex disease.* If the immune complexes lodge in the small, terminal blood vessels of the joints, kidneys, heart and skin, they cause a potentially fatal syndrome, serum sickness, comprising arthritis, glomerulonephritis, oedema, cutaneous vasculitis and carditis (see Ch. 11 on renal disease).
- *Local immune complex disease.* If antigen persists at a site of injection or administration, for example because of indolent infection or autoimmune response, immune complex deposition may be recurrent and the resulting disease long-lasting. Rheumatoid arthritis and polyarteritis are examples of conditions in which

this mechanism is active (see 'Autoimmune disease' below and specific chapters on joint and vascular disease).

Type IV hypersensitivity – cell mediated

Cell-mediated, type IV or delayed hypersensitivity is of crucial importance in determining the cellular injury and tissue lesions of infection by bacteria such as *Mycobacterium tuberculosis*, by fungi, and by some viruses, for example the measles virus. Type IV hypersensitivity is responsible for many examples of transplant rejection and for skin reactions to important, small molecules such as the antibiotic neomycin, paraphenylenediamine (in hair dyes), and nickel and chromates which bind to protein and act as haptens. Type IV hypersensitivity is exemplified by the Mantoux reaction for tuberculosis.

SUMMARY BOX
HYPERSENSITIVITY

- An exaggerated response on second and subsequent exposure to an antigenic stimulus (may be humoral or cell mediated).
- Type I hypersensitivity (anaphylaxis) may be local, e.g. asthma and hay fever, or general; it is mediated by IgE.
- Type II hypersensitivity is a humoral response where antibodies bind to cell surfaces, e.g. in haemolytic reactions to incompatible blood transfusions and some drug reactions.
- Type III hypersensitivity is immune complex mediated where antigen–antibody complexes are formed in or deposited on vessels and may be systemic or localized.
- Type IV hypersensitivity is cell mediated and is of delayed type; examples are infection with *Mycobacterium tuberculosis* and some aspects of transplant rejection.

AUTOIMMUNE DISEASE

Tolerance

Before it is possible to understand autoimmune disease it is important to know why our lymphocytes do not recognize and attack our own antigens. The failure to react to 'self' antigens constitutes a process called natural tolerance. Tolerance can also be acquired or transmitted, and lost or 'broken', changes that provide a key to understanding autoimmunity. Although both T and B cells can be 'tolerized', T cells do so more easily.

Tolerance is generally the result of suppression of the immune responses through production of T suppressor cell clones. Thus suppressor T cells that recognize self antigens predominate over helper cells and the reaction to self antigens is thus inhibited. Very young, immunologically immature animals are readily tolerized to many antigens, for instance newborn mice can even be induced to tolerate skin grafts from foreign donors. It is probable that tolerance to our own molecules is induced in utero. The state of tolerance is usually specific, that is, confined to the antigen used and persists into adult life. The T cells that effect this change can be transferred passively to other hosts.

Adult animals can be tolerized by suppressing or depleting the lymphocyte population when antigen is given, or by giving antigen that cannot effectively be processed by antigen-presenting cells. Other protein antigens can cause tolerance if given in very low or high doses. Between these doses, intermediate amounts of antigen cause antibody formation.

Autoimmunity

Natural T cell suppresser activity diminishes with age. The increased tendency to recognize self antigens as foreign in the old may be as a result of this change.

Some tissues, such as the lipoproteins of the central nervous system, the cornea, the lens, and the colloid of thyroid follicles, are effective antigens but do not normally establish contact with the immune mechanism because there is a blood–tissue barrier or lack of a vascular supply, both of which prevent access to lymphocytes. These molecules do not, therefore, have the opportunity to induce tolerance. Thus, should they come into contact with the immune system at any time after birth, through, for instance trauma or some other disease process, they are recognized as foreign and can induce an immunological reaction. This is clearly different from a loss of tolerance.

Failure of tolerance with age and emergence of normally hidden antigens are only two ways in which the immune system comes to attack self antigens, a process known as autoimmunity. Autoimmune disorders can also be initiated by infections, particularly virus infections which can corrupt host genes to produce a hybrid molecule of viral and autoantigens. These can stimulate the immune system into producing antibodies against epitopes which are normally the subject of tolerance. Drugs, acting as haptens, can also bind to host molecules producing complexes that bypass normal tolerance mechanisms.

The processes leading to autoimmunity are made more likely if the host possesses certain types of HLA molecule, particularly those expressed at the HLA-D locus. Autoimmune disorders therefore tend to be familial.

It is usual to describe autoimmune disorders as either organ specific or organ non-specific. Organ-specific disorders are caused by autoantibodies directed at specific components of the organ. They include autoimmune thyroiditis (Graves' and Hashimoto's diseases) (Fig. 4.6), autoimmune gastritis (pernicious anaemia) and auto-immune adrenalitis (Addison's disease). Organ non-specific disorders are caused by tissue deposition of immune complexes, consisting of mixtures of antigens and antibodies. These tend to be deposited on the epidermal basement membranes, vascular basement membranes and within joints where they lead to complement activation and tissue damage. These diseases include rheumatoid arthritis, systemic lupus erythematosus and polyarteritis nodosa.

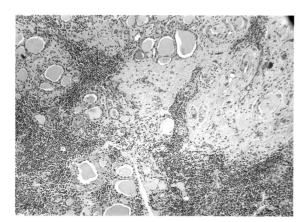

Fig. 4.6 **Autoimmune thyroiditis.** Section of thyroid tissue in which there is a dense lymphocytic infiltrate with occasional germinal centres and associated oncocytic change in thyroid follicular cells. The appearances are typical of autoimmune thyroiditis in Hashimoto's disease.

SUMMARY BOX
AUTOIMMUNITY

- The failure to react to self antigens is called natural tolerance which can be acquired or inherited.
- With increasing age, natural suppressor T cell activity diminishes, while antigens which have previously been 'hidden' may also become recognized.
- Certain human leukocyte antigen (HLA) types predispose to autoimmunity which may be accelerated by viral infections or by drug exposure.
- Autoimmunity may be either organ specific where antibodies are directed against specific organ components, e.g. thyroiditis, or non-organ specific where immune complexes are deposited at various sites and where the antigen may be a cellular component, e.g. systemic lupus erythematosus.

5 Microbes and infection

Microbes are organisms that are too small to be seen with the naked eye, but may be viewed using microscopes to magnify the image. The size of microbes is generally described in terms of micrometres (μm) and nanometres (nm). Many of these organisms colonize and live their lives on the surfaces (skin and mucus membranes) of humans, animals and other life forms. Others live in the environment, e.g. in soil and water. Of the millions of microorganisms surrounding us, only some can cause diseases in humans. The study of these agents and all aspects of the infectious diseases they produce (including prevalence, diagnosis, treatment and control of transmission) constitutes the field of medical microbiology.

Routes of infection

Infective agents may be transmitted from one human to another or from animal to human or from the environment to human. Many such agents may remain in the environment in a viable and infective form for varying periods of time – even years. Human-to-human transmission occurs as result of shedding of infective microbes by the initial host in skin scales, faeces, vomit, urine, respiratory, oral and genital secretions and blood. These infections are acquired in different ways:

- Ingestion of infected food, or food or water contaminated with faeces of infected humans or animals.
- Inhalation of aerosols containing infective particles coughed or sneezed by a patient, or released in other ways by animals or the environment.
- Injection into the body as in insect and animal bites or trauma. Exchange of blood products, e.g. during transfusions, or accidental mingling of blood as occurs following needlestick injuries in health care, and also in transplantation of infected tissues. Infected skin scales in dust settling on broken or incised skin can cause wound infections.
- Direct contact with skin or mucosa including sexual intercourse.
- Vertical transmission from mother to fetus in utero, or the baby may be infected during birth.

Methods used to destroy these infective particles before they are transmitted to a fresh host and cause disease include sterilization, i.e. ensuring the destruction of all living forms on any object, e.g. instruments or equipment, that has come in contact with a person or the environment, by using steam or dry heat at very high temperatures or chemical agents; and disinfection where chemical agents are used to destroy or reduce the numbers of infective agents on surfaces.

During the course of an infection microbes may be destroyed in the body by the immune defence mechanisms of the host. This process may be accelerated by the use of chemotherapeutic agents like antibiotics which either kill bacteria or prevent their multiplication, so that they may be cleared by the host defences. Many microbes have now developed systems of resistance to these chemotherapeutic agents and in some cases no suitable drugs are available for the treatment of these multi-resistant microbes.

- Ingestion of infected food or water.
- Inhalation of aerosols.
- Injection by bites or needlestick injuries.
- Direct contact of skin or mucous membranes.
- Vertical transmission from mother.

MEDICALLY IMPORTANT MICROBES

These may be conveniently classified into three broad groups, as follows.

1. Eukaryotic cells:
   – cestodes
   – nematodes
   – trematodes
   – protozoa
   – fungi
2. Prokaryotic cells:
   – bacteria
   – chlamydia
   – rickettsia
   – mycoplasma
3. Noncellular – viruses.

In recent years much interest has been focused on a group of atypical agents known as prion proteins, with speculation on their possible role as transmissible infective agents. They lack both DNA and RNA, and consist mainly of self-replicating proteins that are able to survive high temperatures. The diseases associated with prion proteins are called transmissible encephalopathies. They have a long incubation period (many years) and show a characteristic slow progression of chronic degenerative changes, which are usually in the nervous system, e.g. bovine spongiform encephalopathy (BSE) in cattle and the new variant Creutzfeldt–Jakob disease (nv CJD) in humans.

Infective agents relevant to the mouth and pharynx are mainly bacteria, viruses and the fungus *Candida albicans*.

Eukaryotic cells share many of the characteristic features of animal and plant cells, e.g. the presence of a membrane-bound nucleus containing separate chromosomes. Prokaryotic cells, on the other hand, have all their genes on a single tightly coiled thread of DNA. This nuclear body is not surrounded by a membrane.

Reproduction is by a simple process of cell division (binary fission) yielding two identical daughter cells. Prokaryotes also have a cell wall containing peptidoglycan, which maintains the integrity and shape of the organism. Mycoplasma, however, are bacteria that are devoid of a cell wall. Eukaryotes do not have peptidoglycan and generally lack cell walls. Although fungi possess cell walls, these are strengthened with chitin rather than peptidoglycan. Whilst most bacteria may be grown in laboratory culture media, chlamydia and rickettsia are obligate intracellular parasites. Viruses are not cellular in structure and are strict intracellular parasites that can only replicate themselves after entering a living cell of the preferred host, e.g. human, animal, plant or bacterium. They are much smaller than bacteria and an electron microscope is needed to visualize them. They possess few enzymes and survive by subverting the enzyme systems of the host cell to produce more viral particles.

Eukaryotes

Metazoans

Cestodes (flat or tapeworms), nematodes (roundworms) and trematodes (flukes) are metazoans, i.e. multicellular organisms with complex life cycles. Although the eggs and larvae (which are the infective forms) are microscopic, the adults in most cases are large enough to be clearly visible to the naked eye.

Protozoa

These are unicellular organisms that are generally larger than bacteria. Each cell is composed of cytoplasm surrounding a well-defined nucleus. Reproduction usually involves replication of the nucleus by mitosis followed by simple division of the surrounding cytoplasm into two identical cells. Some protozoa reproduce by sexual means, for example the *Plasmodium* species (agents causing malaria) express both sexual and asexual phases of reproduction during the course of their complex life cycle.

Fungi

These are usually larger than bacteria, and have thick cell walls containing chitin but no peptidoglycan. Within the cell wall lies the cell membrane which contains sterols and is susceptible to attack by some antifungal drugs. Fungi may be:

- Yeasts, which are round or oval cells that reproduce by budding e.g. *Cryptococcus*.
- Yeast-like fungi which grow mainly as yeasts but can also grow as long chains of filamentous cells – pseudomycelium. *Candida albicans*, an important fungus in the mouth can exist in two forms – a yeast-like form of oval or spherical cells 2–5 μm in diameter or it may produce filaments of the pseudomycelial form which may give rise to yeast cells by budding. This is differentiated from true mycelium of other fungi by the cross-walls in the filaments.
- Filamentous fungi grow as interlacing filaments of mycelium and reproduce by asexual spores, e.g. *Aspergillus*.
- Dimorphic fungi grow as filaments in the saprophytic form at room temperature, but in the yeast form as a parasite in the body at 37°C, e.g. *Histoplasma*.

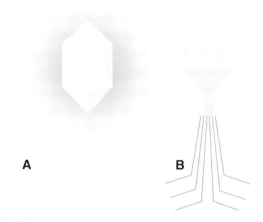

Fig. 5.1 Structure of virus. A. Capsid of herpesvirus showing icosahedral symmetry. **B.** Bacteriophage.

SUMMARY BOX
FUNGI

- Usually larger than bacteria, containing thick cell walls with chitin.
- May exist in several forms including yeasts, e.g. *Cryptococcus*; yeasts with pseudomycelia, e.g. *Candida albicans*; filamentous fungi, e.g. *Aspergillus*; dimorphic forms (both yeast and filamentous at different temperatures), e.g. *Histoplasma*.
- Fungi of particular dental significance are *Candida albicans* causing oral disease and *Aspergillus* which may colonize nasal sinuses after some oral procedures.

Viruses

These are classified on the basis of their size, shape and structure. Small viruses, e.g. poliovirus, are approximately 20–30 nm in diameter while poxviruses measure 200–300 nm in diameter. The shape of viruses seen by electron microscopy is a useful means of identification. They form regularly shaped particles. Many are polyhedra, others are filamentous (influenza virus) or brick-shaped (poxvirus). Bacterial viruses are called bacteriophages (phages) and are shaped like tadpoles with a polyhedral head and a tail (Fig. 5.1).

Each particle of infective virus (virion) consists of a nucleocapsid, i.e. a core of nucleoprotein surrounded by a protein shell (the capsid). Many viruses have, in addition, an envelope acquired from the host cell, e.g. herpesviruses, and when this is destroyed by a fat solvent the virion loses its infectivity.

The virion may contain RNA, DNA or transcriptase enzymes that instruct the host cell to synthesize, assemble and release many copies of the infective virus. These infective virions enter fresh host cells, and the intracellular replication cycle continues. The host cell may be lysed in order to release the virus particles. This is called a cytopathic effect and results in the disease process, e.g. influenza virus. Alternatively the virus may be released from the cell by a process of budding so that the infected cells take longer to die. Some viruses accumulate inside host cells to produce characteristic intracellular structures about 30 μm in diameter called inclusion bodies. These are of value in histological diagnosis. Certain viruses are able to remain dormant for years within host cells. They may then be reactivated at a later stage by conditions that lower the host's immunity.

This is typically seen with human herpesvirus type 1 (herpes simplex virus type 1 – HSV-1) and the varicella zoster virus (VZV). HSV-1 is a very common infective agent. Most people are infected in infancy and childhood and develop painful vesicular lesions in the mouth (acute vesicular gingivostomatitis). The symptoms soon resolve but some of the virus makes its way to the sensory ganglia, especially of the trigeminal nerve, having tracked up along the sensory nerves. HSV can remain dormant in the ganglion for many years. When it is reactivated by conditions like cold, stress, etc., the infective virus particles are released and travel down the nerve to establish the painful lesion called 'cold sore', i.e. blisters on the margin of the lips or nose. The infective virus is released from the lesions and also intermittently in the saliva. It is transmitted by direct contact, e.g. kissing. A similar dormant state occurs in chickenpox (caused by VZV) where the virus remains dormant for years in the nerve root ganglia and when reactivated cause 'shingles', i.e. painful blisters on the skin, characteristically distributed in the segment or dermatome supplied by the nerve concerned. The dormant forms of these viruses are inaccessible to host immune mechanisms or chemotherapy.

Persistent infection of host cells may also occur where the cell is not destroyed but its function may be impaired. Some viruses are able to transform host cells which can then rapidly multiply to form cancerous tumours.

Just as animal viruses infect living human cells as noted above, so bacteriophages infect specific bacteria. Here also, intracellular replication occurs and may lead to rapid lysis of the bacterium after exposure to the phage. Alternatively phages may integrate with bacterial chromosomes and be reproduced along with them thus transferring new properties and characteristics to the bacterial progeny. This is called transduction and is involved in the transfer of ability to produce toxins, e.g. diphtheria bacillus, and also in the transfer of resistance to antibiotics. The question of whether specific phages may be used for therapy of some infections caused by antibiotic-resistant bacteria is a field of experimental interest.

When host cells are infected simultaneously with two distinct but similar viruses, genetic recombination can occur and new strains of viruses may be produced with some properties of each. Thus, from time to time, new pandemic strains of influenza virus make an appearance. It is believed that these arise by a process of recombination following co-infection by virus strains of human and avian origin. This happens when humans and their poultry live together in very close contact.

SUMMARY BOX
VIRUSES

- Strict intracellular parasites which only replicate after entering living cells.
- Classified on size, shape and structure.
- Each particle of infective virus (virion) contains a core of nucleoprotein (nucleocapsid) with surrounding capsid (protein shell) with many also having an envelope.
- Infected cells may die from a direct cytopathic effect, or viral inclusions may accumulate within cells; some may persist for many years.

Bacteria

These have cells that are generally bound by a rigid protective cell wall composed of peptidoglycan, a polymer of *N*-acetyl muramic acid and *N*-acetylglucosamine

cross-linked by peptide chains. The cell wall may be surrounded by a capsule of polysaccharide or protein material. The presence of a capsule is often linked to the virulence of the organism in the human or animal host, since capsules can inhibit phagocytosis. Within the cell wall lies the semipermeable cytoplasmic membrane containing all the cell cytoplasm (Fig. 5.2). An intact cytoplasmic membrane is essential for the well-being of the microbe, as it is associated with enzymes required for respiration and transport of essential materials into the cell. Inside the cytoplasm may be seen the nuclear body – a simple coiled filament of double-stranded DNA containing all the genetic material, ribosomes, storage granules, etc., and in some cells there are pieces of extrachromosomal DNA called plasmids. Plasmids may code for important characteristics like the ability to produce toxin or the expression of antibiotic resistance. These characteristics may be passed on not only to the progeny of that cell during binary fission but also to other bacterial cells by a process called conjugation. Here two bacterial cells are linked to each other by a sex pilus (see below) through which plasmid DNA is exchanged.

Some bacteria are able to move themselves from place to place. Motile bacteria may have long filamentous processes called flagella which rotate to propel the cell forward. Flagella may be single or multiple and attached to one or both poles of a cell or all around it. Some genera of bacteria (spirochaetes) though non-flagellated, show

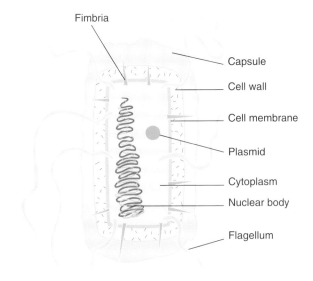

Fig. 5.2 **Structure of bacterium.** (See text for details.)

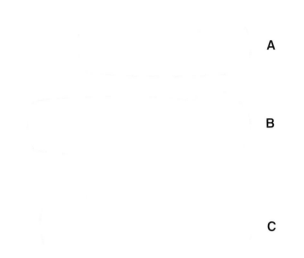

A

B

C

Fig. 5.3 **Bacterial spores. A.** *Bacillus anthracis* – central oval spore. **B.** *Clostridium tetani* – terminal spherical spore. **C.** *Clostridium sporogenes* – subterminal oval bulging spore.

motility by flexion and extension of their bodies. In addition to flagella, many bacteria carry short stiff hair-like processes called fimbriae or pili which help the cell to adhere to mucous surfaces or to other cells. A modified long form of a fimbria is referred to as the sex pilus and is involved with sexual conjugation between bacterial cells.

Certain bacteria are able to produce tough spores which help them to survive unfavourable conditions for long periods of time. The ability to form spores, their shape, position within the vegetative cell and size relative to the cell, provide useful information for identifying these species (Fig. 5.3). Spores are dormant forms which can resist heat, dryness and absence of nutrients. Spores of the organism causing tetanus, *Clostridium tetani*, can survive in the dormant state for many years in the soil. When they are introduced into a suitable environment, e.g. a dirty skin wound following a road traffic accident, the spores germinate into the vegetative forms which multiply rapidly, producing the tetanus toxin. Cell division does not occur in the spore. A spore gives rise to a single bacterial vegetative cell.

Classification of bacteria

Bacteria are classified according to their characteristics (Fig. 5.4). The most basic is the shape of the organism, e.g. when spherical cells about 1 μm in diameter are produced the bacterium is described as a coccus, whereas rod-shaped cells approximately 0.5–1 μm wide and

2–5 μm in length are described as bacilli (sing. bacillus). Comma-shaped rods are called vibrios, long spindle-shaped rods are fusiforms, spiral slender filaments up to 20 μm long are spirochaetes and branched filaments include the Actinomycetales. The arrangement of cells in relationship to each other helps to describe them further, e.g. streptococcus where the spherical cocci are arranged in a chain, like a string of beads, or staphylococcus when the cells are in a cluster, like a bunch of grapes. When cocci are seen in pairs they are called diplococci: for example, the pneumococcus, meningococcus and gonococcus are arranged in pairs.

Another method used for classification depends on the staining characteristics. Here the Gram stain is used, and bacteria described as Gram-positive if they stain violet or Gram-negative if they stain pink/red. Gram-positive cells have a thick layer of peptidoglycan in the cell wall. Gram-negative cells on the other hand have a narrow layer of peptidoglycan and an outer membrane of lipopolysaccharide with an intervening periplasmic space.

Bacteria are denoted by the generic name starting with a capital letter followed by the species name (in lower case), e.g. *Streptococcus pneumoniae* (the pneumococcus). This is a Gram-positive diplococcus that can cause pneumonia, meningitis and other septic conditions.

Bacterial growth

Bacteria require water, sources of carbon, energy, nitrogen, inorganic salts and other factors for growth and survival. Some bacteria, called aerobic organisms, only grow in the presence of oxygen, while others are strict anaerobes growing only in the total absence of oxygen – in fact they are rapidly killed in the presence of small amounts of atmospheric oxygen. A group of bacteria that are able to grow either in the presence or in the absence of oxygen are termed facultatively anaerobic. Bacteria that prefer low concentrations of oxygen (5%) are microaerophilic. Most bacteria require the presence of carbon dioxide for growth, but some require higher concentrations of CO_2 and are described as capnocytophilic. Optimum temperature is another factor that is essential for the growth of bacteria. Most medically relevant bacteria grow within a temperature range that includes human body temperature. In the laboratory they are usually cultured at 36–37°C.

When all the nutritional and cultural conditions are provided, bacteria multiply by binary fission, i.e. the nucleus replicates and the cell then divides into two daughter cells each with one copy of the nucleus

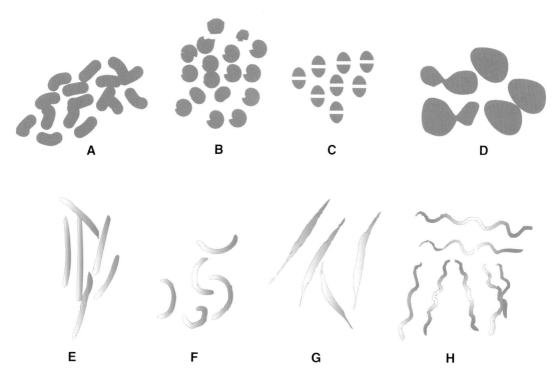

Fig. 5.4 Classification of bacteria. A. Staphylococcus. **B.** Streptococcus. **C.** Diplococcus. **D.** Budding yeast form of *Candida albicans*.
E. Bacillus. **F.** Vibrio. **G.** Fusiforms. **H.** Spirochaetes. (See text for details.)

(Fig. 5.5). The time taken for this replication varies between different genera, but many pathogenic organisms, e.g. salmonellae, double in around 15–20 minutes. Others, e.g. the organism causing leprosy, may require several hours. Thus in a period of around 15–20 hours, clearly visible growth may be observed as colonies on solid agar plates or, in the former case, turbidity in liquid broth. For the slow growers, e.g. tubercle bacillus, several weeks may be required.

Each colony contains many billions of identical organisms. Genetic variability is introduced in bacteria by mutation or by gaining DNA from other organisms by the process of conjugation, transformation or transduction.

When the growth of bacteria in a nutrient liquid medium is monitored over a period of time, the growth curve obtained (Fig. 5.6), shows an initial lag phase (with no increase in numbers) lasting a few hours, followed by a phase of exponential growth called the log (logarithmic) phase. Having acclimatized themselves to the new environment and produced the necessary enzymes for growth and replication in the lag phase, the cells divide rapidly in the exponential growth phase. This phase lasts for as long as the nutrients are available and at the end of this period the number of live bacteria remains stationary

for several hours before it starts to decline. During the exponential phase while the bacteria are intensively synthesizing new cell materials, antibiotics like penicillin are able to attack and kill them by interfering with the normal synthesis of the peptidoglycan cell wall. These defective cells are unable to maintain their integrity and soon die. Penicillin is thus highly active on growing cells in the log phase and not on cells that are static or resting. Other antibiotics act at different sites on the cell, e.g. tetracycline interferes with bacterial protein synthesis, ciprofloxacin acts on DNA gyrase preventing replication, while metronidazole acts specifically on anaerobic organisms.

If the viable counts of an initial 100 bacteria growing in the log phase are monitored every 20 minutes over a period of 4 hours, they progress thus:

$100 \rightarrow 200 \rightarrow 400 \rightarrow 800$ in 1 hour
$800 \rightarrow 1600 \rightarrow 3200 \rightarrow 6400$ in 2 hours
$6400 \rightarrow 12\,800 \rightarrow 25\,600 \rightarrow 512\,00$ in 3 hours
$51\,200 \rightarrow 102\,400 \rightarrow 204\,800 \rightarrow 409\,600$ in 4 hours,
i.e. 4×10^5 organisms.

Thus, if a piece of cooked chicken contaminated with 100 *Salmonella typhimurium* is left in a warm room,

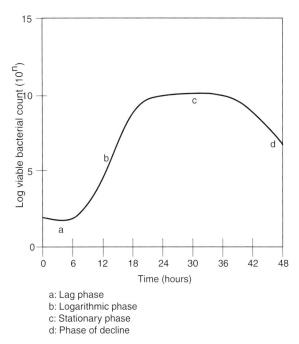

a: Lag phase
b: Logarithmic phase
c: Stationary phase
d: Phase of decline

Fig. 5.6 Bacterial growth curve. (See text for details.)

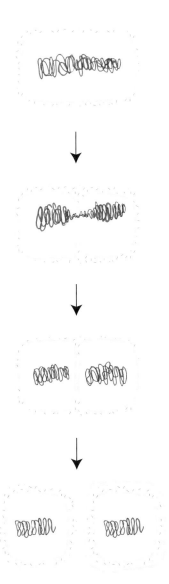

Fig. 5.5 Bacterial cell division. (See text for details.)

within a few hours it will contain sufficient numbers of the organism to cause symptoms of food poisoning (gastroenteritis) if ingested. The infective dose required to induce symptoms in this case is around 10^5–10^6 organisms, and if the chicken with 10^2 organisms had been consumed immediately, it is unlikely to have caused symptoms in healthy individuals. In cases of food poisoning the food containing the infective dose of microbes or their toxins usually looks and tastes perfectly normal and appetizing.

A similar example is the rapid growth of *Pseudomonas* species in dilute disinfectants or in water. These organ-

isms are relatively resistant to the disinfectant and can multiply rapidly, so that within a few hours a very large population is produced which may cause severe infection when brought into contact with susceptible patients, e.g. skin in burns units. Furthermore these bacteria are also very resistant to many antibiotics. It is therefore important that disinfectant solutions should be made up fresh every day.

SUMMARY BOX
BACTERIA

- Structure: rigid cell wall, capsule, cytoplasm, nucleus containing plasmids, mechanisms of motility, and the capacity to produce spores.
- Classified on shape, on Gram staining characteristics, and on growth in nutrients.
- Bacteria divide by binary fission with a lag phase followed by an exponential phase of rapid division; antibiotics may act in the actively dividing phase or elsewhere in the cycle.

Normal body flora

Many different microorganisms colonize various sites of the human body – skin and mucous membranes – living in a dynamic state of equilibrium without causing disease. The normal human fetus, in the uterus, is maintained in a sterile environment, but during and after birth, the baby is rapidly colonized by microbes acquired from the mother and others in its immediate surroundings. Some of these strains persist for many years while others are transient residents. When these stable relationships are disturbed, as happens following use of broad-spectrum antibiotics to treat various infections, the normal flora may also be killed and disease may be produced owing to colonization by exogenous pathogens or overgrowth of drug-resistant microbes at the site. Thrush caused by *Candida albicans* infections in the mouth and colitis due to *Clostridium difficile* in the colon frequently follow the use of antibiotics in the patient. The prevalence and distribution of microbial flora at a particular site may vary from time to time as a result of various causes other than the use of antibiotics. For example, in acute necrotizing ulcerative gingivitis there is an unusual overgrowth of a mixture of some normal flora including *Treponema vincenti, Leptotrichia buccalis, Prevotella melaninogenica, Campylobacter* and *Vibrio* species, which may be demonstrated in stained smears of the gingival crevicular fluid. The condition is caused by poor oral hygiene in addition to stress and is more commonly seen in students, army recruits and vagrants.

Sometimes pathogenic microbes may colonize a clinically normal host. Such a person is termed a carrier, since he or she may transmit the agent to others. The word carrier is also used to describe those harbouring the organism for variable periods of time following recovery from a disease (e.g. following recovery from typhoid, carriers may continue to excrete the organism intermittently for many years in their faeces or urine). With respiratory viruses, transmission of infection may occur during the incubation period prior to the symptomatic phase – incubational carriers.

Oral cavity

In the oral cavity the normal resident flora includes viridans streptococci, lactobacilli, neisseria and various anaerobic organisms of the genera *Prevotella, Porphyromonas,* and *Fusobacterium,* and Spirochaetes as well as *Campylobacter,* etc. *Candida albicans* is also found in small numbers in the normal mouth, although it may overgrow and cause oral disease following use of antibiotics or in immunosuppressed individuals. It is therefore referred to as an opportunistic pathogen.

Dental plaque

Dental plaque is an example of a biofilm developing on the surface of teeth. Oral microbes adhere to a salivary pellicle deposited on the tooth surface, and to each other, colonize the site and form a dense film. Large amounts of extracellular polysaccharides produced from dietary carbohydrate by organisms like *Strep. mutans* are an important factor in development of plaque by gluing the bacteria together. Whilst aerobic bacteria may survive on the surface of the film, facultatively anaerobic organisms can inhabit the deeper levels. As they utilize the available oxygen in this area, the strict anaerobes are able at last to colonize in this environment of reduced oxygen tension. This process occurs over a few weeks. Stable relationships are formed here, e.g. the corn-cob appearance seen, where spherical oral streptococci adhere to the tip of an elongated rod-shaped organism. If dental plaque is permitted to accumulate without control, it eventually calcifies forming tartar. This is now more difficult to remove by normal methods, e.g. tooth brushing.

Dental caries and periodontal disease

Strains of *Strep. mutans* in plaque are implicated in the aetiology of dental caries. They utilize dietary sucrose to produce large amounts of lactic acid which demineralizes the enamel and initiates the caries process. Late plaque is associated with the development of periodontal disease. Here the gingiva become inflamed, bleed easily and the point of attachment of the junctional epithelium to the tooth recedes apically producing a periodontal pocket (Fig. 5.7). This becomes colonized by advancing plaque

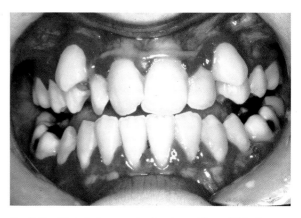

Fig. 5.7 Clinical photograph of patient with established acute gingivitis.

bacteria resulting in further deepening of the pocket. In time, the periodontal ligament and neighbouring alveolar bone are destroyed leading to loss of the tooth. Anaerobic Gram-negative plaque bacteria, e.g. *Porphyromonas gingivalis* and *Acinobacillus actinomycetemcomitans* are primarily implicated in this progressive process. The host's own immune inflammatory response to the products of these bacteria is an important factor in the pathogenesis of this condition.

Bacteraemia and infective endocarditis

Whilst dental caries and periodontal disease are not life-threatening conditions, resident microbes from the oropharynx or other sites can, on occasions, lead to the severe, potentially fatal condition called infective endo-carditis. This occurs primarily in people with pre-existing damage to the heart valves, e.g. following rheumatic fever, and congenital or degenerative valvular defects, or those with a valve prosthesis. Infective endocarditis often follows surgery, including dental extraction or deep scal-ing. The organisms involved are often the viridans group of streptococci, e.g. *Strep. sanguis*, although other species may also be involved. It is therefore important that a thorough history should be taken before invasive proce-dures are undertaken on this group of patients. Further-more, such procedures should only be undertaken while the patient is being given prophylactic antibiotic cover starting ½–1 hour prior to surgery and continuing for up to 24–48 hours after completion of the surgery. Penicillin or amoxycillin is usually used. Patients allergic to penicillin may be given an alternative drug like erythro-mycin. The short period of antibiotic cover is necessary in order to prevent the development of antibiotic-resistant strains.

Microbial pathogenicity

Virulence

Organisms capable of causing disease are referred to as pathogenic species, e.g. staphylococci and salmonellae. Among the pathogenic species certain strains are capable of causing more severe disease than others and the word virulence is used to describe this quantitative difference, e.g. *Mycobacterium tuberculosis* and *Mycobacterium bovis* cause tuberculosis in humans and they are patho-genic species. However, variations in virulence among these organisms may be noted. The BCG strain (bacille Calmette–Guérin) has been derived from the virulent

---

SUMMARY BOX
NORMAL FLORA

- After birth, the body is rapidly colonized by organisms from the mother and the environment; the use of broad-spectrum antibiotics can disturb the balance achieved.

- In the mouth, large numbers of organisms survive without causing damage; however, in antibiotic usage or poor oral hygiene, mixed organisms may overgrow, producing trench mouth or oral thrush.

- Dental plaque is an example of a biofilm on the surface of teeth with deeper facultative anaerobes, which ultimately calcifies producing tartar.

- Dental caries occurs when lactic acid is produced, capable of demineralizing enamel; the process is facilitated by *Strep. mutans*.

- Periodontal disease occurs in late plaque, associated with gingivitis which damages the attachment of teeth to junctional epithelium.

- In susceptible individuals with pre-existing valvular heart disease, the release of organisms into the bloodstream during extractions or deep scaling causes a bacteraemia which may lead to infective endocarditis.

- At-risk individuals should be identified and given antibiotic prophylaxis before any dental procedure.

Mycobacterium bovis. It was attenuated by growth under artificial conditions so that it could no longer cause disease in the normal human body, even though it can grow and multiply in the host. It is thus of lower viru-lence than *Mycobacterium bovis* and so can be utilized to immunize people against infection with the fully virulent strains of mycobacteria that cause tuberculosis.

Microbes that are adapted for ready transmission from person to person, like the measles virus, generally require only a small infective dose to effect this. Similarly, inges-tion of a few hundred typhoid bacilli may cause the disease, whereas millions of salmonellae are needed to cause food poisoning.

Toxins

Microbes cause disease using various different mecha-nisms. Not all the mechanisms are known but in some cases toxins are produced by bacteria. These protein sub-stances are able to cause symptoms of the disease when introduced in purified form into the host even in the absence of the bacteria, e.g. the toxins that cause diphthe-ria, cholera, tetanus or botulism. The cholera toxin acts locally at the site of bacterial colonization, i.e. the mucosal cells of the small intestine, but the other three toxins invade the body and cause damage at distant sites. In other cases, microbial invasion with growth and multiplication in the host is a prerequisite, e.g. pneumococcus.

Host factors

Host tissues may be damaged not only by microbial growth and its by-products but also by the associated inflammatory response set up in self-defence. The resulting pathology is responsible for the clinical presentation of the disease. The lesions produced depend on the microbe involved. Some bacteria (*Staphylococcus aureus*, *Strep. pyogenes*, meningococcus, pneumococcus) typically cause pus-containing lesions due to an acute inflammatory response, and are called pyogenic organisms. With staphylococci, the lesions take the form of abscesses, while streptococcal infections spread along tissue planes. Bacterial capsules are known to be a factor linked to virulence. In the case of *Strep. pneumoniae* the presence of capsule is associated with greater virulence as the noncapsulate strains are rapidly removed from the body by phagocytes. However, when eventually the host produces antibody to capsule, the virulent strains are also phagocytosed and removed.

Adhesion factors

Adhesion factors that help organisms colonize the site of infection are also an important feature associated with the ability to cause disease. Fimbriae are well known for their adhesive properties. However, many other bacterial surface structures, e.g. cell wall, capsule and flagellar antigens, also serve this function, enabling adhesion to and colonization of epithelial surfaces and biofilms. The possession of specialized fimbriae known as colonization factor antigens (CFA) are an essential feature of pathogenicity in some strains of *Escherichia coli* that cause gastroenteritis by production of toxin in the gut. In order to cause disease in this situation, the organism must possess colonization factors as well as the ability to secrete enterotoxin.

Opportunistic infections

Microbes of relatively low virulence may cause disease under certain conditions, e.g. when immunity or resistance to infective agents is lowered following (a) chemotherapy for cancer or (b) certain infections, e.g. human immunodeficiency virus (HIV), measles, etc. Such agents are termed opportunistic pathogens. e.g. *Candida albicans*

and *Pseudomonas* infections in immunosuppressed individuals. Patients who are immunocompromised are highly susceptible to all infections including opportunistic pathogens.

SUMMARY BOX
PATHOGENICITY

- The ability of microorganisms to cause disease is their pathogenicity.
- Virulence is the extent of disease caused.
- Some microorganisms cause disease through toxins.
- Many microorganisms cause problems through the extent of the provoked inflammatory response.
- Adhesion factors are important in determining an organism's ability to cause damage at a particular site.
- In opportunistic infections, low-virulence organisms can cause disease.

Preventive strategies

Microbes may also have strategies to prolong their stay in a host by subverting the immune defence mechanisms. These include:

- Production of capsules to avoid or delay phagocytosis.
- Destruction of phagocytes by secreting leukocidins, e.g. *Staph. aureus* and *Strep. pyogenes*.
- Antigenic variation to avoid recognition by the immune response, e.g. influenza virus and HIV. These organisms are constantly changing their surface antigens so that antibodies and T lymphocytes produced against the initial form are no longer effective against the new variants.
- Destruction of antibodies by secreting proteases that cleave the immunoglobulin molecule, e.g. the proteases secreted by *Bordetella pertussis* and *Neisseria meningitidis* are able to cut up the IgA molecules in mucosal secretions. Other immunoglobulin classes may also be damaged. As a result, the antibody is no longer able to damage or remove the microbe. Furthermore, it is possible that the fragments of antibody may then enhance the infection by combining with the surface of the organism and protecting it from the lethal effects of complement, cytotoxic cells and phagocytes.
- Destruction of T lymphocytes, e.g. HIV. This leads to a profound level of immunosuppression associated with recurrent reinfection which eventually leads to death.
- Avoid recognition by:
  a. Intracellular position, e.g. viruses, and the tubercle bacillus survive and multiply within the host cell.

The immune mechanisms are unable to attack them until they emerge from the cell or until bacterial antigens are expressed on the surface of the infected cell.

b. Acquisition of host protein antigen, e.g. the larvae of schistosomes and other helminths coat themselves with host-derived proteins such as serum albumin, immunoglobulin etc. and are thus able to avoid recognition.

- Avoid killing mechanisms within phagocytes, e.g. tubercle bacillus and legionella, by:

a. Avoiding fusion of lysomes with phagosomes.

b. Preventing the oxidative burst that normally follows phagocytosis and helps to kill the microbe. Some microbes appear to be able to withstand these toxic free radicals quite effectively.

c. Emerging from the phagosome to lie free in the cytoplasm safe from the killing mechanisms.

- Production and release of large amounts of bacterial surface antigens leads to competition for antibody-combining sites and receptors on phagocytes and cyto-toxic T lymphocytes.

- General immunosuppression is produced in many infections, e.g. measles, malaria and HIV.

SUMMARY BOX
STRATEGIES OF MICROORGANISMS TO SUBVERT THE IMMUNE RESPONSE

- Development of capsules to delay phagocytosis, e.g. pneumococcus.
- Ability to destroy phagocytes, e.g. *Staph. aureus*.
- Capacity for antigenic variation, e.g. influenza virus, HIV.
- Destruction of antibodies, e.g. meningococcus.
- Destruction of T lymphocytes, e.g. HIV.
- Ability to avoid recognition, e.g. viruses, tuberculosis.
- Ability to avoid killing mechanisms.
- Releasing large amounts of surface antigens to promote competitive binding with antibodies.
- Some organisms promote general immunosuppression, e.g. HIV, measles, malaria.

IMMUNITY TO INFECTIVE AGENTS

Innate non-specific immunity

The natural innate immune mechanisms are the first to detect and attack or withstand microbes. This system includes non-specific factors like the intact skin and mucosa. When these barriers are breached microbes invade and cause disease. Secretions on mucosal surfaces and their flow lead to the mechanical removal of microbes, e.g. tears and saliva. The secretion of mucus at these sites also helps to trap microbes which may then be readily removed. In the respiratory tract the action of ciliated epithelium helps to waft the trapped microbes and mucus upwards so that they may be coughed out.

The presence of normal flora plays an important role in preventing colonization of skin and mucous membranes by harmful microbes. Not only do they compete for receptor sites here, but the metabolites secreted by some commensal organisms are damaging to would-be invaders. When broad-spectrum antibiotics are used, normal flora is often disturbed, and in this situation thrush may develop, i.e. white patches of *Candida albicans* growing on the oral and intestinal mucous membrane.

Acidic pH in the stomach kills many ingested microbes. In conditions where there is an absence of or low levels of gastric acidity (e.g. following gastric surgery) smaller numbers of ingested organisms are sufficient to cause disease, e.g. cholera and typhoid.

On the skin, sweat and fatty acids in sebum are bactericidal.

The acute phase proteins (APP) are a series of naturally occurring substances that are produced in large amounts, and secreted into body fluids like serum, tears, saliva, etc. within 24 hours of infection. They include factors like complement, C-reactive protein (CRP), lysozyme, trans-ferrin, lactoferrin, lactoperoxidase, etc. Lysozyme is able to attack peptidoglycan in the cell wall of Gram-positive bacteria. Complement factors are activated either by microbial components or by APP like CRP or mannose-binding protein. They are mediators of inflammation, promoting chemotaxis and phagocytosis. Transferrin and lactoferrin trap and withhold iron from bacteria which require iron for growth. Lactoperoxidase helps to kill microbes. Phagocytosis is an important early non-specific defence mechanism. Macrophages and neutrophils ingest the microbes into phagocytic vacuoles which then combine with lysosomes. The bacteria are killed by the generation and release of highly reactive oxygen intermediates into the phagolysosome. Molecular oxygen is converted into highly toxic products such as H_2O_2, NO and OH, which damage the microbe.

An additional defence mechanism seen with virus infections is the production of interferon by the infected cell. This is able to prevent viral invasion of neighbouring cells, and is important in recovery from diseases like the common cold. Natural killer (NK) cells are a population of cells that can attack and lyse infected cells in the early non-specific stage of immunity to infection.

Acquired specific immunity (see also Ch. 4)

When microbes enter the body, they are phagocytosed and their antigens presented to lymphocytes. The specific immune response is expressed as production of antibody and sensitized T cells, and both factors can help recovery and resistance to infection. Humoral immunity is the arm of the immune response dealing with antibody production by B lymphocytes and its functions. Thymus-derived CD4 lymphocytes of the Th2 category are important in helping to stimulate B cells to produce antibodies to protein antigens (T-dependent antigens). Here a good immunological memory is registered with subsequent IgG secretion due to immunoglobulin class switch. Some bacterial polysaccharide antigens are able to directly stimulate B cells (T-independent antigens) without help from T cells but here, memory is poor and a short-lived IgM response is seen. Cellular immunity on the other hand is dependent on production of sensitized CD4 thymus-derived lymphocytes of the Th1 type that produce cytokines promoting T cell activation of macrophages, and also cytotoxic CD8 T cells which damage infected cells. Cellular immunity is important in recovery from infection with intracellular pathogens, e.g. viruses and the bacilli causing typhoid and tuberculosis. Humoral immunity on the other hand helps recovery from pyogenic infections, e.g. pneumococcal pneumonia, and is also important in prevention of reinfection following recovery from disease or following vaccination. In preventing reinfection, humoral immunity plays a very important role even with intracellular pathogens like viruses and the typhoid bacillus, but fails to do so in tuberculosis. The presence of preformed memory cells is pivotal in helping the rapid and sustained synthesis and release of antibodies when the pathogen is encountered for the second time, i.e. a secondary immune response.

An important feature of the immune response is the ability to produce an augmented specific output of immune factors (both humoral and cellular) on subsequent exposure to the same organism or antigen. This is implemented by the production of relatively long-lived memory B and T cells which are able to rapidly produce a greatly augmented response on meeting specific antigen at a later date. The response lasts for a long period of time (months or years). The nature of this secondary immune response renders a useful function in recovery from infection and prevention of reinfection on subsequent exposure to the pathogen.

Immunoglobulins (see Ch. 4)

Each of the five classes of immunoglobulins (antibodies) produced plays an important role in recovery from or prevention of infection.

- Immunoglobulin G (IgG) can act by neutralizing toxins and viruses, activating complement and thus aiding chemotaxis and opsonization for phagocytes, and lysis of infected cells. IgG also helps some cytotoxic cells (ADCC) to recognize and kill virus-infected cells. Activation of complement can also help lyse and destroy a limited range of Gram-negative bacteria (*Neisseria* and *Vibrio cholerae*), by acting synergistically with lysozyme. However, its main defensive role against Gram-positive bacteria and many Gram-negative species, is through opsonization. IgG is the only class of antibody that is transmitted from a mother to her fetus in the uterus and helps to protect the baby through the first few months of life. IgG is extremely important in the long-lived secondary response that prevents reinfection either following recovery from disease or vaccination.

- Immunoglobulin M (IgM) is the first antibody to be produced (early antibody) and is able to combine with more antigen and activate complement. It is therefore able to promote inflammation with chemotaxis, phagocytosis, etc. It is a short-lived response lasting only a few weeks compared to the long-lived IgG response.

- Immunoglobulin A (IgA) is secreted onto mucosal surfaces in its secretory form (SIgA) and mediates mucosal immunity by preventing organisms adhering to the mucosal epithelial cells. It binds to the microbes which are then trapped in the mucus and removed. SIgA can also activate complement by the alternative pathway and can act synergistically with complement and lysozyme to lyse some Gram-negative bacteria. It is the predominant immunoglobulin found in secretions like tears, saliva, colostrum, and respiratory, genitourinary and gastrointestinal fluids. However, IgG predominates in serum, gingival crevicular fluid and other internal secretions such as synovial and cerebrospinal fluid.

- Immunoglobulin E is involved with the release of histamine and other vasoactive substances from mast cells. This causes the inflammatory response attracting eosinophils to the site. Some microbes, e.g. larval

forms of certain parasitic helminths including schistosomes, are damaged by the activity of the eosinophils
and IgE antibody. IgE is particularly associated with
the type I hypersensitivity reaction seen as allergy to
pollen and house dust mite, e.g. hay fever and asthma.
Microbes also stimulate the IgE response.

Humoral immunity

Microbial structural components and secretions are
recognized as antigens by cells of the immune system.
The immune response mounted by the host is directed
against specific microbial antigenic determinants. The
antibody directed against bacterial surface antigens
will combine specifically with the organism and may
prepare it for removal by phagocytes – a process called
opsonization. This process is augmented by activation of
complement by the classical pathway, resulting in the
inflammatory process. Combination of antibody with
organisms also prevents the microbe adhering to host cell
surfaces prior to entry, e.g. secretory IgA acts on mucosal
surfaces, and IgG in serum prevents viruses from invading fresh tissue cells (referred to as virus neutralization). Antibody directed against bacterial exotoxin
combines with and neutralizes the toxin by preventing
its adherence to the preferred receptor sites on host
cells. Humoral immunity is particularly important for
recovery from pyogenic infections, e.g. by staphylococci,
streptococci and meningococci.

Cellular immunity

T cell-mediated immunity is also directed specifically
against microbial antigens expressed on the surface of
infected cells. Cell-mediated immunity plays an important role in recovery from infection with microbes that
are obligate or facultative intracellular pathogens, e.g.
viruses, fungi and the tubercle bacillus. The Th1 class
of cells are activated. The released cytokines attract
and activate macrophages which can ingest and destroy
pathogens and produce an inflammatory response of the
granulomatous type. This may serve to localize the infection while it is being overcome, e.g. tuberculosis. It
appears that when Th1 cells are activated they can inhibit
Th2 cells, and vice versa. Cytotoxic T cells of the CD8
type can directly attack and lyse infected cells bearing
microbial antigens on the surface. Although antibodies
are unable to enter host cells, they do play a part in
defence against intracellular pathogens. They may
combine with antigen on the surface of infected cells and

promote destruction of the cell either by activating complement or by aiding a population of killer cells called
antibody-dependent cytotoxic cells (ADCC). Once the
host cell is lysed and the pathogens released, circulating
antibody can combine with and neutralize virus particles
that are free in the bloodstream, tissue fluids or secretions
on mucosal surfaces. All the released microbes are then
phagocytosed and cleared from the site. Pre-existing antibodies are also important in preventing reinfection with
the same organism.

Knowledge of the antigens carried by pathogens is
made use of in production of vaccines used for inducing
artificial immunity against infectious disease. It is also
very helpful in the laboratory diagnosis and epidemiological investigation of infection and in the assessment
of prognosis.

SUMMARY BOX
IMMUNITY TO INFECTIVE AGENTS

- Innate non-specific immunity relies on mechanisms which existed before exposure to an organism.
- Acquired specific immunity develops after antigen presentation with either a specific antibody response or sensitized T cells.
- The humoral response is effected by B lymphocytes helped by CD4/Th2 cells.
- Cellular immunity is effected by T cells including CD4/Th1 helper and CD8 cytotoxic cells.
- Subsequent exposure causes an augmented response through the long-lived memory T and B cells.
- Immunoglobulins have different roles depending on the organisms; hypersensitivity responses may also have a role to play.

Prevention of infection

Ever since it was observed that one attack of a severe
infection like measles conferred life-long immunity to
subsequent infection it was only a matter of time before
deliberate induction of artificial immunity came into its
own.

Immunization

Active immunization with vaccine as we know it was
first described by Sir Edward Jenner in 1796 with the
successful demonstration of a vaccine against smallpox.
With appropriate use of this vaccine it has been possible
to eradicate from the earth the disease caused by small-

pox virus. This was brought about not only by the effective vaccine and the excellent immunization policy funded largely by the World Health Organization but also owing to the fact that the virus is transmitted only from person to person, there is no other animal host or reservoir of infection and there is no carrier state. Diseases with similar characteristics, e.g. poliomyelitis and measles, are currently being targeted for eradication. Transmission of an infection from person to person occurs when the number of immune individuals in the community falls below a critical threshold level. If herd immunity is maintained at a high level, by effectively immunizing about 90% of the community, it should be sufficient to break the chain of transmission and to eliminate the disease. The ability to maintain this level of herd immunity throughout the world is essential, if the disease is to be eradicated. Following eradication, the vaccine can be withdrawn from use – as with smallpox vaccine. Vaccines induce specific active immunity so that on subsequent exposure to the microbe the individual is immune to infection or only suffers a minor or subclinical form of the disease. In order to produce effective immunity, the vaccine used should contain the designated microbial protective antigens and it should be given in repeated doses so as to stimulate a good secondary type response with immunological memory. When eventually over a period of time, the level of immunity starts to decline, it can be restimulated by administration of small doses of vaccine called booster doses, given for example 5–10 years after the initial course of vaccine.

Vaccines

Vaccines in common use may be prepared in different ways.

- *Killed whole cell vaccine.* Here the whole bacterial cell or virus is killed/inactivated and injected into a host. Several doses are necessary, given several weeks apart, e.g. the whooping cough or pertussis vaccine.
- *Live attenuated vaccine.* Here bacteria or viruses are grown under adverse conditions in the laboratory until mutant strains of low virulence are obtained. These are able to grow and stimulate immunity in the host without causing disease. Such live attenuated organisms are used in the vaccine against tuberculosis (BCG) and poliomyelitis (Sabin). Where BCG vaccine is concerned, long-term immunity is conferred and boosters are not given. The dangers of using live vaccines include the possibility of spontaneous reversion to fully

virulent strains (sometimes seen with Sabin) and also the possibility of causing severe disease if given to immunosuppressed individuals, e.g. pregnant women.

- *Acellular vaccines.* The first acellular vaccine used was that against diphtheria. Here the toxin is entirely responsible for the disease process as is also true for the disease tetanus. If these toxins are treated with formalin they are altered to toxoids which are still antigenic but no longer toxic. They can be injected into people to stimulate the production of antitoxin antibodies. In order to increase the antigenicity of these weak antigens they are combined with an adjuvant, aluminium hydroxide, which potentiates their immunogenicity. Killed vaccines also need adjuvants. Vaccines against infections by pneumococci, meningococci and *Haemophilus influenzae* type b (Hib) contain the capsular polysaccharide of the organisms concerned since it has been identified as the protective antigen. The Hib vaccine is unique in that the polysaccharide is conjugated with the protein diphtheria toxoid or tetanus toxoid to render it more immunogenic. Proteins are in general better immunogens than polysaccharides. The conjugated vaccine is thus able to recruit T helper cells to ensure a good IgG antibody response. Most polysaccharides stimulate only a short-lived IgM response and are particularly poor in children under 2 years of age.
- *Recombinant vaccines.* The vaccine against hepatitis B is a recombinant vaccine. In this disease the protective antigen is a surface antigen of the virus. The gene coding for this antigen is cloned into yeast cells which are then cultured to yield large amounts of hepatitis B surface antigen which is purified and used as vaccine.

Immunization strategies

Routine immunizations are started in early childhood and repeated doses of vaccine are administered to produce good immunological memory so as to protect the child against future infection. The human fetus acquires maternal IgG across the placenta during pregnancy, so that at birth, babies have a full complement of their mothers IgG. This protects them from infection in the initial months of life. Since the half-life of IgG molecules is 19–21 days, this passive immunity is soon lost. The baby starts to produce its own IgG after birth but this does not reach adult levels until many years later. There is thus a gap in immunity after about the third month of life when babies could be most susceptible to common infectious diseases. The current vaccination schedule in the UK starts immunization of babies at the age of 2 months with a combined triple vaccine against diphtheria, pertussis and tetanus (DPT) given by injection, mixed with Hib vaccine in the same syringe, i.e. really a quadruple vaccine. The Sabin polio vaccine is given orally at the same time. Immunization with DPT, Hib and Sabin is repeated at age 3 months and 4 months. There is some concern regarding administration of vaccines at too early an age. Firstly, any pre-existing antibody (acquired from the mother) would combine with the vaccine and remove it rapidly thus reducing the potency. Secondly, the baby's immune mechanisms may not be fully mature and this may lead to immune tolerance so that subsequent infection could cause a more severe presentation of the disease. There is at present insufficient evidence to support this. At the end of the first year babies are given a live triple vaccine (MMR) consisting of live attenuated vaccine strains of measles, mumps and rubella. At school age (fifth year) boosters are given – DT (pertussis component is not required), Sabin and MMR vaccine. During the 14th year children are tested for skin sensitivity to tuberculin, and BCG is given only to tuberculin-negative individuals. At school-leaving age (around 16 years) a further booster for tetanus and diphtheria (adult low dose) and poliomyelitis is given. Further boosters every 10 years for tetanus are recommended. If going to areas where poliomyelitis and diphtheria are endemic, then boosters 10-yearly are recommended, as are vaccines for other diseases that are prevalent in the area.

Certain vaccines are given to groups of people at particular risk of infection, e.g. hepatitis B vaccination of health care workers (see below), injected-drug abusers, inmates of prisons, etc. Other such hazard groups include institutionalized old people who are given influenza vaccine during epidemics and individuals who are to have their spleens removed surgically who are given pneumococcal vaccine. Immunosuppressed individuals are especially at risk of contracting all forms of infections. Travellers to areas with endemic disease need to be immunized against the prevalent diseases before travel.

A vaccine for dental caries has been extensively researched and tested. The *Strep. mutans* vaccine was found to reduce the incidence of dental carries but it is believed that there may be a possibility that the vaccine could damage the heart. Although this has not been proved, concerns regarding the safety of the vaccine in humans have stayed its progress, especially since caries is not a life-threatening disease. Above all, it is imperative that a vaccine intended to prevent a disease should not cause any unwanted damage or toxic symptoms.

Health care workers

Hepatitis B vaccination is given to all health care workers including medical and dental students, owing to the ease with which the virus may be transmitted in accidental blood contact. Asymptomatic ambulant carriers are common with this disease and they may also readily transmit infection. Therefore in the field of health care it is necessary to treat all patients with maximum care to avoid cross-infection. The vaccine against hepatitis B is given intramuscularly in three doses at intervals of 1 and 6 months. 2–4 months after completion of the full course, antibody levels are checked, and if found to be less than 100 milli-international units (IU) per ml a booster is given. If less than 10 mIU/ml is recorded, then the whole course of vaccine is repeated. A level of 100 mIU/ml or above is regarded as protective. It is necessary to maintain immunity with a booster after 5 years.

Passive immunization

Whilst vaccines give good active immunity, this may take several weeks or months to be effective. It is also possible to confer artificial passive immunity. Here preformed antibodies obtained from animals or humans are injected into a person and give immediate protection against the disease even though this wears off within a few weeks. Human antitetanus serum is obtained from the blood of people immunized with tetanus toxoid. The purified immunoglobulins concentrated from the serum may be used prophylactically to protect unimmunized individuals following a dirty wound obtained in a road traffic accident. This may also be administered therapeutically, in addition to antibiotics, to a clinical case of tetanus in order to neutralize any further toxins that may be produced in the patient. It is particularly important that all individuals should be actively immunized with a sufficient number of doses of tetanus toxoid in order to avoid contracting this life-threatening disease which may be acquired from even small wounds obtained in the garden or playground, especially when soil or dirt has been introduced into a penetrating wound. The principles of herd immunity do not apply in this case, and a 100% vaccination rate is advocated.

Hyperimmune gamma-globulin from a convalescent case of chickenpox may be used to treat a severe case of chickenpox or shingles in immunosuppressed individuals. In the context of hepatitis B, an unimmunized person who has been exposed to the blood of a carrier, e.g. following needlestick injury, or splashes in eyes, mouth or cuts on skin, is immediately given hyper-immune hepatitis B immunoglobulin and is also started on a full course of vaccine. Immunized individuals are given a booster dose of vaccine unless they are known to have adequate levels of antibody.

The main drawback to the use of passive immunization is the possible occurrence of hypersensitivity reactions. These are caused by an immune response of the host, directed against the antigenic determinants on the donated serum proteins. They may be very severe and life-threatening when animal sera are used, but are generally mild and reversible if human serum preparations are used. A further concern is the possibility of transfer of undetected or unknown infective agents in such preparations.

SUMMARY BOX
PREVENTION OF INFECTION

- Vaccination is an important public health measure since transmission of infections occurs if numbers of immune individuals fall below a critical level.
- Vaccines contain the microbial protective antigens given in repeated doses, producing a good secondary response with immunological memory, and restimulation with booster doses.
- Types of vaccine include killed whole vaccines, acellular vaccines, and recombinant vaccines such as to hepatitis B virus.
- HBV vaccination should be offered to all health care workers including dental and medical students.
- Passive immunization may be considered in certain situations such as acute infections in non-immune individuals.

LABORATORY DIAGNOSIS

In addition to observing the clinical features and clinical history, the laboratory findings play a relevant role in the diagnosis and management of infectious disease. Here, samples of material collected aseptically from patients are dispatched in sterile containers to the microbiology laboratory, where they may be cultured to isolate the organisms involved. The specimens sent to the laboratory could be samples of urine, faeces, blood, pus, tissue or swabs taken from infected sites. The isolated organism is identified by microscopy, cultural and biochemical characteristics, or tests for toxigenicity may be performed. Antibiotic sensitivity assays then indicate the drug of choice for treatment. Serum samples may be examined

to detect microbial antigens or DNA. This is relevant when cultures are negative, either because of prior use of antibiotics or for other reasons. Serum may also be screened for the presence of raised levels of specific antibody. During the course of an infection, antibody is produced and the level will rise progressively. Therefore the detection of a more than fourfold increase in the titre of specific antibodies in the second of a pair of serum samples taken 7–10 days apart is significant. The presence of specific IgM antibodies also denotes current infection, since IgM production is an early short-lived response. IgG, once formed, remains in the body for longer periods, and a high level of specific IgG on its own is not sufficient justification for making a firm diagnosis, since it may represent residual antibody from a previous infection. Serodiagnosis suffers from a serious problem in that troublesome non-specific reactions are frequently seen as a result of sharing of antigens by different microbes of various genera or species. When interpreted with care, however, serology has a useful role to play. Histological study of tissue samples may also be employed in laboratory diagnosis of infection.

Typing of microbes by further tests, e.g. serotyping, phage typing, plasmid analysis, DNA typing, etc., is useful in epidemiological studies so as to establish the common source of infection and lines of transmission in outbreaks. It also helps differentiate between reinfection with a different strain of the same species of microbe on the one hand and relapse or recurrent infection with the same strain on the other.

TREATMENT OF MICROBIAL INFECTION

Antibiotics

The availability of antibacterial agents since 1935, first sulphonamides and then penicillin and other antibiotics, has succeeded in transforming the management and control of infection. These agents act rapidly at different sites on the bacteria either killing them outright or preventing replication, thus restricting numbers to a level that can be dealt with by the host's own immune defences. In general, it is sufficient to use drugs that prevent further replication of bacteria (bacteriostatic agents). However, in severe systemic infections like infective endocarditis or infections in the immunocompromised it is necessary to use bactericidal drugs to bring the infection under control rapidly. In such cases combinations of drugs are used where synergism is known to occur, i.e. the augmented effect of the drugs in combination is greater than an additive effect. It is necessary to be aware of the actions of each drug used in combination since some may result in antagonism, i.e. lowering the potency. Furthermore, use of combination drug therapy helps to overcome the development of resistant strains of the bacterium during the course of the treatment. This is especially relevant in the treatment of diseases like tuberculosis, where the prolonged course of therapy required permits the slow-growing bacteria to develop resistance to the antibiotic, as was seen in the days when monotherapy was practised. Therefore therapy with a three-drug combination is routinely used in this case. However, patient compliance is poor, therefore directly observed therapy under supervision is now recommended.

Resistance

Resistance to antibiotics may be acquired by bacteria during the course of treatment, either by mutations occurring in the bacteria during replication or by transfer of plasmids coding for resistance from other bacteria. In many organisms multiple resistance to several antibiotics may be acquired via one plasmid. Resistance genes may also be transferred from one bacterium to another by bacteriophages or by acquiring the free DNA of the resistant bacteria from the surroundings. Many bacteria are now resistant to commonly used antibiotics and some are multiply resistant, posing a major problem in treatment of infection, e.g. methicillin-resistant *Staph. aureus* (MRSA) and multidrug resistant agents that cause tuberculosis and typhoid fever. The more widespread the use of an antibiotic the sooner the appearance of resistant bacteria. In the hospital environment resistant microbes are frequently isolated and may be the cause of serious outbreaks of infection. It has been noted that strict restrictions to the use of an antibiotic for a few years allows susceptible strains to re-establish themselves in the community.

It is now increasingly being recognized that where antibiotics are used in animal farming either for veterinary treatment of infection or as growth-promoting agents, resistance develops rapidly and then spreads to humans. As each new antibiotic is used for farmyard animals and poultry, so the resistant microbes emerge. The latest in this list is ciprofloxacin, hailed as the new wonder drug. A related compound has already been used for farming poultry and food animals and resistant strains are now well established, e.g. the multidrug-resistant typhoid bacillus in Pakistan.

In addition to having a deleterious effect on the microbes, antibiotics may also show toxic effects on host cells, some more so than others. Their ability to damage e.g. kidneys, bone marrow, has been noted. Another danger is development of hypersensitivity to particular drugs, e.g. penicillin allergy may result in symptoms ranging from fever and rash to arthralgia, haemolytic anaemia and anaphylactic shock. In such cases the drug and its related compounds cannot be used again in these patients.

Alteration of the host's normal bacterial flora following the use of powerful antibiotics with a broad spectrum of activity, i.e. against both Gram-positive and Gram-negative bacteria, may lead to the selection of and subsequent infection of the site with opportunist bacteria. These may be naturally resistant to that drug and normally reside in only small numbers at these regions. Furthermore, antibiotic-resistant mutants of the original infective agent may develop during the course of treatment and will be able to establish themselves in this situation and cause a prolonged and more severe disease.

The smallest concentration of drug required to prevent multiplication of the bacteria is referred to as the minimum inhibitory concentration (MIC). The minimum bactericidal concentration (MBC) refers to the smallest dose required to kill the organisms. It is necessary to ensure that the correct dose of antibiotic is given to achieve these levels at the site of infection and that they are maintained over the period of time required to bring the infection under control. Prolonged use of antibiotic, or inadequate dosage, increases the chances of survival and growth of resistant bacteria which may not only harm the patient but may be transmitted to others. This transmission may occur as outbreaks in hospital wards or may even occur in the community. Strains of *Staph. aureus* resistant to multiple drugs are usually treated with vancomycin. In Japan vancomycin-resistant MRSA are now being isolated. Enterococci which cause severe infection in neutropenic patients have now acquired resistance to vancomycin, probably following use of the drug in farming.

Mechanisms of action

The penicillins, cephalosporins and clavulanic acid, all possess a β-lactam ring in the basic structure. Bacteria that secrete the enzyme β-lactamase (penicillinase) are able to withstand the effect of β-lactam antibiotics since the enzyme breaks open the β-lactam ring. These drugs act by interfering with the synthesis of bacterial peptidoglycan in cell walls, leading to lysis of the organism.

Benzylpenicillin (penicillin G) and phenoxymethyl-penicillin (penicillin V) are useful in infections caused by many Gram-positive bacteria, e.g. *Strep. pyogenes* and *Actinomyces israeli*. Penicillin is also useful in the treatment of infections caused by Vincent's organisms, *Neisseria meningitidis, N. gonorrhoeae,* and *Treponema pallidum*. However, many strains of *Strep. pneumoniae* and *N. gonorrhoeae* have now acquired resistance to penicillin.

Ampicillin and amoxycillin are broad-spectrum penicillins, i.e. act against Gram-positive and Gram-negative organisms. They can be given by mouth, whereas benzylpenicillin has to be given by injection. Clavulanic acid is a β-lactam drug with little antibacterial activity on its own. It is, however, a powerful inhibitor of many bacterial β-lactamases. It is therefore given in combination with amoxycillin for the treatment of β-lactamase-producing bacterial infection. Methicillin and flucloxacillin are penicillins that are resistant to staphylococcal penicillinase and the drug mecillinam is a penicillin that is more active against Gram-negative bacilli than against Gram-positive organisms. Whilst penicillin is of relatively low toxicity, hypersensitivity to the drug does occur. Hypersensitivity to one brand of penicillin indicates a sensitivity to the others. If a patient gives a history of a severe reaction to one dose of penicillin, then none of these drugs should be used again.

Metronidazole is a drug that acts specifically on all strictly anaerobic bacteria and also on protozoa, by entering the microbial DNA and interfering with replication.

Prophylactic use of antibiotics

Whilst the use of antibiotics to prevent the development of infection incurs the risk of producing symptoms of toxicity in the patient, or the selection and spread of resistant organisms, these arguments are overcome in situations where the risk of infection is particularly dangerous to the patient. In such cases, the drugs are chosen on the grounds that they show the most action against the organisms responsible for the infection. During dental procedures, oral streptococci and other normal flora usually enter the bloodstream but are effectively removed by the normal individual. However, in patients with pre-existing abnormalities of the heart, these organisms can establish themselves on the damaged valves leading to infective endocarditis. In order to avoid this, all patients with a history of damaged heart valves should be given chemoprophylaxis before the dental procedure, such as deep scaling or extractions. A single dose of amoxycillin may be given orally before the intervention. Erythromycin and clindamycin are often used as alternative drugs and clinicians should consult appropriate guidelines.

Antiviral agents

There are far fewer antiviral agents available as compared to the number of antibacterial agents on the market. Many agents that inhibit viral multiplication within host cells are also toxic and cause damage to the host cell. Acyclovir (acycloguanosine) is active against herpesviruses and is of low toxicity to the host. It acts only on viral DNA not on host DNA, and is useful in treatment of life-threatening infections caused by these agents in patients with the acquired immunodeficiency syndrome or those on immunosuppressive therapy. Mutant strains resistant to acyclovir are now recognized. Topical creams are available for local application for lesions on skin or mucous membranes, e.g. cold sores. While it may shorten the duration of the presenting symptoms if started very early, it will not prevent recurrence since it only acts on replicating virus and not on the latent forms. Foscarnet, vidarabine and gancyclovir also act against the herpes group of viruses. Amantadine is a drug used for prophylaxis against influenza A. Many more antiviral agents are emerging now for management of HIV infection. AZT (azidothymidine, zidovudine) is one such anti-retroviral which can reduce the severity and incidence of opportunist infections in such patients. Side-effects of nausea, vomiting and bone marrow toxicity are a problem. Other drugs more active against HIV than AZT are available and alternating courses with combinations of drugs may be used to avoid development of resistance.

Antifungal agents

Many of these agents have extremely toxic side-effects when used to treat severe systemic and generalized fungal infections. Localized infections on oral mucosa can be treated with nystatin lozenges and topical application may be used, e.g. for skin infections. The polyene group of drugs damage fungal cells by acting on the sterol content of fungal cell membrane. Amphoteracin B has a broad spectrum of activity but produces nephrotoxicity as a side-effect.

The imidazole group of drugs act by inhibiting synthesis of ergosterol while flucytosine inhibits synthesis of proteins. Griseofulvin is concentrated in the stratum corneum of skin and is active against dermatophytes by inhibiting fungal cellular microtubules.

- Antibiotics may be bactericidal (kill bacteria) or bacteriostatic (prevent replication).

- Resistance may be acquired during a course of treatment, either by mutation or by plasmid transfer; resistant bacteria are now seen more frequently.

- Some antibiotics contain a β-lactam ring which leads to lysis of the organism; some bacteria have developed β-lactamase to prevent this action.

- Fewer antiviral agents are available; they inhibit viral multiplication but may also be toxic to host cells.

- Antifungal agents may be used topically or systemically in severe infections; they are often toxic to host tissues.

STERILIZATION AND DISINFECTION

Microbial infections may be transmitted from person to person by articles that have been contaminated by infected secretions from a patient, a carrier, animals, dust, soil or water. It is therefore necessary to remove potential pathogens from articles like surgical instruments, dressings, equipment, soiled linen, cutlery, crockery and surfaces. Many microbes are killed by heating to about 60°C for half an hour. However, many other potential pathogens are able to survive at temperatures higher than this and some bacterial spores can survive boiling for several hours. Furthermore, the presence of dried dirt, blood, secretions, food, etc. on articles will to some extent protect microbes from the heat or chemical treatment. It is therefore necessary to clean objects before sterilization or disinfection. Sterilization refers to the absolute killing of all life forms on or in an object. Thus a sterile object should contain no bacterial spores or vegetative cells, viruses, fungi protozoa or other life forms. This is particularly important in the case of instruments, dressings, etc. that are to be used in invasive procedures.

Sterilization

Common methods used for sterilization include heat, irradiation and chemicals. Heat is commonly used and may involve dry heat or steam under pressure. In either case the principle of 'hot enough for long enough' is critically important. Dry heat is obtained in a hot-air oven, and items to be sterilized must be heated to 160°C for 1 hour or alternatively 180°C for 20 minutes. For moist heat, an autoclave, in which steam under increased

pressure achieves a higher temperature, is used. Here the temperature, time and pressure necessary are 121°C for 15 minutes at 15 lb/in² pressure or alternately 134°C for 3 minutes at 32 lb/in² pressure.

It is important that the hot air or steam at the determined temperature is able to penetrate all parts of the item to be sterilized for the critical duration of time. These articles are pre-wrapped to ensure that they do not get contaminated after heat treatment.

Heat-sensitive items may be sterilized in other ways. Gamma irradiation using a cobalt-60 or caesium-137 source is used on a commercial basis to sterilize disposable plastic syringes, hypodermic needles, etc.

Heat-sensitive equipment may also be sterilized with chemicals like glutaraldehyde or the gases ethylene oxide and formaldehyde. Glutaraldehyde and formaldehyde are both effective against bacterial spores.

Disinfection

Disinfection refers to the elimination of most harmful bacteria from an article so as to render it safe for use. Contaminated work surfaces, floors and utensils may be cleaned and disinfected. Soiled dressings, swabs and other materials may be safely disposed of by incineration. Many chemical substances, suitably diluted and made up to the appropriate pH, are used for disinfection, but here again, it is necessary to clean articles prior to treatment as many disinfectants are inactivated by organic material like vomit, blood and tissue debris. This is particularly true of hypochlorite and chlorhexidine. Phenolic disinfectants show markedly less inactivation in the presence of organic matter containing bacteria, e.g. faecal contamination. They are, however, poor at inactivating viruses. Hypochlorite is particularly useful in destroying viruses, so is used at a very high concentration for disinfection of blood spillages. Sufficient chlorine then remains to overcome the quenching effect of organic material.

Pasteurization is a process where milk for human consumption is heated for 30 minutes at a temperature of 64–66°C or for 15 seconds at 72°C and then maintained at 4°C. This kills all vegetative pathogens and renders the milk safe for human consumption. Bacterial spores are not destroyed but do not present a problem here. Some heat-resistant vegetative bacteria survive in the milk as evidenced by the souring of pasteurized milk when stored for a few days. Sterilized and ultra-heat-treated (UHT) milk (132°C for 1 second) have a longer shelf life owing to removal of the souring bacteria. Only a few bacteria remain in the UHT milk.

Control of infection in health care

In the setting of the dental surgery, potential routes of transmission of infection include (a) from patient to staff, (b) from staff to patient, (c) staff to staff and (d) from patient to patient via the staff or contaminated equipment, instruments, surfaces, etc. Such infections may be minimized by strict attention to details of hygiene, cleaning, sterilization and disinfection of instruments and equipment, zoning and disinfection of work surfaces, wearing of gloves, masks and goggles, immunization of personnel and safe practice regarding disposal of used needles, sharps and other infected material. Transmission of blood-borne virus diseases is particularly relevant here. Hepatitis B is readily transmitted in small amounts of blood following needlestick injuries. The human immunodeficiency virus (HIV) and hepatitis C are other blood-borne viruses. Herpes virus is shed in the saliva of carriers or from cold sores and may enter cuts on ungloved hands to give a painful destructive lesion called herpetic whitlow, or it may enter the eye causing recurrent distressing herpetic keratoconjunctivitis. Other infections spread by inhalation of respiratory droplets, or infected aerosols may also occur, and routine vaccination of all staff and students is recommended, e.g. against tetanus, diphtheria, polio, measles, mumps, rubella, tuberculosis and hepatitis B. The recent increase in transmission of diphtheria in the countries of the former Soviet Union has led to reports of the disease in travellers returning to the UK from that region. Hence full immunization with the toxoid and maintenance of immunity with boosters every 5–10 years is recommended.

Since hepatitis B may be transmitted by unidentified asymptomatic carriers, it is necessary to pay scrupulous attention to all routine infection control procedures for each and every patient. These measures would then be effective against other microbial agents as well.

It is vital that sterile disposable needles and syringes are used for each patient, and that after use they are discarded safely into stout bins that should only be two-thirds full before incineration. Although hepatitis B is the major agent transmitted by accidents with needles and sharps, HIV has also been reported. Resheathing of used needles is the major cause of needlestick injuries and should be avoided or only done using safe needle guards or bayonet technique. Gloves, goggles and masks should be worn for all procedures and also when handling used instruments that are to be cleaned and sterilized for later use. All cuts and abrasions on the skin should be sealed with waterproof dressings. The use of goggles and mask prevents splattering of blood and bodily fluids onto the mucosa of eyes and mouth. Masks have a disadvantage in that when they are saturated with vapour from the breath they are able to transmit microbes with ease. They should be changed at intervals.

The immunization status of all health care staff should be monitored and adequate immunity maintained with timely administration of booster doses of vaccines. Reporting of all accidents and maintenance of an accident log book is helpful, so that immediate prophylactic measures may be instituted.

SUMMARY BOX
STERILIZATION, DISINFECTION AND CONTROL OF INFECTION

- Sterilization is the absolute killing of *all* life forms and is particularly important for instruments, dressings, etc. used in invasive procedures; it may be accomplished by heat, gamma irradiation and chemical sterilization.

- Disinfection refers to the elimination of *most* harmful organisms allowing safe use, e.g. work surfaces, floors and utensils.

- Pasteurization uses heat to kill off most significant bacteria in milk for human consumption.

- Routes of infection in dental practice include from patients to staff, staff to patients, staff to staff and patients to patients via contaminated equipment, instruments and surfaces.

- Practices should be established to minimize such occurrences with clearly defined policies; particular consideration should be given to needlestick injuries, viruses including HIV, HCV and HBV, aerosol spread and the use of goggles and masks.

6 Growth disorders and neoplasia

GROWTH DISORDERS

Growth disorders may be systemic or localized to a tissue or organ. Cell growth is stimulated by hormones and growth factors. The action of these agents requires the presence of specific cellular receptors which are mostly located on the cell membrane. Regulation of growth depends to some extent on the concentration of hormone or growth factor, but receptor concentration is critical in determining whether a cell will react to the chemical signal. If the specific receptor is absent, then the cell cannot respond to a hormone or growth factor.

- Hormones are synthesized and stored in endocrine glands and are released into the blood to act on distant target cells.
- Growth factors are synthesized by many types of cells. They act upon the cell which produced the factor (autocrine action) or on adjacent cells (paracrine action). Growth factors can be sequestered in the extracellular matrix and are often secreted in latent form to be activated by enzymes. They may also act on distant cells in endocrine fashion by travelling through the bloodstream.

Control of cell proliferation

Hormones and growth factors often act in concert in a series of complex feedback loops. Cell proliferation is a closely regulated process in which a balance is maintained in adult tissues between the number of cells generated by mitosis and destroyed by apoptosis. The balance is achieved by inhibitors and inducers of both processes (Ch. 1). Growth factors can recruit quiescent (G_0) cells into the cell cycle, for instance to achieve regeneration after injury. The cell has several inbuilt mechanisms which can inhibit proliferation, including p53 which acts as the 'guardian of the genome' by directing cells with faulty DNA into apoptosis rather than mitosis. Other tumour suppressor gene products such as p16 and pRb also control proliferation. The suppressors and inducers of apoptosis are discussed in Chapter 1.

SUMMARY BOX
CONTROL OF CELL PROLIFERATION

- Growth factors recruit quiescent cells into mitosis.
- Growth inhibitors, e.g. p53, p16, pRb, control proliferation.
- Apoptosis inhibitors and inducers determine the fate of post-mitotic cells.

Disorders of growth control

Fetal growth

Locally acting growth factors such as epidermal growth factor, nerve growth factor, platelet-derived growth factor and transforming growth factor beta are important in embryonic and fetal growth. The most important hormone in fetal growth is insulin. Production of the intermediate somatomedin growth factors, insulin-like growth factors 1 and 2 (IGF 1 and 2), is stimulated by insulin directly and they have a major role in stimulating growth by autocrine and paracrine interactions. Placental and other fetal hormones are involved also.

Postnatal growth

Hormonal control of postnatal growth is mediated by hypothalamic and pituitary hormones. Central to growth control is the production of growth hormone. Release of growth hormone from the pituitary is stimulated by growth hormone releasing factor from the hypothalamus and inhibited by somatostatin. Growth hormone acts via the intermediate somatomedin hormones, IGF 1 and 2, which are synthesized mostly in the liver. Other factors such as insulin, thyroid hormone, sex-steroid hormones and nutritional factors can stimulate somatomedin release directly.

- Reduced postnatal growth (dwarfism) may result from reduced growth hormone production or reduced growth hormone receptor levels. Reduction in thyroid hormone levels can lead to undersecretion of IGF 1 and a form of dwarfism where the head is of normal size, but the limbs reduced. Various disorders may lead to failure of interaction of growth hormone and somatomedin, for example malnutrition and emotional disorders. Postnatal growth can also be inhibited by corticosteroids produced endogenously (e.g. Cushing's syndrome) or administered therapeutically.
- Increased growth can result from increased growth hormone secretion, either as a result of overactivity or a pituitary tumour. In puberty, before skeletal maturity has been reached, excess growth hormone secretion produces gigantism. After fusion of the epiphyseal bone plates, growth hormone will reactivate growth in the hands, feet and head, causing acromegaly. The facial appearance tends to become coarse and the mandible enlarges resulting in prognathism.

Genetic factors such as parental height and gender are major determinants of postnatal growth patterns. Disproportional skeletal growth is seen in certain chromosomal disorders and in the rare genetically mediated osteochondrodysplasia syndromes. Environmental factors such as starvation and emotional deprivation, e.g. in children from unstable home backgrounds, may cause reduction in growth rate.

SUMMARY BOX
DISORDERS OF GROWTH CONTROL

- Fetal growth is regulated by insulin and growth factors.
- Reduced postnatal growth can be due to reduced growth hormone, growth hormone receptors, thyroid hormone, or nutrition, and to emotional causes.
- Excess growth hormone causes gigantism before puberty and acromegaly in adults.

Abnormal growth in tissues and organs

Alteration in growth in a single organ or tissue may occur as an adaptive change to physiological circumstance, ageing or a pathological process.

Increased growth (Fig. 6.1)

Hyperplasia is defined as an increase in the size of an organ or tissue by increase in cell number. This is generally effected by stimulation of mitosis but inhibition of apoptosis can also contribute. Hyperplasia is dependent upon a stimulus and is reversible on its withdrawal.

Hypertrophy is defined as an increase in the size of an organ or tissue by increase in cell size. It is a response to a stimulus for increased functional activity and is the only cellular adaptation possible in permanent cells, e.g. muscle cells.

It should be noted that the processes of hyperplasia and hypertrophy often coexist. Examples of physiological hyperplasia and hypertrophy are well known and include:

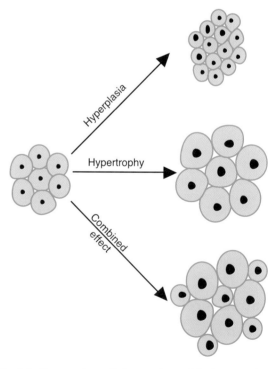

Fig. 6.1   Increased growth. Increased growth in tissues can be achieved through an increase in the number of cells (hyperplasia), an increase in the size of individual cells (hypertrophy) or a combination of the two.

- compensatory hyperplasia and hypertrophy of an organ (e.g. salivary gland or kidney) following surgical removal of its counterpart
- muscle hypertrophy in athletes
- breast hypertrophy at puberty and for lactation
- bone marrow hyperplasia as a response to reduced oxygen tension at high altitudes.

Pathological hyperplasia and hypertrophy are processes which are frequently involved in a wide variety of diseases. Although some disorders are self-perpetuating and characterized by increased cell production over destruction, growth control is maintained overall and this distinguishes such disorders from neoplasias.

Pathological hypertrophy

The best-known example of pathological hypertrophy relates to myocardial cells. Enlargement of a cardiac ventricle occurs in response to an increased requirement for work to maintain cardiac output. Hypertrophy of the myocardium is common following infarction or valve disorders. Left-sided ventricular hypertrophy may ultimately lead to pulmonary hypertension and subsequently to right-sided hypertrophy (see Chapter 7).

Arterial smooth muscle cells may undergo hypertrophy in hypertension.

Pathological hyperplasia

The process of pathological hyperplasia is involved in a wide range of disorders. Hyperplasia in endocrine glands can have widespread and major effects due to excess secretion of hormones. Some important examples are:

- Adrenal cortical hyperplasia may result from excess ACTH secretion. The hyperplasia can result in excess secretion of glucocorticoids (Cushing's syndrome) in which there is a characteristic 'moon face' and 'buffalo hump' due to oedema, hypertension, osteoporosis, peptic ulceration and many other effects.
- Thyroid follicular hyperplasia can result from autoimmune disease. Hyperthyroidism can lead to exophthalmos, hair loss, anxiety, myxoedema and numerous other features.
- Parathyroid hyperplasia induces hypercalcaemia, renal stones, thirst and lytic areas in bone known as brown tumours, which may present in the jaws.

Hyperplasia is an important process in immune responses and disorders where lymphoid cells undergo hyperplasia when stimulated by cytokines and interleukins. Myointimal cell hyperplasia in response to platelet-derived growth factor is a key process in atheromatous plaque formation (see Chapter 7).

Localized hyperplasia is a common problem in the oral cavity where the stimulus is chronic irritation. Dental plaque, calculus or mechanical trauma results in fibrous hyperplasia. Elimination of the stimulus will tend to reverse the process, but scar formation may necessitate removal of the hyperplastic overgrowth.

SUMMARY BOX
INCREASED GROWTH IN TISSUES

- Hyperplasia is mediated by increase in cell number by mitosis.
- Hypertrophy is mediated by increase in cell size.
- Hyperplasia and hypertrophy may occur simultaneously.
- It can be physiological or pathological.

Decreased growth

Hypoplasia can be defined as a failure of an organ to achieve normal size or shape during development. Hypoplasia (or aplasia, complete failure of development) of salivary glands causes dry mouth. Dental enamel hypoplasia can arise as a result of genetic or acquired disease during the period of tooth development and is a rare example of a hypoplastic process which may commence well into the postnatal period.

Atrophy may be defined as a decrease in the size of an organ, tissue or cell by reduction in cell size, cell number or a combination of both. Atrophy is an adaptive response to a decreased functional requirement. Often there is a failure of cell production, active reduction in cell size and cell deletion by apoptosis.

Physiological atrophy may be due to 'disuse', for example wasting of a limb which is temporarily immobilized by a splint. When the splint is removed, the muscle can regain its normal size owing to resumption of normal function. Atrophy is also a feature of the ageing process and can be multiorgan in nature. Atrophy of the cerebrum, skin and bone (including the jaws) can cause problems associated with senescence.

Pathological atrophy can occur in numerous situations. Sometimes pathological atrophy is reversible initially but the effects may become irreversible because of tissue damage or persistence of stimulus. Some important examples of pathological atrophy are:

- Reduction in endocrine stimulation may cause atrophy of the target cells, e.g. atrophy of the adrenal cortex may follow decreased ACTH secretion as part of a feedback loop when corticosteroids are given therapeutically.
- Hypoxic atrophy occurs when vessels are obstructed by external or internal pressure, or when the circulation is impaired. Chronic ischaemia and in particular hypoxia results in tissue atrophy.
- Denervation of muscle will lead to atrophy through disuse. If a whole limb is involved, bone atrophy may lead to local osteoporosis. Physiotherapy treatment may be used to minimize the effects of atrophy in this circumstance.
- Nutritional atrophy may be caused by protein deficiency (kwashiorkor), protein and calorie deficiency (marasmus) and cachexia in cancer patients. There is generalized wasting, with loss of adipose tissue. Tumour necrosis factor (TNF) is a cytokine thought to be responsible for cachexia in wasting illnesses.

SUMMARY BOX
DECREASED GROWTH IN TISSUES

- Atrophy is a decrease in size of tissue or organ.
- It may involve decrease in cell size, number or both.
- It can be physiological or pathological.
- It is often related to loss or diminution of function.
- Hypoplasia is a failure of attainment of normal size or shape of an organ.

ABERRANT GROWTH AND DIFFERENTIATION

Hamartoma

A hamartoma is a congenital tumour-like lesion composed of two or more mature cell types normally present in the area affected. The growth of a hamartoma is coordinated with that of the body, though many regress in the first few years of life. Hamartomas are benign and show normal cellular differentiation but abnormal gross architecture. Incomplete removal before growth cessation tends to be followed by recurrence. Pigmented moles, odontomes and vascular malformations are common examples of hamartomatous lesions. Some genetic syndromes, for example neurofibromatosis and tuberous sclerosis, are characterized by multiple hamartomas.

Cyst

A cyst is a pathological cavity, other than an abscess, containing fluid or semi-fluid material. Cystic change is seen in a variety of pathological lesions arising by different processes, and the term 'cyst' is imprecise. Some cysts do arise spontaneously and these are often lined by epithelium. They often originate from embryonic rests or ectopic inclusions and are relatively common in the neck and jaws. The radicular cyst, which is the most common type in the jaws, arises from odontogenic epithelial rests stimulated by inflammation.

Metaplasia

Metaplasia is the transformation of one differentiated cell type to another differentiated cell type. It is a reversible process and often represents a functional adaptation to altered environment. Epithelial cell metaplasia is seen for example in:

- respiratory lining where glandular, ciliated epithelium undergoes metaplasia to squamous epithelium in response to smoking
- jaw cyst linings where mucous metaplasia of the squamous epithelium is commonly seen
- exocrine ducts in the salivary and pancreatic glands, which show mucous metaplasia in response to obstruction and stone formation
- oesophagus, where gastric reflux stimulates metaplasia of the normal squamous lining to glandular type. This is known as Barrett's oesophagus.

Osseous metaplasia is the best-known example of metaplasia in connective tissue and it is seen in areas of dystrophic calcification and degenerative extracellular matrix.

Dysplasia

The term 'dysplasia' has many uses in pathology but is now generally accepted to imply a premalignant state characterized by increased cell proliferation, aberrant differentiation and sometimes cellular atypia. The use of the term to indicate disordered differentiation during development or local persistence of fetal phenotype (in conditions such as dentine dysplasia and fibrous dysplasia) is confusing and the term 'dysgenesis' is considered more appropriate. Dysplasia is almost always an acquired condition and the early forms are probably reversible if the causative agent is eliminated. If, on the other hand, the stimulus persists, dysplasia may intensify and eventually progress to malignant neoplastic growth (cancer).

Microscopically, dysplasia may be recognized by such features as increased mitotic activity, cellular atypia, increased nuclear-to-cytoplasmic ratio, nuclear and cellular pleomorphism, nuclear hyperchromatism, abnormal maturation and differentiation patterns, leading to atypical morphology and increased thickness. The best-known example is cervical intraepithelial neoplasia (CIN) which can precede the development of cervical cancer by many years and can be detected by cytological screening. Epithelial dysplasia is also an important prognostic indicator in premalignant lesions in the oral cavity and in other tissues. Dysplasia may coexist with metaplasia, the classic example being dysplasia arising in areas of squamous metaplasia in the respiratory tract, in smokers.

SUMMARY BOX
DISORDERS OF DIFFERENTIATION AND GROWTH

- Hamartomas are congenital tumour-like lesions whose growth is coordinated with the body growth.
- Cysts are pathological cavities containing fluid or semi-fluid material.
- Metaplasia is the transformation of one mature cell type to another; it is a reversible response, e.g. squamous metaplasia of the bronchi in smokers.
- Dysplasia is a potentially pre-neoplastic change; increased mitosis, atypical morphology and abnormal maturation may be present; it may be reversible but only in the early stages, e.g. epithelial dysplasia in leukoplakia.
- Neoplasia is uncontrolled, excessive and abnormal growth associated with cellular genetic abnormalities.

Neoplasia

The term neoplasia means 'new growth' and can be defined as an abnormal and uncoordinated tissue growth which persists after the initiating stimulus has been removed. A neoplasm is a lesion resulting from such growth and is often referred to as a tumour, though strictly speaking the term tumour can be used to denote any abnormal swelling. Broadly speaking, neoplasms can be divided into two groups.

- benign, with autonomous local growth and potential to cause damage by pressure effects or secretions such as hormones in some cases
- malignant, with lethal potential and the ability to invade and spread (metastasize).

Malignant neoplasia is referred to generally as cancer, a term sometimes best avoided in certain clinical situations because of its alarming implications. The process of conversion of a normal cell to its neoplastic counterpart is known as neoplastic transformation and it is associated with a series of genetic events which enable the cell to avoid normal growth restraints.

Epidemiology

It is estimated that around 25% of the population will develop some form of malignant neoplasm and the frequency of benign neoplasia is thought to be even higher. Individual risk increases with age, but some neoplasms, for example leukaemia and CNS tumours, have a high incidence in childhood. In the aged, the risk of developing certain neoplasms is high, for example the risk of developing prostate cancer is over 90% in men over 90 years of age.

Incidence is the frequency of new cases arising in the population and most data on incidence relate to malignant neoplasia. Cancer registries and records are the source of such information and it is acknowledged that these underestimate the true incidence. There are sex differences and geographic variations in cancer incidence. Oral cancer, for example, is more common in men and, whilst it accounts for around 2% of all cancers in the UK, it makes up to 40% of all cancers in Southern India.

SUMMARY BOX
EPIDEMIOLOGY OF NEOPLASIA

- Around 25% of individuals will develop a malignant neoplasm.
- Benign neoplasms are extremely common.
- The risk of malignant neoplasia increases with age.
- Wide geographical and sex differences in incidence are known.

Classification of neoplasms

As mentioned previously, neoplasms can be divided into benign and malignant categories. Some neoplasms do not fit into this scheme and are classified as 'intermediate or borderline tumours'. The main characteristics of benign and malignant neoplasms are summarized in Table 6.1.

Benign neoplasms

Benign neoplasms are generally slow growing and they

TABLE 6.1

CHARACTERISTICS OF BENIGN AND MALIGNANT NEOPLASMS

Characteristic	Benign	Malignant
Rate of growth	Usually slow	Usually rapid
Border	Circumscribed or encapsulated	Usually irregular and poorly defined
Differentiation (resemblance to tissue of origin)	Usually good	Variable, often poor
Mitotic activity	Low, normal appearances	High, often abnormal
Nuclear features	Generally normal	Hyperchromatic, pleomorphic, often contain nucleoli
Necrosis	Usually not	Often present
Local (stromal) invasion	No	Yes
Distal metastases	No	Possible

SUMMARY BOX
CLASSIFICATION OF NEOPLASMS

- Benign neoplasms are non-invasive, slow growing and well differentiated.
- Malignant neoplasms are invasive, capable of distant spread, grow rapidly and show variable differentiation.
- Carcinoma arises from epithelium, is the most frequent malignant neoplasm and tends to occur mostly in those over 50 years of age.
- Sarcoma arises from connective tissue and occurs over a wide age range.

remain localized, without invasion of adjacent tissue. In solid organs they form well-circumscribed masses often surrounded by a compressed fibrous tissue capsule, or sometimes a true capsule. When benign neoplasms form on surfaces, they may grow outwards to form a polyp. Such polypoid neoplasms may develop a stalk (pedicle) or simply bulge outwards.

It should be remembered that benign neoplasms can damage or even cause death, particularly if they occur in a critical site. The principal effects of benign neoplasms are:

- Most are non-symptomatic and may be removed for cosmetic reasons or to establish diagnosis and allay anxiety.
- Pressure on adjacent structures may cause major clinical problems, for example a benign CNS tumour may cause epilepsy.
- Obstruction of a vessel or duct may cause problems, for example benign salivary gland tumours can block

ducts and cause recurrent swellings at meal times. Obstruction may also predispose to chronic infection.

- Malignant transformation may occur and there is, for example, a significant risk of cancer arising in long-standing benign salivary gland neoplasms and colonic polyps.

Production of a hormone can have widespread effects when a benign neoplasm arises in an endocrine gland, for example a benign thyroid neoplasm causing thyrotoxicosis.

At a cellular level, benign neoplasms are generally well differentiated, i.e. the neoplastic cells closely resemble their normal counterparts and often retain their biochemical characteristics.

Malignant neoplasms

Malignant neoplasms are typically rapidly growing and are, by definition, invasive. They are poorly circumscribed and often form claw-like extensions into the underlying tissue. This is the reason for the generic term cancer, which likens this pattern to a crab. Invasion into the underlying tissue often results in a fibrous (desmoplastic) reaction. The neoplastic cells tend to invade lymphatic channels and blood vessels and then spread to distant sites. This process is called metastasis and the tumours which form in the distant sites are known as secondary or metastatic deposits. Malignant neoplasms may disseminate widely to produce the condition termed carcinomatosis. Cachexia, a wasting condition characterized by weight loss, anaemia and loss of appetite, is often a feature of carcinomatosis and is thought to result from production of tumour necrosis factor (TNF) by the neoplastic cells.

Malignant neoplasms in solid organs are poorly circumscribed and often show central necrosis, which is due to failure of vascular ingrowth to keep pace with cell proliferation. Often the malignant cells extend into adjacent tissues and the desmoplastic response may cause them to be matted together and distorted (indurated). When malignant neoplasms arise in mucosa and skin, they initially form a raised (exophytic) mass, but with extension into the deeper tissue, central necrosis, infection and ulceration are common. Often the periphery of the neoplasm remains as a raised margin but eventually cavitation may occur because of inward invasion resulting in an endophytic neoplasm. As with benign neoplasms, malignant neoplasms may cause pressure and obstruction, which often lead to clinical presentation. Malignant neoplasms can also secrete hormones, sometimes in an unexpected fashion. The principal effects of malignant neoplasms are:

- destruction of adjacent tissue causing loss of function, for example nerve invasion may cause pain, paraesthesia or palsy
- pressure on adjacent tissue, which may cause obstruction to ducts predisposing to infection or local damage to vital structures
- haemorrhage, which may occur from ulcerated surfaces leading to acute or chronic blood loss
- secondary deposits (metastatic tumours), which may cause localized damage or become widespread leading to cachexia
- obstruction of flow, for example inability to swallow in malignant neoplasms arising in the oesophagus
- production of hormones which may be normal in malignant tumours of endocrine glands or inappropriate, for example some lung cancers secrete ACTH and ADH
- pain, anxiety and anorexia
- paraneoplastic disorders including pigmentation, skin rashes, weight loss and general debility.

At the microscopic level, cells in malignant neoplasms exhibit a range of differentiation. Well-differentiated neoplasms may retain a number of structural and biochemical features of the cell of origin, for example well-differentiated squamous cell carcinoma cells often form keratin. At the other end of the spectrum some malignant cells are anaplastic, i.e. show no identifiable features of specialization. Often, poorly differentiated malignant neoplasms retain sufficient of their biochemistry to be identified by tumour markers in the laboratory. In certain cases, the degree of differentiation can be used to determine the tumour grade and this can be used prognostically.

SUMMARY BOX
CLINICAL EFFECTS OF TUMOURS

- Destruction of adjacent tissue may cause loss of function, e.g. nerve invasion may cause pain, paraesthesia or palsy.
- Pressure on adjacent tissue may cause obstruction to ducts predisposing to infection or local damage to vital structures.
- Haemorrhage may occur from ulcerated surfaces leading to acute or chronic blood loss.
- Secondary deposits (metastatic tumours) may cause localized damage or become widespread leading to cachexia.
- Obstruction of flow, e.g. inability to swallow in malignant neoplasms arising in the oesophagus.
- Production of hormones that may be normal in malignant tumours of endocrine glands or inappropriate, e.g. small cell lung cancers secrete ACTH and ADH.
- Pain, anxiety and anorexia.
- Paraneoplastic disorders including pigmentation, skin

Histogenesis

Neoplasms can also be classified by consideration of their cell of origin, which is determined by the pattern of differentiation and site, and is usually divided into three groups:

- epithelial origin
- connective tissue origin
- haemopoietic and lymphoid tissue origin.

Malignant neoplasms arising from epithelium are known as carcinomas and those arising from connective tissue are known as sarcomas. The term haemopoietic malignancy is generally applied to malignant neoplasms in the third group. Malignant neoplasms arising from melanocytes are termed 'malignant melanomas'. It should be borne in mind that neoplasms originate from stem cells and are genetically aberrant. They may exhibit features of differentiation which are inappropriate to their origin and often fetal characteristics are re-expressed.

Nomenclature

Neoplasms are named by addition of the suffix '-oma',

but it should be noted that there are a number of exceptions, such as granuloma and tuberculoma which refer to inflammatory lesions. Malignant neoplasia of the bone marrow and circulating white cells is also an exception and is known as leukaemia. Individual neoplasms are given separate names because each type of neoplasm has a distinctive set of features in terms of appearance and clinical behaviour. Accurate classification of every neoplasm is essential for diagnosis, research and clinical management. Some neoplasms are classified by generic means and others have quite specific names such as Kaposi's sarcoma, Burkitt's lymphoma, Ewing's sarcoma and Wilms' tumour. The term 'carcinoma' is used to denote a malignant epithelial neoplasm and 'sarcoma' to denote a malignant connective tissue neoplasm. Again, there are exceptions, for example the term 'myeloma' is used to denote a malignant neoplasm of plasma cells. Sometimes, to avoid confusion, the word malignant is used as a preceding adjective, e.g. malignant lymphoma, malignant mesothelioma. Histopathologists and oncologists (cancer specialists) refine and update classifications and almost every neoplasm is now regarded as a 'pathological entity', i.e. associated with a specific set of histopathological and clinical features. Follow-up of large patient series helps to define clinical outcomes and sometimes subclassification is necessary.

With these exceptions and provisos, the generic rule for nomenclature of neoplasms is a prefix denoting the cell or tissue of origin added to the suffix -oma (-carcinoma or -sarcoma for malignant neoplasms). As an example, a benign tumour of bone is known as an osteoma and its malignant counterpart as an osteosarcoma. Further examples are given in Table 6.2. Note that in many cases the word benign or malignant precedes the name. Traditional (often Latin) and modern names for tissue and neoplasms are used.

Epithelial neoplasms. Two groups of benign epithelial neoplasm are recognized:

- papilloma, arising from a non-secretory epithelial lining
- adenoma, arising from glandular or secretory epithelium.

The tissue of origin is prefixed by the tissue or cell of origin and some examples are given below:

- squamous cell papilloma – benign neoplasm arising from squamous epithelium

---

TABLE 6.2
NOMENCLATURE OF COMMON NEOPLASMS

Tissue of origin	Benign	Malignant
Epithelial		
Squamous cell	Squamous cell papilloma	Squamous cell carcinoma
Glandular	Adenoma	Adenocarcinoma
Transitional	Transitional cell papilloma	Transitional cell carcinoma
Basal cell	Basal cell papilloma	Basal cell carcinoma
Mesenchymal		
Smooth muscle	Leiomyoma	Leiomyosarcoma
Striated muscle	Rhabdomyoma	Rhabdomyosarcoma
Blood vessels	(Haem)angioma	Angiosarcoma
Connective tissue	Fibroma	Fibrosarcoma
Nerves	Neurofibroma	Neurofibrosarcoma (Schwannoma)
Adipose tissue	Lipoma	Liposarcoma
Cartilage	Chondroma	Chondrosarcoma
Bone	Osteoma	Osteosarcoma
Lymphoid cells		Malignant lymphoma
Haemopoietic cells		Leukoaemia
Melanocytes		Malignant melanoma
Embryonic tissue		
Totipotential cells	Benign teratoma	Malignant teratoma e.g. retinoblastoma, nephroblastoma
Unipotential cells		(Wilms' tumour)

- salivary adenoma – benign neoplasm arising from salivary gland epithelium
- colonic adenoma – benign neoplasm arising from colonic epithelium (which is glandular)
- pituitary adenoma – benign neoplasm arising from the pituitary gland.

Similar rules apply to the naming of a malignant epithelial neoplasm, which is always referred to as carcinoma. Those arising from glandular tissue or mucosa are termed adenocarcinoma and the cell or tissue of origin is added as in the following examples:

- squamous cell carcinoma – malignant neoplasm arising from squamous epithelium
- urothelial carcinoma – malignant neoplasm arising from the genitourinary tract (transitional) epithelium
- salivary adenocarcinoma – malignant neoplasm arising from salivary gland epithelium
- colonic adenocarcinoma – malignant neoplasm arising from the colonic epithelium.

Connective tissue neoplasms. Benign neoplasms of connective tissue origin (often referred to mesenchymal origin in this context) are also named by combining their cell or tissue of origin with the suffix -oma. Some common examples are given below:

- lipoma – benign neoplasm of fatty tissue
- osteoma – benign neoplasm of bone
- leiomyoma – benign neoplasm of smooth muscle
- rhabdomyoma – benign neoplasm of striated muscle
- chondroma – benign neoplasm of cartilage.

A malignant neoplasm of connective tissue (mesenchymal) origin is termed sarcoma. Again, the prefix relating to the tissue or cell of origin is added and examples corresponding to those above are given below:

- liposarcoma – malignant neoplasm of fatty tissue
- osteosarcoma – malignant neoplasm of bone
- leiomyosarcoma – malignant neoplasm of smooth muscle
- rhabdomyosarcoma – malignant neoplasm of striated muscle
- chondrosarcoma – malignant neoplasm of cartilage.

Mixed tumours. A few neoplasms contain more than one neoplastic cell type and these are referred to as mixed tumours. They can generally be classified by the dominant cell type. A well-known example is the pleomorphic salivary adenoma, which is a benign neoplasm of salivary gland origin that contains epithelial, myoepithelial and connective tissue elements. Odontogenic tumours can also be mixed and particular patterns of differentiation dependent upon epithelial–mesenchymal interactions may only be seen when both elements are present. Rare malignant mixed tumours also exist.

Teratomas. Teratomas are germ cell neoplasms which include all three embryonic layers. Benign teratomas may include fully differentiated structures such as teeth, hair, gland, bone and other tissues, but malignant teratomas are often poorly differentiated. Most benign teratomas arise in the ovary.

Embryonal tumours. In early childhood, a distinctive group of neoplasms may arise known as 'blastomas' or more correctly embryonal tumours. They include retinoblastoma, nephroblastoma (Wilms'), sialoblastoma, hepatoblastoma and others. Often there is a hereditary basis and such tumours have provided important clues to understanding the genetic basis of cancer, for example mutation of the retinoblastoma gene (Rb) is important in many neoplasms (see p. 3).

Neoplasms of the diffuse endocrine system. Cells of the diffuse endocrine system, such as the islets of Langerhans, gastrin-secreting cells and others are collectively known as APUD (amine precursor uptake and decarboxylation) cells on the basis of their histochemistry. Neoplasms arising from these cells often cause distinctive clinical syndromes due to excess secretion of peptides. Examples include:

- insulinoma, associated with episodes of hypoglycaemia
- gastrinoma, causing hyperacidity and peptic ulceration
- carcinoid tumours, may not secrete or they produce 5-hydoxytryptamine (5-HT) causing sweating and flushing
- phaeochromocytoma, associated with hypertension and diabetes.

Oncogenesis

The process which leads to neoplastic transformation is known as oncogenesis. Most research in the area of oncogenesis has been undertaken in relation to malignant neoplasms, where the process is termed carcinogenesis. An agent known to participate in the process is known as a carcinogen. There is good evidence that carcinogenic agents ultimately act on the DNA and that neoplastic transformation is the result of accumulation of genetic damage. This is often referred to as the theory of multistage carcinogenesis.

Epidemiological studies have enabled cancers to be linked to environmental factors such as geographic area, occupation, diet and lifestyle, whilst genetics has established the role of inherited factors and susceptibility in some neoplasms. Well-known epidemiological links have been made between some cancers and environmental factors:

- smoking and lung cancer
- hepatitis B and C infection and liver cancer
- radioactive iodine and childhood thyroid cancer
- tobacco and alcohol use and oral cancer.

There are three main groups of carcinogenic agents, although several cofactors are known. These are chemical carcinogens, radiation and viruses.

Chemical carcinogens

A variety of agents have been implicated in cancer by epidemiological studies, animal experiments and accidental exposure. Some chemical carcinogens act directly at the site of contact. Many others, known as procarcinogens, require active metabolic conversion into active carcinogen. Genetic factors may determine the rate at which procarcinogens are metabolized in individuals and 'metabolizer status' may account for variation in susceptibility to carcinogens. Metabolic conversion accounts for patterns of neoplastic change in some instances. Bladder cancer has been attributed to beta-naphthylamine used in the dye and rubber industry. After uptake it is converted in the liver to 1-hydroxy-2-naphthylamine, the active carcinogen. The active carcinogen is masked by glucuronic acid which is deconjugated in the urinary tract exposing the bladder epithelium to active carcinogen. In other situations the metabolizing enzyme is ubiquitous and cancers tend to arise at sites of exposure to carcinogenic agents. Tobacco smoke contains 3,4-benzpyrene which can be metabolized by hydroxylating enzymes such as aryl carbohydrate hydroxylase, which is ubiquitous. Tobacco smoke is strongly associated with cancer of the mouth, larynx and bronchus, but there is also an increased incidence of cancer of the cervix and bladder in smokers, presumably owing to systemic absorption and metabolism of carcinogens.

Carcinogens are chemically diverse and the major classes include:

- polycyclic aromatic hydrocarbons, e.g. lung cancer, oral cancer, skin cancer
- nitrosamines, associated with liver cancer in animals

- azo dyes, e.g. bladder and liver cancer
- vinyl chloride, associated with liver angiosarcoma
- aromatic amines associated with bladder cancer.

Other known carcinogenic agents include asbestos fibres, metal and wood particles, and fungal toxins.

Radiation

Both ultraviolet light and ionizing radiation are known to play a role in carcinogenesis.

Ultraviolet radiation. Ultraviolet light, particularly UVB, is a major cause of skin cancer. The risk is greatest for basal cell carcinoma and malignant melanoma, both of which arise more commonly on sun-exposed skin than in other sites. Fair-skinned persons living in tropical latitudes and in mountain areas show a particularly high incidence. Genetic deficiency of DNA repair enzymes in the condition xeroderma pigmentosum predisposes to multiple skin cancers.

Ionizing radiation. Associations between ionizing radiation and malignant neoplasia are well established and precautions are taken to avoid exposure. Many examples arise from the time when the risks were not known, e.g. the increased incidence of leukaemia and skin cancer in radiologists who were occupationally exposed. Thorotrast was an alpha-emitter contrast medium used in imaging in the 1930s. It was taken up by macrophages and later shown to be associated with cancers of the liver.

More recently, accidental leakage of radioactive material from Chernobyl has been associated with an increased incidence of thyroid, bone, haemopoietic and breast cancer.

Viruses

The first associations between viruses and carcinogenesis were made in animal studies, where cell-free filtrates of tumours were found to be able to transmit the neoplastic stimulus. Epidemiological studies have identified clusters of cancers, which suggests a possible viral aetiology. In humans, tumours associated with viruses tend to be linked to immunosuppression, e.g. human herpesvirus 8 and Kaposi's sarcoma in AIDS, or occur at an unusually young age.

The main associations between viruses and human neoplasia are:

- Epstein–Barr virus (EBV) – Burkitt's lymphoma and nasopharyngeal carcinoma

- human papillomavirus (HPV) (types 16 and 18) – cervical carcinoma
- hepatitis B and C viruses (HBV, HCV) – hepatocellular carcinoma
- human herpesvirus 8 (HHV8) – Kaposi's sarcoma
- human T-lymphotropic viruses (HTLV) – T cell leukaemia/lymphoma.

Often a cofactor is required (such as malaria with Epstein–Barr virus) and genetic predisposition is also relevant. Studies from animal cancer-causing viruses (oncoviruses) led to the discovery of oncogenes and also provided insight into molecular mechanisms in carcinogenesis.

SUMMARY BOX
CARCINOGENESIS

- Chemical carcinogens often require metabolic processing to the active form.
- Radiation inducers include ultraviolet light and ionizing radiation.
- Oncogenic viruses in man include EBV, HPV, HBV, HBC, HHV8 and HTLV.
- Asbestos, nickel, fungal toxins and other environmental factors are carcinogenic.

Multistep carcinogenesis

The effects of carcinogens ultimately are manifested in the DNA, where genes can be activated or inactivated by a number of mechanisms. Cancer can be considered to be a result of natural selection among somatic cells. If a mutation confers a selective growth advantage on a cell, then its progeny may form a clone which has the potential to take over the body. During evolution many sophisticated controls to prevent such an event have emerged and cancer results only when several independent controls have been lost. Mutation rates in DNA have been estimated at 10^{-7}–10^{-9} per gene per generation. It is widely accepted that between six and eight successive mutations are required to develop a normal cell into its neoplastic counterpart. The probability of any single cell undergoing so many mutations is $1:10^{22}$, which is practically negligible. Two mechanisms exist which make stepwise progression possible.

- Some mutations enhance cell proliferation creating an expanded target population for subsequent mutations (see Fig. 6.2).
- Some mutations affect the entire genome and increase the mutation rate.

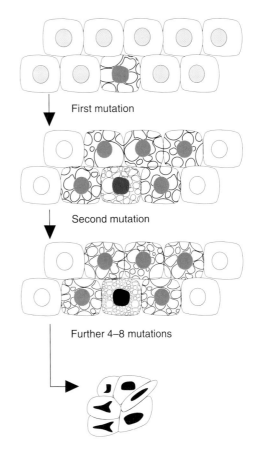

First mutation

Second mutation

Further 4–8 mutations

Malignant neoplasm

Fig. 6.2 Multistep progression of neoplasia. (See text for details.)

There are three groups of genes which are implicated in multistage carcinogenesis:

- oncogenes, whose action is to promote cell proliferation
- tumour suppressor genes, whose products inhibit cell proliferation
- mutator genes, responsible for maintaining the integrity of the genome.

Mutant versions of oncogenes are excessively or inappropriately active and a single mutant allele may alter the cell in this way. Mutant tumour suppressor genes and mutator genes require loss of both alleles to render them inactive (Fig. 6.3).

A useful analogy has been proposed by A P Read and N S Thakker in which the cell is likened to a bus with two accelerators, two sets of brakes and two mechanics. Jamming on one accelerator (one mutant oncogene allele,

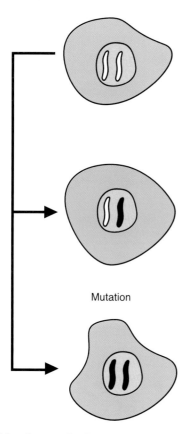

Mutation

Fig. 6.3 **Mutations may involve one allele or both alleles of a particular gene.** The effect of such changes will depend on whether the gene involved is a mutator gene, tumour suppressor gene or an oncogene (see text for further details).

dominant gain of function) will cause the bus to speed out of control. Failure of one set of brakes would allow control to be maintained, but if both sets failed (both alleles in a tumour suppressor gene inactivated) then the bus would run out of control. In a similar way, if one mechanic attended to the servicing then all would be well, but if both failed (both alleles in a mutator gene inactivated) then faults would occur in many systems, including the brakes and accelerators.

SUMMARY BOX
MULTISTEP CARCINOGENESIS

- Oncogenes are activated in cancer and act in dominant, gain of function mode.
- Tumour suppressor genes act in recessive, loss of function mode. Inactivation promotes cell proliferation.
- Mutator genes act in recessive, loss of function mode. Inactivation causes genetic instability and increases mutation rate.

Oncogenes

Animal tumour viruses led to the discovery of genes which could induce cancer. These became known as oncogenes. It was quickly discovered that oncogenes have counterparts in normal mammalian cells, correctly referred to as proto-oncogenes. Usually this distinction is ignored and the term oncogene is used for the normal genes in cells. Mutated oncogenes are generally referred to as activated oncogenes. In normal cells, oncogenes control the types of cell function that may be altered in cancer and five groups of cell activity controlled by oncogenes are identified:

- secreted growth factors
- intracellular signal transducer components
- cell surface receptors
- DNA-binding nuclear proteins and transcription factors
- cell cycle regulators.

Activation of oncogenes is a key event in malignant transformation and is seen in sporadic neoplasms. Only one familial cancer is associated with a hereditary onco-gene defect, the RET oncogene which is associated with multiple endocrine neoplasia syndrome and thyroid cancer.

Activation of oncogenes may occur by at least three mechanisms:

- amplification, where the cell possesses multiple copies of the gene
- point mutation, where biochemical deregulation increases activity
- translocation, where the oncogene is moved to an area of high transcription (Fig. 6.4).

Tumour suppressor genes

Evidence for tumour suppressor genes first came from the observation that fusing a normal cell to a neoplastic cell could correct its behaviour. This implied that recessive genes acting by loss of function were involved in neoplasia. Many tumour suppressor genes have been identified by studies of rare familial cancers.

Retinoblastoma is an aggressive childhood tumour of the retina which is hereditary in 40% of cases. When DNA samples from tumour tissue and blood (constitutional) were compared in retinoblastoma family patients, it was found that the constitutional DNA was hetero-zygous for chromosome 13 markers whereas the tumour tissue was homozygous. One copy of the mutant tumour

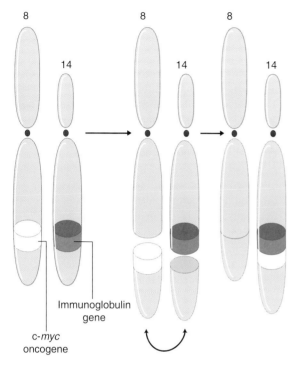

Fig. 6.4 Example of a translocation where part of chromosome 8 (the c-*myc* oncogene) is translocated to chromosome 14, close to the immunoglobulin gene region, at a point of high transcription.

Immunoglobulin gene

c-*myc* oncogene

neoplastic transformation can only occur if there is an accumulation of six to eight events. Mutator genes are directly involved in the cell cycle control errors involved in cancer. Loss of function of mutator genes leads to inefficient repair and replication of DNA resulting in a 100- to 1000-fold increase in mutation rate. It is likely that mutator genes are responsible for general genetic instability in cancer cells, which often display major chromosomal losses, gains and translocations. Some authors consider the distinction between tumour suppressor genes and mutator genes to be artificial.

Multistage models of carcinogenesis

Although oncogenes, tumour suppressor genes and mutator genes have differing roles, they act together in stepwise fashion during carcinogenesis. Models of the multistage process have been proposed for many cancers, where early and late-stage genetic events have been identified. The best known is that of Fearon and Vogelstein for colorectal cancer, in which patterns of genetic alteration can be related to progression through formation and development of adenomas to adenocarcinoma. A similar model of multistep progression has been described for oral squamous carcinoma (Fig. 6.5).

suppressor gene had been inherited and mutation of the other normal allele had occurred in the tumour cells.

This work fitted with Knudson's two-hit hypothesis, that two successive mutations (hits) are required for neoplastic transformation. The locations of tumour suppressor genes can be determined using the loss of heterozygosity method, as well as linkage analysis and comparative genome hybridization.

The functional roles of tumour suppressor genes are not all known, but the two best-known, Rb1 product and p53 product, act as inhibitors of cell cycle progression. In the rare Li-Fraumeni syndrome, p53 mutations are inherited and affected family members suffer from multiple primary tumours including breast, sarcoma, CNS tumours and leukaemia. It is thought that p53 prevents cells with damaged DNA from replicating by inducing apoptosis. It can be inactivated by a number of mechanisms.

Mutator genes

Although oncogenes and tumour suppressor genes produce expanded target populations in carcinogenesis,

Invasion

Malignant cells spread through the tissues in amoeboid fashion and invasion of tissue is a key criterion for diagnosis of malignancy in a neoplasm. It has been known for many years that neoplastic cells show abnormal motility and lose their contact inhibition. Cancers spread in the local tissue along lines of least resistance, particularly natural cleavage planes. Some tissue components resist invasion including the capsules of the kidney, liver, salivary gland and periosteum. Movement of malignant neoplastic cells is recognized to be mediated by three factors:

- secretion of proteolytic enzymes, in particular matrix metalloproteinases
- acquisition or increase of cell motility
- loss or decrease in cell attachment, often by downregulation of adhesion molecules.

The process of invasion allows the neoplastic cells to reach lymphatic and blood vessels and from there more distant spread can occur.

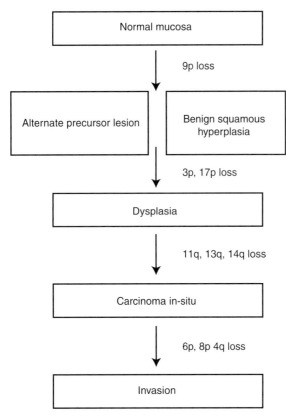

Fig. 6.5 Schematic representation of the multistep progression of oral squamous carcinoma.

SUMMARY BOX
INVASION IN MALIGNANT NEOPLASIA

- Invasion is a key feature in diagnosis of malignancy.
- Abnormal cell motility, secretion of proteases and loss of adhesion molecule are important.
- Invasion is limited by dense tissue planes and some organ capsules.

Metastasis

Metastasis is the process by which neoplastic cells spread from the primary tumour to form tumour deposits at distant sites. These are termed secondary deposits or metastases. The metastatic process involves invasion of lymphatic or blood vessels, detachment, transportation as emboli and finally extravasation and growth at the distant site. Neoplastic cells in lymphatic vessels tend to arrest in regional lymph nodes and those in blood vessels may reach more distant sites. Neoplastic cells can also be implanted or spread across body cavities. Recognized metastatic routes are:

- *Lymphatic spread.* Neoplastic cells may grow directly down afferent lymphatic channels or travel as emboli. The neoplastic cells grow at the periphery of the node and gradually obliterate the normal structure. Central necrosis may occur. Extracapsular extension may eventually fix the node to adjacent tissues.
- *Haematogenous spread.* Metastatic deposits are often multiple and anatomy influences their pattern of distribution. For example, adenocarcinoma of the colon frequently spreads through the blood to the liver (Fig. 6.6). Haematogenous metastases often involve the brain, liver, lung and adrenal gland, sometimes occur in the skin but rarely involve skeletal muscle or spleen. Also, primary carcinomas in the lung, breast, thyroid, kidney and prostate have a particular tendency to metastasize to bone, where they may cause pathological fractures. The non-random distribution of metastatic deposition may be explained by vascular heterogeneity and preferential growth advantage in certain tissues. Some metastatic deposits appear to remain clinically dormant for many years.
- *Transcoelomic spread.* The mesothelial-lined cavities provide a surface upon which secondary deposits can form. Neoplastic cells can spread directly in a protein-rich exudate in the pleural, peritoneal and pericardial cavities. Detection of such effusions and sampling by cytological analysis is important in diagnosis, especially of ovarian, breast and lung cancer.

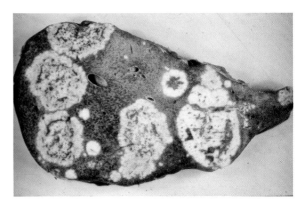

Fig. 6.6 **Metastatic carcinoma.** Slice of liver in which there are numerous deposits of white tumour, some showing central necrosis. These are the typical appearances of metastatic carcinoma in the liver, and in this case the primary tumour was in the bronchus.

- *Implantation.* Accidental implantation of neoplastic cells may occur at the time of surgery or biopsy. Precautions such as placing a ligature around a tumour pedicle or removing the tract of a needle biopsy site at definitive surgery aim to avoid this risk.

SUMMARY BOX
METASTATIC SPREAD

- Routes are lymphatic, via blood vessels, transcoelomic and implantation.
- Metastases can remain clinically dormant for years.
- Distribution of metastases is influenced by anatomy, tumour type and growth advantages in particular tissues.

SYSTEMIC PATHOLOGY

7 Cardiovascular disease

ATHEROMA

Atheroma is one of the commonest causes of death in the western world, mainly by causing ischaemic heart disease and cerebrovascular disease. There are numerous well-recognized factors in the causation of atheroma, many of which are capable of amelioration through changes in lifestyle.

Atheroma is a disease of the intima of arteries (Fig. 7.1) caused by the accumulation of lipid material initially in macrophages and later in smooth muscle cells.

The earliest lesion of atheroma is the 'fatty streak' (Fig. 7.2) which is visible as a raised yellow area on the luminal surface of arteries, particularly at the site of branching of larger vessels such as the aorta. They may be seen in young children but are not necessarily the precursor lesion for atheroma itself.

The established lesion of atheroma consists of a fibrous plaque (Figs 7.3 and 7.4), which covers a larger surface area in vessels and has a white appearance. It is this lesion which predisposes to the various complications of atheroma (see below).

Pathogenesis

Lipids, particularly cholesterol bound to low-density lipoproteins (LDLs), derived from circulating blood lipids, accumulate in macrophages in the intima of vessel, producing a foamy appearance of the cells. The macrophages are derived from circulating monocytes, although resident macrophages may also be present. Later, smooth muscle cells, which originate in the media of vessels, migrate into the intima where they are capable

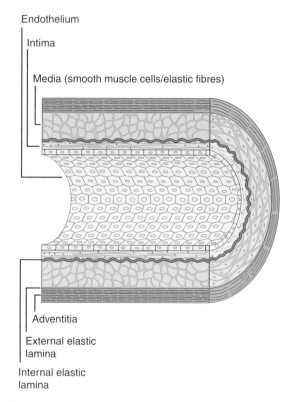

Endothelium

Intima

Media (smooth muscle cells/elastic fibres)

Adventitia

External elastic lamina

Internal elastic lamina

Fig. 7.1 Cross-section of normal artery showing lumen with endothelium, intima, internal elastic lamina, media, external elastic lamina and adventitia.

of ingesting lipid and may also adopt a foamy appearance. These smooth muscle cells develop myofibroblastic activity and thus are also capable of producing collagen. As the lipid load increases, extracellular accumulation of lipid occurs, often in the form of needle-like cholesterol

Foam cells

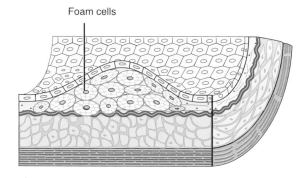

A

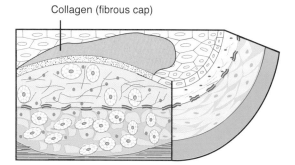

Fig. 7.3 **An established lesion of atheroma where there is continuing expansion of the media by foam cells and smooth muscle cells.** The luminal endothelial surface is covered by fibrous tissue – a collagenous cap. The disease has spread into the media with disruption of the internal elastic lamina and accumulation of foam cells and smooth muscle cells.

Collagen (fibrous cap)

B

Fig. 7.2 **Early lesions of atheroma. A.** Fatty streak, the earliest lesion of atheroma, in which there is accumulation of lipid material within foam cells eccentrically within the intima of an artery. **B.** Aorta removed at autopsy, showing the earliest lesion of atheroma with fatty streaks in the thoracic aorta. Note the raised yellow/white lesions.

crystals, and as an irritant, this lipid induces a chronic inflammatory cell response which in turn may increase the deposition of new collagen in the vessel wall, producing a fibrous cap over the atheromatous plaque. As time progresses, with the increased accumulation of lipid, the internal elastic lamina separating the intima from the media is damaged and the process of atheroma development continues in the media.

Many theories have been postulated for the causation of atheroma and these have been combined in the 'response to injury' hypothesis, which supersedes the two most commonly held theories, the 'thrombogenesis' and 'insudation of lipid' theories:

1. Altered endothelial cell permeability, which may be caused by direct physical damage to the endothelial layer as in hypertension or by chemical effects of hyperlipidaemia or cigarette smoking, allows the movement

of circulating lipids from the vascular lumen into the intima, where the lipid accumulates initially in monocyte-derived macrophages.

2. Platelet adherence, at the site of endothelial damage where subendothelial collagen is exposed, leads to the release of growth factors especially PDGF (platelet-derived growth factor) and cytokines.

3. Smooth muscle migration and proliferation, which is promoted particularly by PDGF, causes the migration of cells from the media to the intima and these smooth muscle cells can store lipid, giving a foamy appearance, and produce collagen, forming a fibrous cap over the atheromatous plaque.

4. An inflammatory response occurs at the site of extracellular lipid accumulation and as part of the healing process, leads to new vessel formation and contributes to the formation of collagen.

Complications

Ulceration. As the amount of atheroma increases, the fibrous cap becomes stretched and ulcerates, predisposing to thrombosis (Fig. 7.4B).

Thrombosis. One of the factors required for the development of thrombosis is damage to the vessel wall, particularly the endothelial layer, and atheroma is one of the commonest predisposing thrombogenic conditions (Fig. 7.4C and D).

Haemorrhage into a plaque. With the accumulation of extracellular lipid and the subsequent inflammatory and repair response, new vessels within the intima and media are prone to easy haemorrhage. When this occurs suddenly, the rapid expansion of material within the

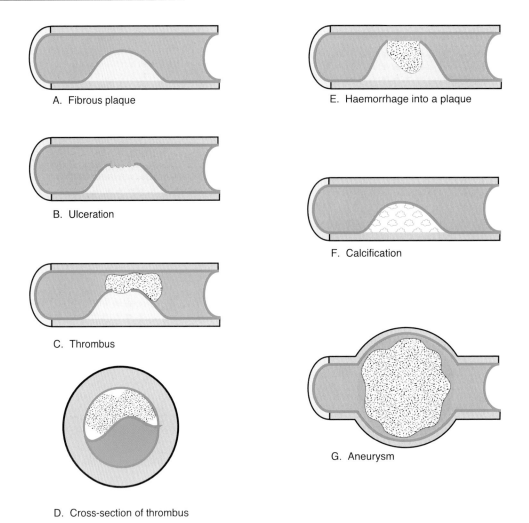

Fig. 7.4 **Lesions of complicated atheroma. A.** Fibrous plaque as in Fig. 7.3. **B.** Ulceration of the endothelial surface, which predisposes to **C.** thrombus formation, which may cause complete occlusion of the lumen, as can **D.** haemorrhage into a plaque. **E.** Calcification leads to hardening of the arteries, and **F.** aneurysm formation, where the atheromatous process extends into the external elastic lamina causing weakness of the wall, making it prone to rupture. **G.** Cross-section of a thrombus (as in **C**).

vessel can cause significant narrowing of the lumen (Fig. 7.4E).

Rupture of a plaque. When the fibrous cap ulcerates, in addition to thrombosis, there is also a possibility that the atheromatous material within the vessel wall will be released into the vessel lumen producing a shower of atheromatous emboli to be carried downstream within the arterial system.

Calcification. The process of atherogenesis produces damaged tissues into which calcium salts may be deposited, so that many vessels affected by atheroma have a brittle, crunchy texture on palpation. Atherosclerosis or arteriosclerosis, the previously commonly used terms for atheroma, also referred to as 'hardening

of the arteries', are produced by such calcification (Fig. 7.4F).

Aneurysm formation. An aneurysm is an outpouching of a vessel wall and occurs in atheromatous vessels when the external elastic lamina separating the media from the adventitia is damaged. This occurs particularly in the lower abdominal aorta below the origin of the renal arteries and above the bifurcation (Figs 7.4G and 7.5).

Aetiology

Much of the information concerning the aetiological factors in atherogenesis is derived from epidemiological

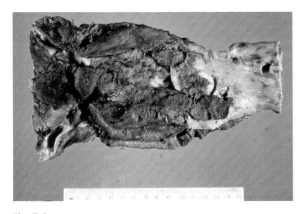

Fig. 7.5 Aneurysm and thrombosis. Photograph of an aorta at autopsy from a patient with an aneurysm of the lower abdominal aorta, below the origin of the renal arteries, which has ruptured producing catastrophic haemorrhage. The lumen of the vessel contains abundant laminated thrombus.

studies, from intervention trials with manipulation of individual factors by changes of lifestyle and/or drug treatment, and from experimental research.

Age. Atheroma is a disease of increasing age and significant disease is rare before the age of 40.

Sex. Atheroma is primarily a disease of men until the latter half of the seventh and eighth decades when the protective effects of the female sex hormones are lost after the menopause.

Hyperlipidaemia. This is the single most important factor in atherogenesis and it is almost impossible to develop atheroma in the presence of normal levels of cholesterol and low-density lipoproteins. The best evidence for the role of hyperlipidaemia in atherogenesis comes from the rare but well-recognized syndrome of familial hypercholesterolaemia. In this condition, affected family members lack or have reduced numbers of low-density lipoprotein (LDL) receptors on cell membranes. This results in high circulating levels of LDL and its main transported lipid, cholesterol, which then leads to the development of atheroma in susceptible individuals in the late teens and early 20s with consequent early sudden death mainly from myocardial infarction. The heterozygous state of hyperlipidaemia, where the numbers of LDL receptors are reduced to 50% of normal, causes increased rates of atheroma in the fourth and fifth decades. Whereas high levels of LDL predispose to the development of atheroma, other lipoproteins particularly high-density lipoproteins (HDL) are protective against its development. Such lipoproteins are found in oily fish, and epidemiological studies have shown that populations who consume large amounts of such fish have a lower incidence of atheroma, e.g. Inuits (Eskimos).

Hypertension. Patients with high levels of systemic hypertension have an increased incidence of the development of atheroma, possibly by causing endothelial damage and allowing the passage of lipids from the lumen into the vessel wall.

Cigarette smoking. This is a well-recognized association with the development of atheroma and is thought to act through the effect of a variety of chemicals within cigarette smoke, damaging the endothelial layer.

Diabetes mellitus. Diabetics are at increased risk of developing atheroma, both insulin-dependent (juvenile onset) and non-insulin-dependent (maturity onset) types, possibly through the microvascular damage associated with diabetes mellitus and partly through the increased incidence of hyperlipidaemia in this condition.

Other factors. The role of diet in the development of atheroma is uncertain but is probably related to the presence of high levels of cholesterol. The effect of alcohol on atherogenesis is variable: at low levels (1 unit, 10 g alcohol/day), there is a protective effect whereas at levels above recommended limits (more than 5 units/day, 35 units/week), there is an increased incidence of atheroma. Exercise is thought to be protective against atheroma whereas sedentary occupations, particularly in obese patients, increase the risk. Similarly, the role of stress is uncertain but is also thought to predispose to atherogenesis. Previously, the higher levels of oestrogen used in the oral contraceptive pill were thought to increase the risk of atheroma but the more recent use of lower levels has reduced this likelihood.

SUMMARY BOX
ATHEROMA

- Disease of large and medium-sized arteries.
- Early lesions are fatty streaks which start in the intima and spread into the media.
- Later, fibrous plaques develop, from which complicated lesions such as ulceration, thrombosis, haemorrhage into a plaque, plaque fissure, calcification and aneurysm formation occur.
- Risk factors include cigarette smoking, hyperlipidaemia, hypertension, diabetes mellitus, increasing age and male gender.
- It is a major cause of morbidity and mortality by causing ischaemia in heart, brain and peripheral vessels.

THROMBOSIS

This is the process of formation of a solid mass in living blood vessels, including the heart, from the constituents of flowing blood. In contrast, a clot is an unstructured mass of material derived from blood vessels, formed outside living vessels or postmortem within blood vessels. Thrombosis can be considered as the pathological counterpart of the normal physiological process of haemostasis/coagulation (see Ch. 8, p. 113).

Three main factors have been shown to contribute to thrombosis. They were originally described by the 19th century German pathologist, Rudolf Virchow, and are known as Virchow's triad.

1. *Changes in the vessel wall*, which refer mainly to changes in the endothelial lining of the vessel which allow the exposure of subendothelial collagen and other matrix proteins. These changes may be caused by micro-trauma in systemic hypertension, chemical agents such as cigarette smoke and high levels of lipids, bacterial toxins, immunological injury, atheroma (Fig. 7.5) and endo-cardial damage. Platelets may then attach to the exposed subendothelial tissues while activation of the coagulation cascade leads to the deposition of fibrin in the region of the platelet plug. Subsequently, red cells derived from the flowing blood may attach to the fibrin–platelet thrombus, although this is more commonly seen in venous rather than arterial or cardiac thrombi.

2. *Changes in blood flow*, which differ between arterial and venous thrombi. The normal flow of blood produces a laminar arrangement of cells in the lumen with the largest cells, mainly leukocytes centrally, smaller cells such as erythrocytes and platelets more laterally, and a plasma-rich, relatively acellular zone peripherally immediately adjacent to the endothelium. In conditions of either turbulence (increased flow) or stasis (reduced flow), the normal laminar arrangement is disturbed and cells come into contact with the endothelial layer. The damaging effect of this contact is enhanced in turbulent conditions, such as in aneurysmal sacs, where exposure of subendothelial tissues is also present. Other conditions which predispose to thrombosis due to vessel wall changes include valvular heart disease, atrial fibrillation (AF) and myocardial infarction (MI) involving the endo-cardium (on the arterial/cardiac side of the circulation) and varicose veins and thrombophlebitis (on the venous side).

3. *Changes in blood constituents*, which refer to the condition of hypercoagulability. This is an increased ten-dency to thrombosis owing to a relative (e.g. in dehydra-tion or hyperviscosity) or absolute increase in individual prothrombotic agents, or a lack of antithrombotic agents. Clinically, these conditions include prolonged bed rest and immobility, the postoperative state, pregnancy and the postpartum state, the nephrotic syndrome, severe burns, major trauma, cardiac failure, disseminated malig-nancy and high-oestrogen-containing oral contraceptive pill use. A common inherited abnormality of coagulation, factor V Leiden, increases the tendency to thrombosis in affected individuals.

There are several mechanisms by which the body under normal circumstances protects against potentially damaging thrombosis. Depletion of the clotting factors present at a particular site may be accomplished simply by dilution. Restoration of normal blood flow may permit the clearance of activated factors or they may be taken up by macrophages or inactivated in the liver. Naturally occurring anticoagulants such as antithrombin III, heparin and protein C have a protease effect on activated clotting factors. At the same time as activation of coagu-lation, the fibrinolytic pathway which promotes the breakdown of fibrin monomers and polymers is also activated.

Fate of thrombosis

Resolution. This may occur by a number of mecha-nisms such as shrinkage, clot retraction, platelet auto-lysis, fibrinolysis or phagocytosis.

Organization. This occurs by the ingrowth of capil-laries, and fibroblasts may lead to recanalization of the thrombus, particularly in completely occluded vessels, or

---

SUMMARY BOX
THROMBOSIS

- Formation of a solid mass in living blood vessels, including the heart, from the constituents of flowing blood.
- Predisposing factors are changes in blood flow, changes in the vessel wall and changes in blood constituents (Virchow's triad).
- The fate of thrombi includes resolution, organization and embolism.
- Venous thrombosis occurs mainly in lower limbs as a result of stasis and clinically may lead to oedema, venous congestion and pulmonary embolism.
- Arterial thrombosis is usually due to underlying atheroma and clinically may cause ischaemia and infarction.

to fibrosis, which is seen particularly in mural thrombosis of large vessels such as the aorta. This latter mechanism is similar to the process of atherogenesis, described above.

Detachment. Detachment of the thrombus may occur, particularly if the thrombus is friable or crumbly, leading to the process of embolism.

EMBOLISM

This is the process in which there is impaction in part of the vascular system of any abnormal undissolved material carried there by the bloodstream. Embolism may take many forms but the commonest and clinically most significant type is that derived from pre-existing thrombosis (see above). However, several other types, although less frequently encountered, may have catastrophic consequences for the at-risk patient.

Thromboembolism

Emboli derived from pre-existing thrombosis are of two main types: venous or arterial/cardiac.

Venous thromboembolism

Venous thromboembolism is a common cause of morbidity and mortality in hospital-based patients, particularly those recovering from operative procedures or who are immobilized for a number of reasons. Thrombosis occurs in the deep veins of the legs or pelvis and fragments of the thrombus detach and are carried along the venous system through the popliteal/femoral/iliac veins to the inferior vena cava and thence to the right side of the heart. The thromboembolus passes across the pulmonary valve into the pulmonary artery (Fig. 7.6). Depending on the size of the embolus, it may impact there as a saddle embolus causing acute right ventricular failure, associated with severe chest pain, breathlessness and collapse and a significant risk of sudden death, or proceed into the major branches of the pulmonary arteries where infarction of the lung tissue supplied by the occluded branch may occur. In general, if more than 50% of the supply of pulmonary vasculature is obstructed by thromboembolus, then acute right ventricular failure is likely to occur. On the other hand, if less than 50% is involved, the more likely outcome is infarction, although other factors, particularly the status of the bronchial arterial supply, are important in determining the effect of embolism. Acute

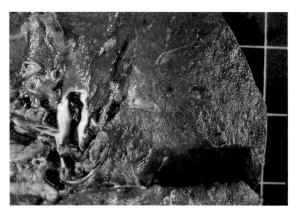

Fig. 7.6 Thromboembolism. Section of lung at autopsy showing occlusion of the pulmonary artery by fresh thromboembolism with an area of infarction in the adjacent lung shown as the dark red/brown material, consistent with previous pulmonary embolism.

episodes may resolve by fragmentation or fibrinolysis, or there may be organization of the thromboembolus with recanalization of the involved vessel. Recurrent embolic episodes may lead to pulmonary hypertension, as the pressure required to permit blood flow is increased through the inevitably narrowed lumina of previously occluded vessels.

Arterial/cardiac thromboembolism

Arterial, including cardiac, emboli arise from thrombi usually on the basis of pre-existing atheroma and are more commonly seen in association with aneurysms. Mural thrombosis within the left ventricle often develops 4–10 days after myocardial infarction. Atrial fibrillation is a disorder of cardiac rhythm where the atria beat at a rate of 160–180 beats per minute and is a common cause of atrial, especially left-sided, thrombosis. Conditions associated with the development of this condition include chronic valvular heart disease, particularly post-rheumatic, ischaemic heart disease, hypertensive heart disease and thyrotoxicosis. The clinical consequences of left-sided thromboembolism include cerebral, splenic, renal and intestinal infarction.

Fat embolism

This condition arises from the release of multiple fat droplets into the bloodstream and is associated particularly with fractures of long bones but may also be seen as a result of trauma to adipose tissue or rarely to fatty liver, in hyperlipidaemia and in sickle cell crises. Fat embolism is a relatively common phenomenon but is much less frequently associated with significant clinical complications. Since the droplets usually enter the venous system, the first signs of fat embolism are seen as a consequence of pulmonary vascular obstruction with the patient complaining of breathlessness and developing a skin rash in the area of distribution of the superior vena cava. The droplets are usually of sufficient size to pass through the pulmonary capillaries and thus reach the left side of the heart where they are carried in the systemic circulation and lead to the potentially fatal effects of cerebral ischaemia. This is associated with disturbances of cerebral function eventually leading to coma and death.

Gas embolism

The two major gases associated with clinical disease are air and nitrogen. Air embolism arises when air is introduced into the circulation where it mimics the effect of pulmonary thromboembolism. This may occur in mismanaged blood transfusions, in head and neck surgery, in haemodialysis, during insufflation of the Fallopian tubes in the investigation of infertility and in criminal abortions where the placental site is damaged. Air may also reach the systemic circulation and lead to cerebral complications. As little as 40 ml of air has been shown to cause fatalities, but more usually, 100 ml or more are required to cause death. Nitrogen emboli occur in decompression sickness, which is also known as 'caisson disease'. A gradual return from high atmospheric pressure, such as in deep-sea divers, is necessary to avoid the release of gas bubbles from interstitial and adipose tissues. If nitrogen enters the bloodstream, the bubbles may coalesce to form larger droplets and cause ischaemic effects on various tissues, particularly around tendons, joints and ligaments and in bones and brain. The pain in this condition may be excruciating and is referred to as the 'bends'.

Tumour emboli

Malignant tumours often metastasize through the bloodstream, usually in capillary and venous vessels, and the presence of intravascular tumour fragments in malignancy is not uncommon. A good example is renal cell carcinoma where the presence of tumour in the renal vein and inferior vena cava is a prognostic factor. These tumour fragments may impact in the lung causing a solitary, so-called 'cannonball', metastasis.

Atheromatous emboli

One of the complications of atheroma arises when there is rupture of an atheromatous plaque with release of showers of atheromatous emboli, which may cause problems downstream of the site of rupture. This may occur naturally in the cerebral or coronary circulations and is a potential complication of procedures such as angioplasty for coronary artery disease, endarterectomy for carotid artery stenosis or aortic surgery such as aneurysm repair. Most atheromatous emboli are of little clinical consequence.

Amniotic fluid embolism

This is an uncommon but potentially catastrophic consequence of normal pregnancy. It was previously seen as a complication of illegal backstreet abortions before the introduction of legal abortions in Great Britain in 1967 but is nowadays seen much less frequently. The danger of this condition lies in the release of potent thromboplastic agents from the amniotic sac into the maternal circulation where they activate the coagulation system, promoting intravascular coagulation and fibrinolysis, rapidly depleting clotting factors and leading to the clinical picture of disseminated intravascular coagulation (DIC). This carries a very high mortality rate and is one of the major causes of maternal death.

Foreign body embolism

This condition arises relatively frequently but is usually of little clinical significance. Small fragments of material are occasionally introduced to the circulation during intravenous injection and infusions, including pieces of plastic venous cannulae. These are usually cleared by macrophages in the lung, liver or spleen and cause no further problems. Intravenous drug abusers may inject larger quantities of materials such as talc used in tablet formation which are solubilized for injection purposes. Much of this material remains in the pulmonary circulation within macrophages and may cause a 'snow-storm' appearance on chest radiography.

'Paradoxical' embolism

This refers to the situation whereby venous thrombosis detaches and forms emboli, which are capable of entering the systemic, arterial circulation through a defect in the cardiac circulation, e.g. patent ductus arteriosus, patent foramen ovale or ventricular septal defect. Most of these conditions are encountered in early childhood but relatively minor congenital defects such as a patent foramen ovale (atrial septal defect) may persist into adult life and serve as a conduit for these 'paradoxical' emboli.

SUMMARY BOX
EMBOLISM

- The impaction in part of the vascular system of any abnormal undissolved material carried there by the bloodstream.
- The most common form is thromboembolism, which is a major cause of sudden death.
- Other types of emboli include fat, gas, tumour fragments, infective fragments derived from infective endocarditis (see below), atheromatous material, amniotic fluid and foreign bodies.

ISCHAEMIA

This is a state of inadequate blood supply to an area of tissue which may lead to harmful effects for that tissue or its component cells.

These harmful effects include:

- hypoxia – a state of impaired oxygenation which may be seen in a number of situations, including:
  - hypoxic hypoxia where there is a low partial pressure of oxygen in the blood, for example in patients with respiratory failure
  - anaemic hypoxia where the oxygen-carrying capacity of the blood is reduced owing to a lack of haemoglobin
  - stagnant/ischaemic hypoxia where the impaired oxygenation at tissue level is due to a reduction in blood supply or venous drainage
  - histotoxic hypoxia where there is competition for the use of oxygen in cells, for example in carbon monoxide or cyanide poisoning
- malnutrition
- failure to remove waste products.

Causes of ischaemia

General. Inadequate cardiac output (shock) may occur, for example in ventricular fibrillation after myocardial infarction or in acute right ventricular failure due to massive pulmonary thromboembolism. These are major causes of generalized ischaemia and are often irreversible.

Local. A number of different causes of local ischaemia may be seen:

- Arterial obstruction, which may be caused by atheroma itself or more commonly by complications of atheroma such as thrombosis or embolism.
- Venous obstruction, which is usually caused by engorgement of vessels, thus impeding venous drainage. This situation is commonly seen in strangulation of bowel in hernia sacs or torsion of organs attached by a loose pedicle, such as testis or ovary.
- Small vessel obstruction, which affects vessels such as arterioles, venules or capillaries and in the case of arterioles particularly may be caused by immune-complex-mediated diseases such as vasculitis in systemic lupus erythematosus or polyarteritis nodosa.

Effects of ischaemia

None. There may be no effects of ischaemia and patients may be unaware of serious underlying conditions until they present with severe disease or even sudden death.

Functional. There may be functional disturbances associated with ischaemia, such as the typical chest pain brought on by exertion or stress and relieved by rest or vasodilator substances (*angina pectoris*) or the leg pains induced by exercise and relieved by rest (*intermittent claudication*).

Sublethal effects. There may be sublethal cellular disturbances where the cell is still intact and viable but undergoes degenerative changes such as fatty change or cloudy/hydropic swelling.

Infarction. The ultimate effect of ischaemia is to cause infarction.

INFARCTION

This refers to the process in which there is a localized area of ischaemic necrosis in an organ or tissue, resulting from sudden reduction of either its arterial supply or its venous drainage. In clinical terms, infarction is far more likely to occur when the arterial supply is obstructed.

A number of factors are involved in determining the degree of injury associated with infarction. These include:

- The general status of the blood, particularly the

haemoglobin level, and of the cardiovascular system, mainly the severity of pre-existing atheroma.

- The anatomical pattern of the blood supply. Infarction is much more likely to occur in a tissue with a single endarterial supply, for example in the kidney, than in a tissue which has a dual blood supply, for example the liver where the hepatic artery supplies oxygen and the portal vein provides nutrients.
- The rate of development of occlusion is important, as gradual obstruction allows the development of collateral supply, for example in the lower limbs, whereas sudden occlusion is more likely to cause infarction.
- The vulnerability of tissues to ischaemia/hypoxia is variable, such that cortical neurons and Purkinje cells in the brain withstand a lack of oxygen for a much shorter time than either skeletal muscle or keratinocytes in the skin.
- The ability of tissues to regenerate is important, not so much in the development of the infarct itself but in the healing and repair response afterwards.

Myocardial infarction

Ischaemic heart disease occurs as a consequence of coronary artery narrowing and produces a range of clinical features including stable angina pectoris (caused by reduced flow in atheromatous arteries), unstable angina pectoris (caused by fissuring of atheromatous plaques) and myocardial infarction.

Gross appearances (Fig. 7.7)

In most instances, infarction arises as a result of thrombus formation which in 25% of cases develops from ulceration of a plaque and in 75% of cases from plaque fissure with or without haemorrhage. If patients present with features of severe ischaemia, thrombolysis may be attempted in the early stages, usually within the first few hours, with agents such as streptokinase or tissue plasminogen activator. The site of infarction in the myocardium is determined by the coronary artery involved, so that the anteroseptal wall of the left ventricle becomes necrotic when the anterior descending branch of the left coronary artery is occluded and the postero-inferior wall of the left ventricle is damaged when the right coronary artery is narrowed. Infarcts may be regional within the area of involvement, up to 2 cm in extent, or may be more global in the subendocardial zone of the left ventricle when there is generalized non-occlusive atheroma, often accompanied by episodes of hypotension.

Histological appearances

Grossly, the heart may not demonstrate any features of infarction in the first 12 hours. Between 12 and 24 hours, the damaged area appears pale and, histologically, the infarcted myocardium becomes eosinophilic and oedematous. Between 24 and 72 hours, the infarct becomes soft and pale and, histologically, there is necrosis of myofibres with polymorph infiltration (Fig. 7.8). Between 3 and 10 days, the infarcted area appears pale with a hyperaemic border which is reflected histologically by granulation tissue infiltration. Over a period of weeks to months, the damaged area is replaced by scar tissue (Fig. 7.9).

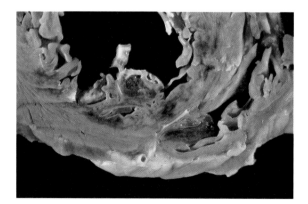

Fig. 7.7 Recent myocardial infarction. Transverse section of the heart showing recent infarction of the left ventricular myocardium shown by a mottled yellow-red area of necrosis with a small amount of overlying mural thrombosis.

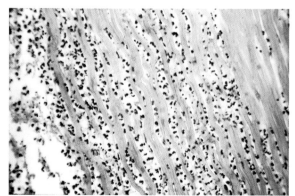

Fig. 7.8 Recent myocardial infarction. Histological section of myocardium showing extensive necrosis of myofibres with interstitial oedema and polymorph infiltration, consistent with a recent MI.

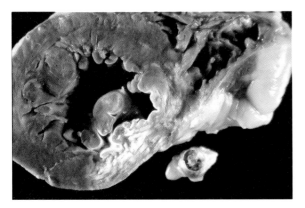

Fig. 7.9   Old myocardial infarction. Transverse section of myocardium showing an area of replacement fibrosis of the anteroseptal wall of the left ventricle, typical of scarring following MI some months or years previously.

Complications

Clinically 35–50% of patients will die in the first week after their first myocardial infarction and, of these, 50% will succumb in the first hour; another 10% will die in the first year. Most of the sudden deaths occur as a result of cardiac arrhythmias, mainly ventricular, and in the first week, death may be due to acute left ventricular failure, cardiac tamponade due to rupture of necrotic myocardium or mitral incompetence due to papillary muscle dysfunction. Mural thrombosis arising on necrotic endocardium may give rise to emboli which can cause cerebrovascular accidents ('strokes'), gut ischaemia or renal infarcts. Pericarditis is another acute complication of infarction. In the longer term, chronic left ventricular failure and left ventricular aneurysm may complicate established infarcts. Patients who have had one myocardial infarction are at increased risk of further infarcts (Fig. 7.9).

SUMMARY BOX
MYOCARDIAL INFARCTION

- Localized ischaemic necrosis of heart muscle, usually left ventricle.
- It is caused by coronary artery atheroma, often with sudden obstruction by thrombosis or haemorrhage into or rupture of a plaque.
- Infarct may not be visible initially, then becomes pale and necrotic; later it undergoes repair with replacement by fibrosis.
- Clinically, it may present with sudden death, cardiac arrhythmias, cardiac failure, pericarditis, cardiac rupture, mural thrombosis and ventricular aneurysm.

ANEURYSMS

An aneurysm is a localized outpouching of a vessel wall which may be symmetrical, producing a fusiform aneurysm, or focal, leading to a saccular aneurysm. Aneurysms usually arise from weakness of the wall, which may be due to atheroma, infection, vasculitis or syphilis.

Atheromatous aneurysms are most commonly seen in the lower abdominal aorta below the origin of the renal arteries but may also occur in the descending thoracic aorta. The aneurysm often accumulates large amounts of thrombus within its lumen which may give rise to emboli, especially to the lower limbs (see Fig. 7.5). Clinically, an aneurysm may be identified as a pulsatile mass in the abdomen and may cause back pain radiating to the legs. If recognized early, surgical intervention by bypass grafting may be successful. However, the larger the aneurysm the more likely it is to rupture, which often causes catastrophic retroperitoneal haemorrhage and sudden death.

Syphilitic aneuryms are much less commonly seen nowadays but were a common cause of aneurysms of the ascending aortic arch. They arise from the typical mesaortitis seen in syphilis and may lead to rupture into the pericardial sac (leading to cardiac tamponade) or into the mediastinum.

Cerebral aneurysms occur at branch points in the circle of Willis, as a result of weakness in the media accompanied by hypertension. Rupture leads to subarachnoid haemorrhage which may be fatal or cause cerebrovascular accidents.

Infective, so-called mycotic, aneurysms occur when there is damage to vessel walls from infected emboli especially in infective endocarditis and particularly affecting the brain and kidneys.

Cardiac aneurysms arise in the left ventricle after myocardial infarction from extensive scar tissue leading to haemodynamic abnormalities and thrombosis.

Traumatic aneurysms may develop from stab wounds but are relatively uncommon.

The term 'dissecting aneurysm' is a misnomer but is often included in the classification of aneurysms. The usual cause is a tear through the intima into the media of the aorta as a result of cystic medial myxoid necrosis, although it may be seen in inherited conditions such as Marfan's syndrome and collagen disorders such as Ehlers–Danlos syndrome. If the tear occurs within the pericardial sac, haemopericardium or cardiac tamponade may result, whereas if the tear occurs elsewhere in the aorta, a re-entry site may be seen causing compression of major ostia or, rarely, a double-barrelled aortic channel may result. Rupture is often precipitated by hypertension.

SUMMARY BOX
ANEURYSMS

- Localized outpouching of a vessel.
- Atheroma is the commonest cause especially involving the lower abdominal aorta.
- Syphilitic aneurysms characteristically affect the ascending thoracic aorta.
- Berry aneurysms occur at the branch points of the circle of Willis in the brain; rupture leads to subarachnoid haemorrhage.
- Mycotic aneurysms arise from infective emboli and usually affect the cerebral vessels.
- Capillary microaneurysms occur mainly in the cerebral circulation and are associated with hypertension and intracerebral haemorrhage.
- Dissecting 'aneurysms' usually occur in the thoracic aorta and rupture through dissection along the media causing haemopericardium and vascular occlusion.

VASCULITIS

This is inflammatory damage to a vessel wall which may affect any size of vessel from capillary to aorta and which may lead to irreversible wall destruction. Three main categories exist: hypersensitivity vasculitis; vasculitis associated with systemic disorders; and giant cell (temporal) arteritis.

- Hypersensitivity vasculitis affects mainly venules and capillaries and is an immune-complex-mediated disease with complement activation and polymorph infiltration. It affects vessels in the skin causing a skin rash with extravasation of red cells leading to purpura. Precipitating factors include infections with viruses and bacteria and specific conditions include Henoch–Schönlein purpura, serum sickness and cryoglobulinaemia.
- Vasculitis may be associated with multi-organ diseases such as systemic lupus erythematosus (SLE) and rheumatoid disease. In these conditions there is often lymphocytic infiltration of vessels in skin and muscle.
- Systemic vasculitis affecting multiple organs is a characteristic of polyarteritis nodosa (PAN). This affects small and medium-sized arteries and is often a patchy, focal disease producing small infarcts in the kidneys,

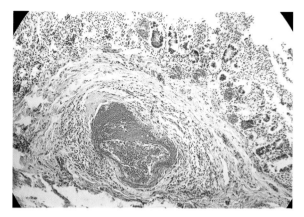

Fig. 7.10 Small bowel: polyarteritis nodosa. Section of small bowel in which there is ischaemic damage to the overlying mucosa owing to occlusion of a submucosal artery by necrosis in PAN.

heart, central nervous system, peripheral nerves, skeletal muscles, skin and gut (Fig. 7.10), where ulcers may be seen including in the oral mucosa. It is thought to be an immune-complex-mediated disease, although a specific antigen is rarely identified (e.g. hepatitis B surface antigen in less than 10% of cases) and antineutrophil cytoplasmic antibodies of perinuclear type (p-ANCA) may be detected in serum. The characteristic histological feature is fibrinoid necrosis of affected vessels with polymorph and eosinophil infiltration within the wall.

- Giant cell arteritis is also known as temporal arteritis since it affects mainly the arteries of the head and neck region, especially the temporal artery. It is a disease of the elderly who present with malaise and tiredness and a very elevated erythrocyte sedimentation rate (ESR). There is an association with the condition of polymyalgia rheumatica and patients may present with sudden blindness which responds well to corticosteroids. Histologically there is disruption of the internal elastic lamina of affected vessels with a giant cell inflammatory reaction.
- Wegener's granulomatosis is a vasculitic condition affecting the nose, palate, gingivae, lungs and kidneys associated with antineutrophil cytoplasmic antibodies of cytoplasmic type (c-ANCA) where there is histological evidence of granulomatous destruction of vessel walls along with polymorph infiltration.
- Buerger's disease is an inflammatory disease of peripheral vessels which is seen particularly in males who are heavy cigarette smokers. It affects both arteries and veins with granulomatous and polymorph inflammation and may lead to gangrene and amputation.

- Less common forms of systemic vasculitis include Churg–Strauss vasculitis affecting vessels in lungs, kidneys, heart and skin with an eosinophil infiltrate, Kawasaki arteritis involving vessels in skin, heart, mouth and eyes with lymphocytic endothelial necrosis, and Takayasu's disease where there is a histiocytic giant cell inflammatory response in the aorta and its main branches.

SUMMARY BOX
VASCULITIS

- Inflammatory change in vessel walls of any size and is usually a result of immunologically mediated damage.
- The common types include hypersensitivity vasculitis such as Henoch–Schönlein purpura and cryoglobulinaemia, vasculitis associated with systemic disorders such as SLE, rheumatoid disease, Wegener's granulomatosis and PAN, and giant cell (temporal) arteritis.
- Commonly, multiple organs are involved, especially kidneys, lungs, skin, joints and the eyes.

CARDIAC FAILURE

This is an abnormality of cardiac function leading to a failure to pump blood at the rate required for normal metabolism. This can be of two main types:

- backward failure where the pump fails, leading to increased venous pressure and oedema formation
- forward failure where there is reduced output to the periphery leading to reduced perfusion, retention of sodium and water and consequent oedema.

Cardiac failure may occur either acutely, as in the case of myocardial infarction and pulmonary embolism, or chronically, as in the case of chronic ischaemic or valvular heart disease.

Left ventricular failure (LVF)

This is the most common form and causes pulmonary oedema, which produces the clinical features of shortness of breath (*dyspnoea*), which may be more pronounced when lying flat (*orthopnoea*) and especially at night (*nocturnal dyspnoea*). Occasionally it may lead to the coughing up of blood (*haemoptysis*).

Right ventricular failure

Right-sided cardiac failure is less common in the first instance and is most usually due to long-standing left ventricular failure, for example post-rheumatic mitral stenosis, causing secondary changes in the pulmonary vasculature. Pure right ventricular failure arising on the basis of chronic pulmonary disease such as primary pulmonary hypertension or pulmonary fibrosis is termed cor pulmonale. The clinical features of right ventricular failure include raised jugular venous pressure, detected by observing the jugular vein of the patient seated at an angle of 45°, congestion of the liver and other abdominal organs, peripheral oedema, either around the ankles if the patient is ambulant or over the sacrum if the patient is less mobile, and pleural, pericardial or peritoneal effusions.

Congestive cardiac failure

When both right and left ventricular failure coexist, the condition is referred to as congestive cardiac failure.

High-output cardiac failure

Most cases of cardiac failure are associated with reduced cardiac output, but occasionally, cardiac failure may be seen as a result of increased output. This may occur in thyrotoxicosis, pregnancy and, rarely, Paget's disease of bone.

OEDEMA

This is the accumulation of excess fluid in interstitial or intracellular tissues or in body cavities. The development of oedema is determined by the forces described in Starling's hypothesis, which include a combination of the hydrostatic pressure of blood and tissues, the oncotic pressure of plasma and the osmotic pressure of tissues. There is a net loss from the arterial to the venular end of the capillary circulation and in normal circumstances, any excess is cleared by the lymphatic system.

A number of different pathogenic mechanisms may give rise to clinically significant oedema:

- Inflammatory oedema which occurs as part of the inflammatory response and is caused by increased permeability of vessels induced by the release of chemical mediators.
- Venous oedema which is the form seen in cardiac failure (see above), associated with increased hydrostatic pressure, and may also be caused by obstruction of

venous drainage, as in thrombosis or extrinsic compression of vessels.

- Lymphatic oedema which occurs when the lymphatic system is blocked either by tumour, as in metastatic disease, or by parasitic infestation of lymph channels, most commonly seen in the Third World, e.g. as elephantiasis in infestation with the filarial worm.
- Hypoalbuminaemic oedema which occurs when the plasma oncotic pressure is reduced, since albumin is the most important contributory factor to the plasma oncotic pressure. Significantly low levels of plasma albumin (i.e. less than 20 g/l, normal range 35–50 g/l) are seen in severe protein malnutrition, chronic liver failure, the nephrotic syndrome and protein-losing enteropathy.

SYSTEMIC HYPERTENSION

This is a condition in which there is a sustained increase in systemic arterial blood pressure, although the clinical definition of the condition is more difficult. The normal level of blood pressure depends on the age of the patient but generally is less than 140/90 mmHg (systolic/diastolic). Hypertension may be either primary, also known as essential, where there is no known cause, or secondary, where an identifiable cause may be found.

Essential hypertension

This is the commonest form of hypertension, responsible for over 95% of all cases. It usually occurs over the age of 40 years and there may be an inherited familial predisposition. It may be related to high dietary sodium intake in a genetically predisposed individual, although the evidence for this is not absolutely certain. Other associated risk factors include stress, obesity, cigarette smoking, high alcohol intake, increasing age and male gender.

Secondary hypertension

In this form, there is a recognizable cause which is most usually of renal origin, possibly as a result of renal arterial disease but also associated with renal parenchymal or glomerular disease. The mechanism is through a stimulation of the juxtaglomerular apparatus causing a release of renin which converts angiotensin I to angiotensin II, leading to an increase in systemic blood pressure. The adrenal gland may also cause secondary hypertension in a number of ways, including tumours of the adrenal medulla (phaeochromocytoma), hyperaldosteronism

mainly due to tumours of the adrenal cortex (Conn's syndrome), excessive activity of the cortex (Cushing's syndrome) and, rarely, congenital adrenal hyperplasia. Some prescribed drugs may cause hypertension (iatrogenic disease) including corticosteroids and the oral contraceptive pill.

Clinical features

In the early phases of systemic hypertension, the great majority of patients are asymptomatic. Most of the symptoms of hypertension are relatively non-specific and include headaches, dizziness and tiredness. Most usually, hypertension is diagnosed incidentally when patients undergo medical examination for other reasons.

Pathology

The organs particularly involved are the heart, arteries, kidneys, brain and eyes.

Heart. The heart shows concentric left ventricular hypertrophy due to the increased pressure load. This increases the risk of ischaemic heart disease, and hypertensive patients are at risk of sudden death, possibly due to arrhythmias.

Blood vessels. The main effects of hypertension on blood vessels are related to vasoconstriction of arterioles associated with smooth muscle contraction. In arteries, this leads to medial hypertrophy, hyaline degeneration and intimal fibrosis. There is an increased rate of development of atheroma. In the accelerated form of hypertension, also known as malignant hypertension, the vessels develop marked intimal fibrosis associated with fibrinoid necrosis (Fig. 7.11).

Kidneys. The vessels in the kidneys are similarly affected and as these are end arteries, with progressive disease, the kidneys become scarred with cortical narrowing and this in turn increases the development of hypertension. This may ultimately lead to renal failure.

Brain. In the brain, hypertension leads to the production of microaneurysms in the deep cerebral cortex near the pons, basal ganglia and cerebellum. Rupture of these microaneurysms causes often fatal intracerebral haemorrhages. Although not a cause of berry aneurysms themselves, hypertension may cause their rupture leading to subarachnoid haemorrhage.

Eyes. The main site of damage by hypertension in the eyes is in the retina and the changes include retinal haemorrhages, exudates, narrowing of the vessels and in accelerated hypertension, papilloedema.

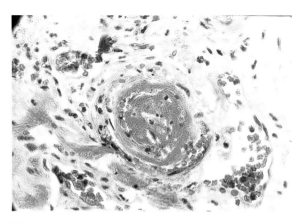

Fig. 7.11 Fibrinoid necrosis (hypertension). Section of a blood vessel showing fibrinoid necrosis (bright pink material in vessel wall) in a patient with accelerated (malignant) hypertension.

SUMMARY BOX
SYSTEMIC HYPERTENSION

- Sustained increase in arterial blood pressure.
- Most cases are primary in which there is no recognizable cause, whereas secondary causes include renal and adrenal disease and drugs such as corticosteroids.
- Organs commonly involved include the heart, arteries, kidneys, brain and eyes.
- In most cases, damage occurs gradually but accelerated (malignant) hypertension is associated with fibrinoid necrosis of vessel walls.

DISEASES OF THE ENDOCARDIUM AND HEART VALVES

Primary diseases of the endocardium apart from the heart valves are rare. Endocardial fibroelastosis in western societies and endomyocardial fibrosis in Central Africa may predispose to thrombosis and precipitate cardiac failure.

Diseases of heart valves have two main mechanical abnormalities. Narrowing or abnormal rigidity of valves is termed stenosis, whereas an inability to close fully is termed incompetence or regurgitation. Both may coexist. Precipitating factors include congenital conditions that may be lethal, leading to death soon after birth, or less severe, when patients survive into adulthood and may require surgical correction. Heart valves tend to degenerate with increasing age; there may be dilatation of the valve ring, degeneration of the supporting connective tissues or acute destruction due to necrotizing inflammation

(see infective endocarditis below). Post-inflammatory scarring, particularly associated with rheumatic fever (see below), is a major cause of valvular heart disease. Whatever the underlying cause, damaged heart valves are more prone to thrombus formation and colonization by bacteria.

The valves most commonly affected in these conditions are those on the left side of the heart – the mitral and aortic valves. Diseases of the right-sided valves, pulmonary and tricuspid, are rare.

Mitral valve

Mitral stenosis is a cause of left ventricular dilatation, left ventricular failure (LVF) and atrial thrombosis, associated with atrial fibrillation. It is most commonly seen after rheumatic heart disease. Mitral incompetence (regurgitation) is also associated with rheumatic heart disease but is also seen after myocardial infarction where there is involvement of the papillary muscles and in the floppy valve syndrome (mitral valve prolapse). This condition is now a much more common cause of mitral incompetence than post-rheumatic disease. The valve leaflet shows degenerative changes leading to ballooning of the posterior cusp particularly, with a risk of rupture. LVF is common in this condition.

Aortic valve

Aortic stenosis is most commonly due to a congenitally bicuspid valve (the normal valve has three cusps) but can also be due to senile calcification (Fig. 7.12). Its presence is often not detected clinically until severe left ventricular

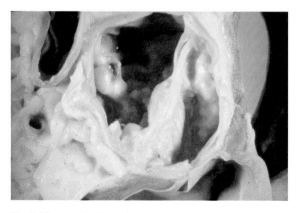

Fig. 7.12 Calcific bicuspid aortic stenosis. An aortic valve viewed from above, showing a bicuspid appearance with extensive calcification.

hypertrophy (LVH) has developed. However, it is a cause of sudden death through myocardial ischaemia or may present with angina pectoris. Aortic regurgitation (incompetence) may also be due to previous rheumatic disease but may be seen with infective endocarditis, senile calcification and dilatation of the valve ring in inflammatory conditions such as ankylosing spondylitis and syphilis. Mixed stenosis and regurgitation are relatively common conditions in the aortic valve.

ACUTE RHEUMATIC FEVER

This is a condition of decreasing incidence which is none the less of great importance in the practice of dentistry because of its potential to cause long-standing cardiac disease many years after its initial occurrence.

Incidence

This condition affects children between the ages of 5 and 15 years and is associated with those in lower socio-economic groups living in overcrowded conditions, particularly in underdeveloped countries. Its incidence has been declining in Western Europe and the USA over the last two to three decades.

Aetiology/pathogenesis

Acute rheumatic fever is an example of an immuno-logical hypersensitivity reaction, in response to Group A streptococcal antigens, occurring 2–6 weeks after a preceding acute tonsillitis or pharyngitis. Typically, there is involvement of all layers of the heart ('pancarditis'). There are usually high levels of circulating antistreptococcal antibodies and a number of theories have been proposed to explain the association between streptococcal infection and cardiac disease in particular. There is thought to be a sharing or cross-reaction between the streptococcal carbohydrate antigens and components of the cardiac tissues. Other tissues in the body may also be involved including synovial joints, skin, subcutaneous tissue and the basal ganglia in the brain. Immune complexes are not themselves thought to be directly involved.

Clinical features

The heart is the site of the most characteristic lesions and all layers may be involved in rheumatic pancarditis (35%). The vast majority of patients with acute rheumatic

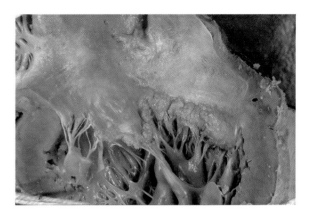

Fig. 7.13 Acute rheumatic endocarditis. Opened mitral valve of a patient with acute rheumatic fever in which there are soft, small, red/brown vegetations on the valve cusps.

carditis do not have symptoms referable to the heart and only if symptoms and signs in other organs lead to the detection of features of carditis, will this potentially damaging component of acute rheumatic fever be recognized. Myocarditis may give rise to cardiac failure and pericarditis leads to features of pericardial effusion with a pericardial rub. Endocarditis (Fig. 7.13) may lead to the appearance of, or a change of character in, a cardiac murmur.

Most patients have joint involvement with an acute migratory polyarthritis accompanied by signs and symptoms of a febrile illness (75%). Subcutaneous nodules may be identified over extensor surfaces and are usually small, pea-sized, painless nodules often unnoticed by patients. The skin may also be involved in acute rheumatic fever, the most characteristic lesion being erythema marginatum. This pink rash occurs on the trunk and extremities and has a clear centre with red round or serpiginous margins, which blanch on pressure and may be brought on by heat. They vary greatly in size and are not itchy or indurated. Erythema nodosum may also occur in acute rheumatic fever but probably represents a response to the preceding streptococcal infection rather than a primary manifestation. The lesions are raised tender nodules occurring usually on the shins but also on the arms and face.

Chorea (Sydenham's chorea, chorea minor, St Vitus' dance) is a disorder of the central nervous system characterized by sudden, aimless, irregular movements, often accompanied by emotional lability and muscle weakness. It is a delayed manifestation of rheumatic fever and other features of the disease may not be apparent, although it may prompt the recognition of previously asymptomatic carditis. It develops gradually and may persist after other manifestations have resolved.

Pathology

Gross appearances

All patients who develop carditis in acute rheumatic fever will have endocardial involvement. The left-sided valves (mitral and aortic) are affected more frequently than those on the right (pulmonary and tricuspid). The initial lesion is the development of oedema followed by the loss of the endocardial lining at the lines of maximum trauma on the free edges of the valves. This leads to the formation of platelet–fibrin thrombi (rheumatic vegetations) which remain firmly attached to the valve cusps and do not become infected. Turbulence over these vegetations (Fig. 7.13) leads to the murmurs noted clinically.

Histological appearances

The most characteristic lesion of acute rheumatic fever occurs in the myocardium, typically in a perivascular distribution within fibrous septa separating bundles of cardiac myofibres. This is the Aschoff body which in its early stages has a non-specific appearance with exudation of plasma proteins and inflammatory cell infiltration. Later, it develops the pathognomonic features of a central zone of altered collagen surrounded by histiocytes and lymphocytes (Fig. 7.14). A characteristic cell is the Anitschkow cell, once thought to be of myocyte origin but now shown to be of macrophage derivation. These lesions may persist for years but are eventually replaced by scar tissue. The clinical feature of left ventricular

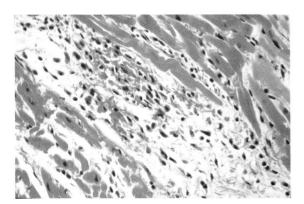

Fig. 7.14 Acute rheumatic fever: Aschoff body. Histological section of myocardium showing an interstitial inflammatory infiltrate composed of lymphocytes and macrophages with central necrosis of collagen, typical of an Aschoff body.

failure occurs when large numbers of Aschoff bodies are present in the myocardium.

Pericarditis in acute rheumatic fever reflects severe fibrinous inflammation leading to the development of a pericardial effusion containing abundant fibrin, producing a so-called 'bread and butter' appearance. This may lead to anterior chest pain and the recognition clinically of a pericardial rub.

Sequelae

The vast majority of patients with acute rheumatic fever recover completely within 6 weeks without any lasting consequences. A small minority with severe myocarditis develops cardiac failure or arrhythmias which may cause death in the acute phase. Those patients with recurrent attacks of acute rheumatic fever are at greater risk of developing significant scarring and subsequent long-term valvular heart disease. The other non-cardiac manifestations usually resolve completely.

The production of fibrosis in the endocardium, typically in the left atrium known as MacCallum's patch, may serve as a focus for the subsequent development of infective endocarditis. The more damaging consequences lie in the progressive fibrosis of the heart valves themselves with the mitral valve alone being affected in 50% of cases, both the mitral and aortic valves in 40%, the aortic valve alone in 8–10% and the tricuspid valve alone in about 2%. This may lead to either stenosis of the valve where there is fusion of the commissures producing a rigid valve with a narrow orifice, described typically in mitral stenosis as being of 'fish-mouth' type (Fig. 7.15), or to incompetence of the valve when the valve cusps are maintained in a dilated, open position allowing regurgitation of blood across the valve and leading to cardiac failure.

The patient is then at risk of developing progressive cardiac failure, predominantly left-sided initially when there is mitral incompetence, aortic stenosis or aortic incompetence, and predominantly right-sided when there is mitral stenosis or much less commonly tricuspid disease. There is also a much greater risk of developing infective endocarditis.

INFECTIVE ENDOCARDITIS

Infective endocarditis is the growth of microorganisms on an endothelial surface, usually a valve, within the heart. The organism is present in vegetations (platelet–

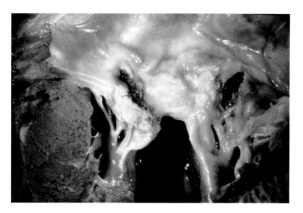

Fig. 7.15 Chronic rheumatic valvular heart disease: mitral stenosis. An opened mitral valve of a patient with long-standing rheumatic valvular heart disease. The valve cusps are thickened and fibrotic and show focal calcification and haemorrhage. The chordae tendineae show shortening and thickening, typical of chronic rheumatic heart disease.

SUMMARY BOX
ACUTE RHEUMATIC FEVER

- Immunological damage to heart and other organs which occurs after streptococcal throat infections.
- It is rare nowadays in western population but common in overcrowded and undernourished populations, especially children between 5 and 15 years.
- Its main effect is to cause carditis which may affect all layers.
- The characteristic cellular lesion is the Aschoff body.
- Long-term effects are associated with chronic valvular damage especially of the mitral and aortic valves.
- It increases the risk of infective endocarditis.

---

fibrin thrombi) on the endocardium from which it can be cultured, in contrast to acute rheumatic endocarditis whose vegetations are sterile. Traditionally, infective endocarditis is classified into the acute form, occurring on previously normal valves and associated with virulent organisms such as *Staphylococcus aureus*, and the subacute form where the endocardium is abnormal for a variety of reasons and where the organisms are of low virulence. However, it is the characteristics of the infecting organism which determine the clinical course and the term 'infective endocarditis' should be simply qualified by the name of the organism (see also Ch. 5).

Pathogenesis

Two factors are required for the development of infective endocarditis: an episode of bacteraemia and the presence of small thrombi on the valve. Alone, neither factor will initiate the disease. Initially, microorganisms are deposited on the surface of the valve and there is then a lag phase of 24 hours while the organism is incorporated into the thrombus, thus being protected from macrophage ingestion, and then proliferating. The virulence of the organism, the load of organisms in the blood and the size of the thrombus all determine whether infection becomes established.

Predisposing cardiac factors

Within the heart, a number of lesions predispose to the establishment of platelet–fibrin thrombi on and in which organisms may attach and proliferate. In general, high-pressure flow leads to endocardial damage and thus regurgitant (incompetent) valves are at greater risk than rigid, stenotic valves. Similarly, high-pressure shunts such as ventricular septal defects are more likely to lead to disease than lower-pressure atrial septal defects. Prosthetic valves of any type are a risk factor. Previously, chronic rheumatic valvular heart disease was the single most important predisposing condition (see above). Nowadays, floppy mitral valve and bicuspid aortic valve are being recognized more frequently as risk factors. While organisms such as *Staph. aureus* can infect apparently normal valves, it is now recognized that normal valves undergo age-related changes such as thickening on which tiny thrombi may develop.

SUMMARY BOX
INFECTIVE ENDOCARDITIS

- Growth of microorganisms on heart valves.
- Vegetations arise from a combination of bacteraemia and thrombi on the valves.
- Most cases develop on previously damaged valves from conditions such as rheumatic valvular disease, degenerative or atherosclerotic valves, congenital defects and prosthetic valves.
- Some cases arise on normal valves, especially in intravenous drug users, when the organisms are more likely to be highly virulent.
- Local complications include valve rupture and incompetence and myocarditis.
- Systemic complications include embolic phenomena to brain, kidneys and spleen, haemorrhages in the skin and mucous membranes, finger clubbing, and immune-complex-mediated glomerulonephritis.

Predisposing factors to bacteraemia

A known cause of bacteraemia is identifiable in about 50% of cases of infective endocarditis. Despite the recognition that antibiotic prophylaxis for dental procedures is advisable, approximately one-third of cases of *Streptococcus viridans* infective endocarditis are preceded by such procedures. Other causes of bacteraemia include naturally occurring disease, such as skin sepsis, wound and lung infections leading to staphylococcal endocarditis, and surgical instrumentation such as cystoscopy, prostatectomy, gastrointestinal endoscopy, especially colonoscopy, and intestinal surgery leading to enterococcal endocarditis. Intravenous drug abuse using contaminated needles leads particularly to tricuspid and pulmonary valve endocarditis, although mitral and aortic endocarditis may also result.

The organisms involved are shown in Table 7.1. The relative proportion of these organisms depends on the patient group involved. In non-immunocompromised patients with native (non-prosthetic) valve involvement, streptococci (60%) and staphylococci (15–25%) are the commonest infective agents, whereas drug addicts and those with prosthetic valves are more likely to have coagulase-negative *Staph. albus*, Gram-negative organisms and *Pseudomonas* infections. The commonest fungus implicated is *Candida* while Q-fever endocarditis is caused by the rickettsial organism, *Coxiella burnetii*. In some cases, no specific organism is cultured (approximately 8–12%) probably because of previously inadequate antibiotic therapy.

Clinical features

Before the introduction of antibiotics, the mortality rate was 100% and even with the use of antibiotics, it is still between 10 and 30%. The clinical course of infective endocarditis relates to the development of cardiac failure, systemic emboli and immunological phenomena.

Cardiac failure results from increasing volume overload on the left ventricle owing to incompetence as valve cusps are destroyed. The more virulent the organism the more rapidly the cardiac failure develops and further myocardial damage may occur as a consequence of small intramyocardial emboli, either bland fibrin–platelet or infective emboli.

The vegetations of infective endocarditis tend to be friable and the combination of friability with high pressure and cusp movement leads to the development of systemic emboli. Emboli of highly virulent organisms may give rise to metastatic abscesses. Cerebral abscesses occur in about 20% of cases, and are the major cause of mortality and morbidity in this disease, while renal abscesses are seen in 50% of patients with infective endocarditis but are less significant in terms of morbidity. Coronary artery emboli are rare but recognized.

Antibodies may be found in up to 100% of patients with infective endocarditis owing to the shedding of bacterial antigens into the circulation. Immune complexes may give rise to arthritis, splinter haemorrhages in the nail beds, skin purpura and glomerulonephritis. Renal failure accounts for about 25% of the mortality in infective endocarditis. The 'mycotic aneurysms' seen in this condition may represent an immunological response rather than direct infection.

Pathology

The characteristic lesion is the vegetation which is a large mass of thrombus adherent to the valve cusp or endocardium (Fig. 7.16). They vary in size, related to the haemodynamic properties of the valve and to the organism, and colour; some may be polypoid such as tricuspid and mitral lesions while aortic vegetations tend to be flatter and more sessile. The more virulent organisms destroy the underlying valve cusp and this is seen particularly with *Staph. aureus* infection where perforation may occur. With the progression of infection, it may not be possible to recognize any underlying cause, although

TABLE 7.1

ORGANISMS RESPONSIBLE FOR INFECTIVE ENDOCARDITIS

Organism	Proportion
Streptococcus viridans, including *Strep. sanguis*, *Strep. mitis*, *Strep. milleri*, *Strep. mutans* and *Strep. salivarius*	40–50%
Group D streptococci, including *Strep. bovis*, *Strep. faecalis* and *Strep faecium*	10–20%
Staphylococcus aureus and *Staph. epidermidis*	15–25%
Gram-negative bacilli	6–8%
Coxiella (Q-fever)	< 1%
Fungal, especially *Candida*	1–5%
Others, e.g. pneumococcus, meningococcus, gonococcus	2–5%
'Culture-negative' endocarditis	8–12%

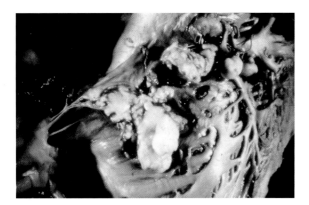

Fig. 7.16 Subacute bacterial endocarditis. Heart valve opened to show a large friable yellow/brown vegetation on the valve surface.

floppy mitral and bicuspid aortic valves tend to remain obvious. Histologically, there is a superficial layer of agglutinated platelets and immediately below this, there is a layer of densely packed fibrin containing micro-organisms (Fig. 7.17). Very few polymorphs are present

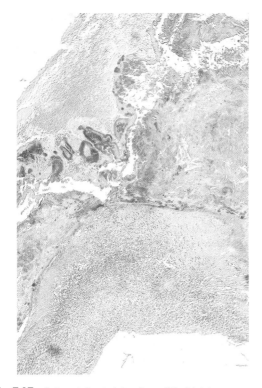

Fig. 7.17 Subacute bacterial endocarditis: histology.
Histological section of a valve in which there is abundant acute inflammatory infiltrate with fibrin, containing bacterial colonies. These are shown as the deeper-staining purple/blue material to the left.

in this layer but beneath the vegetation, the valve cusp is heavily inflamed and contains granulation tissue.

Non-infective vegetations

These vegetations, composed of platelets and fibrin, may occur on the left-sided valves in patients with an increased tendency to hypercoagulability such as patients with disseminated carcinomatosis – so-called marantic endocarditis. A similar condition occurs in patients with systemic lupus erythematosus (SLE) where anticardio-lipin antibodies predispose to thrombus formation; this is referred to as Libman–Sacks endocarditis.

ASPECTS OF CARDIOVASCULAR DISEASE OF PARTICULAR RELEVANCE TO DENTISTRY

- Facial pain may be a presenting feature of both angina pectoris and giant cell (temporal) arteritis.
- Patients with cardiac failure may present an anaesthetic risk.
- Wegener's granulomatosis may present with oral lesions.
- Dentists must be aware of the need for antibiotic prophylaxis in the prevention of infective endocarditis; in particular, they must appreciate which cardiac lesions require prophylaxis and why.

CASE STUDY 7.1
POSTOPERATIVE COMPLICATIONS

A 73-year-old woman was admitted to an orthopaedic ward from a nursing home where she had fallen and sustained a subcapital fracture of the right hip. A total hip replacement was performed and the initial postoperative recovery was satisfactory, although mobilization was difficult because of a moderate degree of obesity and postoperative pain. The site of fracture of her hip was submitted for histopathological examination and was reported as containing, in addition to the usual features of a fracture, metastatic carcinoma suggestive of a primary in the breast.

While recuperating on the ward, this woman asked to use the commode and while sitting on the commode, com-plained of breathlessness and severe chest pain. She then collapsed and was found slumped on the floor cyanotic and pulseless. Despite intensive resuscitation measures including cardiac massage, assisted respiration, and infusion of intravenous fluids along with sodium bicarbonate and adrenaline, this woman died. Her death was reported to HM Coroner who ordered a postmortem examination.

1. What possible complications of surgery may occur in this case, particularly related to immobility?
2. What route of metastasis is the most likely in this case?
3. What type of fracture does this represent and what is the more usual cause of fractures in this age group?
4. What is the likely sequence of events in this case?
5. What are the likely findings at autopsy?

Suggested responses

1. There is an increased risk of the development of deep venous thrombosis. Immobilized patients are also at risk of developing bronchopneumonia.

2. This is an example of blood-borne metastasis and the bones are relatively common sites, after lung and liver (see Ch. 6).

3. This is a pathological fracture, i.e. the fracture has occurred at a site of weakness induced by a lytic bone lesion (see Ch. 6). More usually, hip fractures in elderly women occur as a result of osteoporosis, a metabolic bone disease which is more common in postmenopausal women who lack the protective effect of oestrogen stimulation of their bones (see Ch. 12).

4. Because of her immobility, recent surgical procedure and underlying malignancy, this woman is very prone to developing deep venous thrombosis (DVT) of her lower limbs, particularly on the side of surgery. This is because she has had changes in *blood flow* (stasis due to immobility) and changes in *blood constituents* (increased levels of red cells/platelets post-surgery and increased amounts of thromboplastic agents as a result of her breast carcinoma). In addition, the blood flow changes will almost certainly have caused changes in the *vessel wall* with approximation of platelets in particular to the endothelial layer. Thus, the components of Virchow's triad are present, predisposing this woman to venous thrombosis.

The presence of DVT is the most important risk factor for the development of pulmonary thromboembolism. The thrombus detaches from the lower limb veins and is carried as an embolus through the femoropopliteal system via the pelvic veins to the inferior vena cava, eventually reaching the right side of the heart before impacting on the main pulmonary artery just as it branches into the right and left sides. Here it resembles a saddle and is thus referred to as a 'saddle embolus'. Where more than 50% of the pulmonary circulation is compromised acutely, there is reflex vasoconstriction with complete cessation of venous return and cardiac arrest. Unless the thromboembolus can be moved quickly, then sudden death is almost inevitable.

5. The important findings at postmortem examination will include evidence of deep venous thrombosis with major pulmonary thromboembolism, recent repair of her right hip fracture, and the presence of a breast carcinoma and a search for other sites of metastases including lymph nodes, lungs, brain and other bones. Despite the history of a fall, this death should be considered as due to natural causes because the underlying condition was malignant disease.

CASE STUDY 7.2
ABDOMINAL AND CHEST PAINS

A 65-year-old man presented to his general practitioner complaining of abdominal pain which radiated to the back and down to his legs. He was moderately obese and had been a cigarette smoker of 20–25 cigarettes per day for nearly 40 years. On examination, his pulse was 80 beats per minutes (regular) and his blood pressure was 170/110 mmHg. Palpation of his abdomen revealed a pulsatile mass in the lower abdomen.

On further questioning, the man described pains in his chest which came on with exercise and were relieved by placing a form of medicine under his tongue.

The GP referred this man to hospital for consideration of treatment for both his chest pain and abdominal mass.

1. What is the likely cause of the pulsatile mass in this man's abdomen and what is the condition of chest pain called?
2. What is the underlying condition which links his chest pain and his pulsatile abdominal mass?
3. What factors in this man's history may be of importance in the development of the underlying condition causing both the chest pain and abdominal mass?

Suggested responses

1. The pulsatile abdominal mass represents an atheromatous abdominal aortic aneurysm which has probably leaked a little to produce abdominal pain and pains in his legs. The chest pain is part of the syndrome of ischaemic heart disease and exertional pain relieved by vasodilators such as glyceryl trinitrate, known as *angina pectoris*.

2. The condition which links these two presenting symptoms is atheroma. In the aorta the accumulation of lipid material which begins in the intima has spread through the media to reach the adventitia, having damaged the external elastic lamina. This causes the wall of the aorta to bulge outwards either diffusely over a large segment (fusiform

aneurysm) or focally over a small segment (saccular aneurysm). The presence of atheromatous material in the serosa/adventitia induces an inflammatory reaction which may precipitate rupture. Leakage of aneurysms may cause abdominal pain or pain in the back or lower limbs. If detected early (i.e. at a size of 3–5 cm), surgical treatment may be curative but larger lesions are at great risk of massive catastrophic rupture which has a high mortality rate. Angina develops when there is gradual occlusion of coronary arteries by atheroma so that when the myocardium requires more oxygen the feeding vessels are unable to cope with the demand.

3. In this case, a number of factors are present which may contribute to the development of atheroma, including his age, male gender, his smoking, being overweight and having high blood pressure. There is no history in this man of a familial tendency, of hyperlipidaemia or of diabetes, which may be of relevance especially in a younger age group, but should be considered clinically in the management of this man.

CASE STUDY 7.3
CARDIAC MURMUR

A 40-year-old woman presented to her GP complaining of tiredness and general malaise for a number of months. She also described night sweats and reported a loss of weight over the last few months. On examination, her GP noticed pale mucosae and splinter haemorrhages in the nail beds. On auscultation of the heart, he noted a diastolic murmur at the apex.

She was referred to hospital where a cardiologist elicited more history. She had been told that she had St Vitus' dance at the age of 12 but had apparently been well since that time and had never otherwise consulted a doctor. She was not aware of any heart problems but, on direct questioning, admitted to having palpitations. She was also noted to have poor oral hygiene and on questioning, reported that she had had extraction of six carious teeth several months ago.

Further investigations revealed the presence of splenomegaly. Echocardiography showed vegetations on the mitral valve. Before the results of the investigations were available, the patient was commenced on intravenous antibiotics.

1. What is the likely cause of this woman's symptoms and signs?
2. What are the possible causes of her palpitations?
3. What, if any, is the relevance of her poor oral hygiene and history of dental extraction?

4. Which microorganism is most likely to have caused the problems in this woman's case and how might the problems have been prevented?

Suggested responses

1. The symptoms and initial signs are strongly suggestive of infective endocarditis. The finding of a cardiac murmur should prompt questioning relevant to the cardiovascular system which may reflect underlying cardiac valvular disease or the presence of vegetations on the valves. The description of fever should prompt a search for predisposing events to bacteraemia. Is there any suggestion that she is an intravenous drug abuser or that she has shared hypodermic needles (this question requires considerable tact and discretion)? Patients with any long-standing chronic disease may become anaemic and thus have pale mucosae. The development of immune complexes is common in infective endocarditis. The presence of a persistent infection will lead to fever, particularly at night, and chronic illness tends to cause weight loss through suppression of appetite and impaired metabolism. The underlying cause of her problems is likely to have been previous rheumatic fever.

2. Many people have palpitations which are of no significance or which may be related to diet, e.g. caffeine ingestion. However, in the context of a patient with a cardiac murmur and suspected infective endocarditis, the possibility of atrial fibrillation needs to be considered. There is an increased risk of thromboembolism in this arrhythmia. Other causes, apart from chronic rheumatic valvular heart disease especially mitral stenosis, are ischaemic heart disease, hypertension, constrictive pericarditis and thyrotoxicosis.

3. The presence of poor oral hygiene suggests that increased numbers of bacteria are likely to be present in the mouth and when oral procedures, especially dental extractions, are performed, the likelihood of significant bacteraemia is enhanced. In this circumstance, it is important that dental practitioners be aware of any preceding cardiac condition that may cause small platelet–fibrin thrombi to form on valves, which may then be colonized by microorganisms if bacteraemia is induced by dental procedures. This allows the dentist to arrange for prophylactic antibiotics to be given (see Ch. 5). However, not all cases of bacteraemia are related to dental practice, and the possibility of other procedures, especially in the lower gastrointestinal and genitourinary tracts, should be considered as possible causes.

4. In a patient with probable chronic rheumatic valvular heart disease and a history of bacteraemia related to a dental procedure, the most likely organism is *Streptococcus*

viridans. The diagnosis of infective endocarditis in general requires a combination of clinical, echocardiographic and microbiological features. The problems might have been prevented if the patient had made her dental practitioner aware of her previous history. The dental practitioner should have asked a new patient specific questions relating to cardiac disease. In this case, the patient may not have been in a position to supply relevant information but from a medico-legal point of view, it is important that the dentist be seen to have sought this information. If the appropriate history suggestive of previous cardiac problems had been elicited, the patient could have been referred for cardiological assessment and, before any procedure likely to cause bacteraemia was undertaken, could have been prescribed prophylactic antibiotics.

CASE STUDY 7.4
SHORTNESS OF BREATH

A 58-year-old Polish gentleman developed severe shortness of breath while walking home from the pub with his wife. He was brought by ambulance to the A&E Department where he was noted to be extremely breathless with an increased respiratory rate. On examination, his pulse was 140 beats per minute and irregularly irregular.

After assessment in the A&E Department, he was given diuretics and digoxin. His clinical condition improved and he was able to give a history of having had rheumatic fever as a child in Poland before coming to Britain.

An echocardiogram revealed dilatation of the left atrium with narrowing of the mitral valve and a moderate degree of left ventricular hypertrophy. He was put on the waiting list for mitral valve replacement which was performed 3 months later.

He recovered well postoperatively and went home on the 10th postoperative day. He was well for the subsequent 6 months but developed urinary tract problems with repeated episodes of infection and occasional haematuria.

1. What initial investigations should be performed in this man's case?
2. What is the most likely diagnosis in this man's case?
3. What are the likely appearances of the valve at the time of replacement surgery?
4. Before undertaking cystoscopy, what precautions should be taken in this man's case and why are these precautions necessary?

Suggested responses

1. On initial presentation, this man had features of cardiac failure associated with atrial fibrillation. This would raise the possibility of recent myocardial infarction and, although there is no history of chest pain, these may be 'silent' and biochemical estimation of cardiac enzymes should be performed. Atrial fibrillation detected clinically should be confirmed by electrocardiography (ECG). The causes of AF include ischaemic heart disease, hypertensive heart disease, thyrotoxicosis and valvular heart disease. A chest X-ray (CXR) should be performed to look at heart size, to confirm the presence of pulmonary oedema and to exclude other pulmonary pathology such as pneumonia or pulmonary embolism/infarction.

2. Given the history of rheumatic fever as a child and the echocardiographic findings suggestive of mitral regurgitation (incompetence), the most likely diagnosis is chronic rheumatic valvular heart disease. There are no features in this case to raise the possibility of infective endocarditis, such as fever or embolic phenomena.

3. The valve will show evidence of thickening of valve cusps with fibrosis and calcification and if the chordae tendineae are also submitted, they will also show shortening, thickening and possibly calcification. There should be no evidence of endocarditis. Histologically, there are usually non-specific features only of fibrosis and calcification but, rarely, even 30–40 years later, Aschoff nodules may be seen in which there is central fibrinoid necrosis of collagen with surrounding macrophages.

4. This patient requires prophylactic antibiotic cover for cystoscopy (and other procedures which may cause bacteraemia such as gastrointestinal endoscopies and dental procedures). He is at increased risk of developing endocarditis because of his long-standing rheumatic valvular heart disease which may affect the aortic and tricuspid valves and left atrial endocardium in addition to the known mitral disease. He now also has a prosthetic heart valve which is another potential site for endocarditis to form in the setting of bacteraemia.

8 Diseases of the blood

The bone marrow within the long bones of the body, the vertebrae and sternum is the source of precursor cells for the three main lineages of blood cells: red cells (erythrocytes), white cells (leukocytes/lymphocytes) and platelets. They are all derived from a pluripotential stem cell which is capable of dividing into precursor cells of the above lineages which mature in the marrow before being discharged into the bloodstream where they have their effects. Once released into the peripheral blood, these cells have a variable life span which determines the rate of production within the marrow. The stem cells are responsive to a number of factors including colony-stimulating factors (CSFs), interleukins and growth factors such as erythropoietin which direct the maturation of the stem cell into erythroid, megakaryocytic or myeloid lines. Diseases of blood cells may be caused by primary disorders within the marrow affecting all or individual cell lineages or by disorders outside the marrow affecting mature cells.

ANAEMIA

Anaemia is the commonest haematological disorder affecting the general population. Anaemia is defined as a reduction in the level of circulating haemoglobin which in normal adult males is between 14–16 g/100 ml and in females is between 12–14 g/100 ml. Haemoglobin is a complex substance composed normally of two α and two β globin chains to which are bound haem which carries and releases oxygen in the bloodstream. An important component of haem is iron, deficiency of which for various reasons (see below) is the commonest cause of anaemia. Many patients with anaemia are asymptomatic

and the condition is diagnosed only on routine blood tests. However, symptoms of anaemia include increased heart rate (tachycardia) as the heart seeks to compensate for the lack of oxygen-carrying power, breathlessness (dyspnoea), fainting, tiredness, pallor of skin and mucous membranes including oral mucosa, and smoothness and atrophy of the tongue. Anaemia should always be considered to be a symptom of an underlying disease rather than a disease entity in its own right and a cause should always be found before treatment is instituted. Anaemia can arise from a number of causes including a lack of dietary factors (haematinics) such as iron, vitamin B_{12} and folic acid, diminished production by the bone marrow, and increased destruction of red cells in the peripheral blood.

Anaemia due to deficiency of haematinics

Iron deficiency

Iron is absorbed from the upper small intestine in the ferrous form in small quantities and the normal requirement in adults is 1–2 mg per day. Iron is present in meat and animal products and in some leaf vegetables such as cabbage, spinach and broccoli, but may be deficient in some vegetarian diets. Malabsorption in conditions such as coeliac disease and Crohn's disease may present as iron-deficiency anaemia and there are increased requirements for iron during pregnancy, lactation and growth spurts in childhood. Most western diets can cope with these conditions except in cases of severe malnutrition. The commonest causes of iron-deficiency anaemia are excessive blood loss over a prolonged period. In women of reproductive age this is usually due to menorrhagia, blood loss associated with menstruation. In older men this is most commonly due to colonic neoplasia, especially caecal and ascending colon carcinoma. In younger patients of either sex, blood loss may be due to bleeding from peptic ulcer disease, either duodenal or gastric, and in older patients the possibility of gastric carcinoma must be considered. In the peripheral blood in iron-deficiency anaemia the red cells are smaller than normal (microcytic) and are paler than usual owing to a lack of haemoglobin (hypochromic).

Vitamin B$_{12}$ and folic acid deficiency

Both vitamin B$_{12}$ and folic acid are involved in DNA synthesis generally and in particular are required for maturation of red cell precursors (erythroblasts) in the bone marrow. Lack of either substance leads to a failure of maturation causing the persistence of large cells (megaloblasts) in the marrow and the release of abnormally large red cells in the peripheral blood (macrocytes). Vitamin B$_{12}$ is present in red meats and may be completely absent from vegetarian and vegan diets. It is absorbed in the distal small intestine having been bound to intrinsic factor (IF) which is produced by gastric parietal cells. Intrinsic factor may be absent in patients with pernicious anaemia, which is an autoimmune condition associated with antibodies directed against parietal cells, IF itself or the vitamin B$_{12}$–IF complex. Also, patients with Crohn's disease with predominant terminal ileal involvement, or those who have had previous gastrectomy or right hemicolectomy may develop features of megaloblastic anaemia due to lack of vitamin B$_{12}$. Folic acid is present in leaf vegetables but has a short storage capacity in the human body. Where there is increased demand for DNA synthesis such as in pregnancy, these stores can be exhausted and many pregnant women are given prophylactic folic acid supplements. The diagnosis is made on the characteristic blood film and bone marrow findings and on assays of the blood for both factors. It is important to identify which of the two substances is deficient as the blood manifestations of vitamin B$_{12}$ deficiency may be improved by administration of folic acid but the potentially serious complication of subacute combined degeneration of the spinal cord may progress without vitamin B$_{12}$ replacement.

Anaemia due to failure of production

Failure of red cell production by the bone marrow may occur as part of a generalized failure of bone marrow such as aplastic anaemia or as a single lack of red cells such as pure red cell aplasia. Aplastic anaemia, in addition to anaemia, will also show a reduction in white cells and platelets and is associated with congenital conditions such as Fanconi's syndrome, exposure to radiation, e.g. after the atomic bombs in Hiroshima and Nagasaki, the use of chemotherapeutic agents in the treatment of cancers, some drugs including gold (used for rheumatoid arthritis) and the antibiotic chloramphenicol, environmental toxins such as benzene, and viral infections such as the papovaviruses or human immunodeficiency virus (HIV).

Anaemia due to dyserythropoiesis

Patients with chronic disorders such as non-organ specific autoimmune diseases (including rheumatoid arthritis and systemic lupus erythematosus), infectious diseases (including tuberculosis, malaria and schistosomiasis), and neoplasms (including Hodgkin's disease and some carcinomas) may develop a normochromic or occasionally hypochromic anaemia. This is associated with a lack of normal response to erythropoietin, a failure to release iron from storage macrophages and a reduced life span of circulating red cells.

Myelodysplastic syndromes are diseases in which there are abnormal clones of marrow stem cells. This leads to the production of abnormal defective cells which have a reduced life span leading to increased requirements for transfusion. Such anaemias are refractory to administration of haematinics. In about 40% of cases, myelodysplastic syndromes lead to leukaemia.

Marrow infiltration by conditions such as disseminated carcinomatosis, disseminated lymphoma and myelofibrosis causes anaemia characterized by the presence of circulating precursor red cells (erythroblasts) and primitive white cells; this is referred to as leukoerythroblastic anaemia. A similar picture may develop after severe infections, massive haemorrhage and severe haemolysis.

Anaemia due to destruction of red cells

Red blood cells may be damaged and lost prematurely from the circulation in a number of conditions.

Abnormal cell membrane

Hereditary spherocytosis is the commonest membrane disorder causing haemolysis, and patients with this condition become anaemic, jaundiced (owing to conversion of haem to bilirubin) and develop an enlarged spleen (splenomegaly) because of increased macrophage activity. Marrow spaces are expanded and treatment is by splenectomy to remove the site of lysis.

Enzyme defects

These include defects such as glucose-6-phosphate dehydrogenase (G6PD) deficiency or pyruvate kinase deficiency. G6PD deficiency is an X-linked condition where haemolytic crises are precipitated by infection or exposure to some drugs, e.g. quinine or aspirin, predisposing red cells to damage from oxidative stress.

Abnormality outside the red cell

Red cell damage can be antibody mediated, including warm antibodies in lymphomas/leukaemias, SLE, viral infections or induced by drugs, e.g. α-methyldopa; cold antibodies in some lymphomas, *Mycoplasma* pneumonia or infectious mononucleosis; or isoantibodies due to Rhesus haemolytic disease of the newborn or transfusion reactions. In up to 50% of cases no cause can be found – the so-called idiopathic form. Mechanical trauma can also damage red cells in the circulation and this can be related to prosthetic heart valves, microangiopathy in conditions such as disseminated intravascular coagulation and hypersplenism when the spleen is enlarged and overactive, e.g. in portal hypertension due to hepatic cirrhosis.

Abnormal haemoglobin form (haemoglobinopathy)

Normal adult haemoglobin (HbA) consists of four chains, two α-chains and two β-chains, which are bound together. α-Chains are coded for by two genes on chromosome 16, while β-chains are coded for by two genes on chromosome 11.

Thalassaemia. This is a disorder where there is a reduction or absence of either α-chains (α-thalassaemia) or β-chains (β-thalassaemia). Red cells are smaller and paler than normal (hypochromic and microcytic) with a relative excess of the unaffected chains. The severity of disease depends on the number of abnormal genes present. α-thalassaemia is a disease of Asian and African populations. If all four genes are affected in the embryo then the fetus may not survive (hydrops fetalis). If three genes are involved, an abnormal HbH results where patients have anaemia and an enlarged spleen. If two genes are involved, the patient has the α-thalassaemia trait,

whereas if only one gene is abnormal, the patient has the carrier state; these last two groups are asymptomatic.

β-Thalassaemia. This is a disease of the Mediterranean region along with some parts of Southeast Asia and Africa. The excess β-chains form complexes of abnormal haemoglobin which lead to cell damage during bone marrow maturation, with an increase in fetal type haemoglobin. The severity of disease depends on the number of involved genes with the more severe form (thalassaemia major) requiring frequent blood transfusions and the milder form (thalassaemia minor) being relatively symptom-free. The constant haemolysis leads to increased marrow production by the bones at unusual sites such as the skull, causing deformities, and by extramedullary haemopoiesis, which causes hepatosplenomegaly. Multiple transfusions lead to iron deposition in tissues, particularly liver, pancreas and heart, and these patients are at increased risk of blood-borne viral infections such as hepatitis B and C and HIV.

Sickle cell disease. The other major haemoglobinopathy is sickle cell disease which is caused by a point mutation in the gene coding for the β-globin chain resulting in an abnormal form of haemoglobin, HbS. This form polymerizes at low oxygen saturations producing abnormal rigidity and deformity, giving a sickle shape. The cells are fragile, which predisposes to haemolysis, and clump together in small vessels causing vascular occlusions. Patients with the sickle cell trait are heterozygous for the gene abnormality and have about 30% of their haemoglobin in the form of HbS. Patients with sickle cell disease are homozygotes and have over 80% of their haemoglobin in the form of HbS. They develop sequestration crises where red cells clump and pool in the spleen, causing potentially fatal falls in haemoglobin. They have infarctive crises due to vascular occlusions in sites such as bones, especially the head of femur, spleen and skin. They may have aplastic crises caused by overwhelming infections as a result of a lack of splenic function from repeated infarcts. Other organs may also be involved including the brain (cerebral infarcts), eyes (blindness from small vessel occlusion), gall bladder (stone formation from haemolysis), liver (excess iron deposition from multiple transfusions), kidneys (papillary necrosis), bones (salmonella osteomyelitis) and lungs (pulmonary infarcts and acute chest syndrome). Dentists should in particular be aware of the differences in clinical significance of sickle cell disease (rather than the trait), the potential risks from general anaesthetic in sickle cell disease, and the possible presentation with dental and bone pain from infarcts.

INCREASED MASS OF RED CELLS (POLYCYTHAEMIA)

This is characterized by an absolute increase in the number of circulating red cells. It is most commonly of secondary type where an underlying cause is apparent. This is usually associated with prolonged hypoxia, related to cyanotic congenital heart disease especially in children, and chronic pulmonary conditions in adults. It may also be seen in people who live at high altitudes such as the Andes and Himalayas and less commonly is due to abnormal erythropoietin production in renal disease and cerebellar haemangioblastomas. Primary polycythaemia occurs as part of the myeloproliferative syndromes in a condition called polycythaemia rubra vera (PRV; see below). The danger of polycythaemia is the risk of cerebral infarction when hyperviscosity causes sluggishness or obstruction in cerebral vessels.

SUMMARY BOX
ANAEMIA

- Anaemia is the commonest haematological disorder affecting the general population; it should be considered a symptom of disease.
- It is caused by a lack of various factors (iron, vitamin B_{12} and folic acid), by diminished production, and increased peripheral destruction of red cells.
- Iron deficiency is often due to blood loss from the gastrointestinal and female genital tracts and causes hypochromic microcytic anaemia.
- Vitamin B_{12} and folic acid deficiency are the main causes of macrocytic (megaloblastic) anaemia; associated with pregnancy and poor diet (folic acid) and autoimmune pernicious anaemia (vitamin B_{12}).
- Excessive destruction of red cells may be due to an abnormality of red cell membranes, enzyme deficiencies, antibody-mediated damage or abnormal forms of haemoglobin such as in thalassaemia and sickle cell disease.
- Polycythaemia is an increase in red cells due to bone marrow disease (primary) or secondary to prolonged hypoxia.

PLATELET AND BLEEDING DISORDERS

Normal haemostasis

Normal coagulation requires the interaction of platelets, clotting factors and vessel walls and thus consideration of platelet disorders would not be complete without an understanding of the normal mechanisms of haemostasis. Platelets are released from the bone marrow by extrusion of small particles from megakaryocytes. They are non-nucleated and have a short life span. Their effect is mediated by factors on their cell surfaces and by the contents of the α-granules and dense bodies. When a vessel is damaged, the exposure of subendothelial connective tissues including collagen and the effect of platelet-activating factor lead to the aggregation of platelets at the site with the formation of a primary haemostatic plug. These platelets adhere to the underlying tissues through the action of von Willebrand's factor and become mobile through contraction of actin and myosin filaments. They then release factors from within their cytoplasm including fibrinogen, fibronectin and platelet-derived growth factor (PDGF) from α-granules, and histamine, adrenaline, serotonin (5-HT) and adenosine diphosphate (ADP) from dense bodies. Platelets express platelet factor 3 on their surface, which serves as a focus for the formation of factor X in the intrinsic pathway of the coagulation cascade. The overall effect is to cause vasoconstriction at the site of damage and to convert fibrinogen to fibrin, which merges with platelets to form the secondary haemostatic plug. At the same time as platelets are attracted to a site of vessel damage and initiate haemostasis, naturally occurring antithrombotic factors come into play, including those from endothelium including tissue plasminogen activator (TPA), prostaglandin I_2, thrombomodulin and heparin-like substances. Thus, in normal circumstances, the balance between coagulation and antithrombosis is maintained in equilibrium.

Where vascular damage is extensive, the full extent of coagulation comes into effect by activation of the intrinsic system (from Hageman factor XII) or the extrinsic system by activation of tissue factors III and VII. The cascade mechanism proceeds to the conversion of prothrombin (factor II) to thrombin by the action of thromboplastin (factor X), and in turn thrombin converts fibrinogen (factor I) to fibrin monomer which is then converted to fibrin polymer by fibrin-stabilizing factor (factor XIII). Vitamin K (phytomenadione) and calcium ions are important cofactors in many of the steps in coagulation. The fibrinolytic pathway is activated at the same time as the coagulation cascade mechanism. Plasminogen is converted to plasmin through the effects of TPA and the fibrin degradation products produced also inhibit the polymerization of fibrin through a feedback loop. Poorly formed fibrin is then more susceptible to further fibrinolysis.

Bleeding disorders can then arise from three main causes:

- platelet abnormalities
- coagulation factor deficiencies
- inherent tissue abnormalities.

Platelet abnormalities

Patients with reduced numbers of platelets (thrombocytopenia) have a bleeding tendency and develop petechial haemorrhages and bruising in the skin, bleeding into mucosal surfaces such as gums, and severe bleeding into tissues after trauma including dental extraction (Fig. 8.1).

Thrombocytopenia may be caused by defective production due to marrow suppression, e.g. after chemotherapy, megaloblastic anaemia, or marrow infiltration by carcinoma or lymphoma.

Idiopathic thrombocytopenic purpura (ITP) is caused by premature destruction of platelets due to the presence of antiplatelet antibodies. The disease may follow viral infections especially in childhood when it often resolves spontaneously or after a short course of corticosteroids. In adults it usually follows a more prolonged course and may require treatment with more powerful immunosuppressive agents or splenectomy, which removes the main site of platelet destruction.

Increased platelet consumption occurs when there is excessive thrombosis in conditions such as disseminated intravascular coagulation (DIC), thrombotic thrombocytopenic purpura and haemolytic uraemic syndrome. This leads to increased deposition of platelets in vessels and, in the case of DIC, also to increased loss of clotting factors. DIC results from inappropriate inactivation of the coagulation system in response to overwhelming trauma, infections, burns, blood loss and obstetric catastrophes such as severe haemorrhage and amniotic fluid embolism. Fibrin–platelet thrombi are deposited in small vessels in many organs and tissues causing ischaemia and dysfunction, particularly affecting the kidneys, brain, heart and lungs.

Platelet dysfunction may occur in a number of conditions including chronic renal and hepatic diseases, myeloma and exposure to some drugs such as aspirin and other non-steroidal anti-inflammatory drugs (NSAIDs). Increased platelet numbers known as thrombocythaemia (when due to a neoplastic process in the bone marrow) or thrombocytosis (when it occurs as a reactive process) paradoxically may lead to bleeding tendencies as these platelets are often abnormal and dysfunctional.

Coagulation factor deficiencies

Most of these conditions are inherited and affected patients often have a strong family history. They may describe abnormal prolonged bleeding from a tooth socket following extraction. Haemophilia A is an X-linked inherited disorder where circulating levels of factor VIII, normally produced by the liver, are reduced. This leads to repeated episodes of bleeding into joints and muscles and extensive haemorrhage after superficial injuries, including dental procedures. Treatment is by transfusion of factor VIII and where dental treatment is planned, prophylactic transfusions can be given. Christmas disease is a similar condition where factor IX is deficient. Von Willebrand's factor is required for the attachment of platelets to underlying connective tissues and deficiency is inherited as an autosomal dominant condition. The conditions can be diagnosed by assessment of bleeding time (the time taken for a skin incision to stop bleeding) and clotting times, which are tests of clotting in the laboratory including activated partial thromboplastin time (APTT) and prothrombin time (PT). The commonest cause of abnormalities of clotting times and function is iatrogenic – the use of anticoagulants such as heparin and warfarin in the prophylaxis or treatment of thrombosis.

Inherent tissue abnormalities

These affect mainly vessel walls. This can occur as a result of immune-mediated inflammation, e.g. Henoch–Schönlein syndrome or infection.

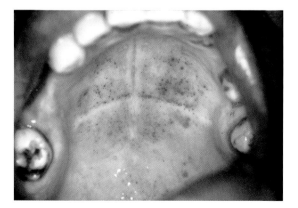

Fig. 8.1 Petechial haemorrhages in the oral mucosa in a patient with idiopathic thrombocytopenic purpura.

WHITE CELL DISORDERS

White blood cells are produced in the bone marrow from myeloid precursors, from which the neutrophil, eosinophil and basophil polymorphonuclear leukocytes are derived, and from lymphoid precursors, from which lymphocytes which are further modified outside the bone marrow into T (from thymus) and B (from bursa of Fabricius, the organ in chickens from which much of this knowledge derives) lymphocytes are produced. White blood cells are responsible for much of the body's response to injury and have a particular role in inflammation, infection and immunity.

An increased number of circulating white cells, known as leukocytosis, may occur in a number of situations.

Reactive leukocytosis

Neutrophil polymorphs

These are the cells responsible for reacting to most common bacterial infections. A rise in the normal neutrophil level in the blood (between 2000–7000 cells/µl, approximately 40–70% of total white cell numbers) to levels in excess of 12 000–15 000 cells/µl indicates that the body is responding to bacterial infection or, in the absence of a recognizable source of infection, to tissue necrosis, e.g. after myocardial infarction.

Eosinophil polymorphs

These cells contribute only a small number to the overall circulating pool of leukocytes (between 100–700 cells/µl, less than 1% of the total) but these numbers can be greatly increased in response to parasitic infestation, hypersensitivity reactions in conditions such as extrinsic allergic asthma or exposure to some drugs, some forms of neoplasia, especially haematological/lymphoid conditions such as chronic granulocytic leukaemia (CGL) and Hodgkin's disease (HD), and other hypereosinophilia syndromes.

Lymphocytosis

Increased numbers of lymphocytes in the peripheral blood from the normal levels of 1500–4000 cells/µl (approximately 30–40% of the total) occur in response to viral infections such as infectious mononucleosis, and less commonly in typhoid and brucellosis.

Monocytosis

These cells are present in the peripheral blood in small numbers (200–1000 cells/µl, less than 1% of the total) but may be increased in response to conditions such as infective endocarditis and some protozoal infections including malaria and trypanosomiasis.

Leukopenia

This is the term for reduced numbers of circulating white cells and it is particularly important when there are reduced numbers of neutrophils (neutropenia). These patients are at increased risk of bacterial and fungal infections and may present with infections in and around the oral cavity, including periodontitis, tonsillitis and pharyngitis. Neutropenia is associated with generalized abnormalities of marrow function, marrow hypoplasia and abnormal autoimmune-associated destruction of white cells. There may also be qualitative defects in circulating cells, especially in association with systemic disorders such as diabetes mellitus, corticosteroid therapy, renal failure and alcoholism. The most significant cause of neutropenia is neoplastic disease of bone marrow, particularly leukaemias.

Neoplastic diseases of white cells

Leukaemia is a neoplastic proliferation of marrow cells which may form one or more cell lines. In turn, the large number of neoplastic cells formed may spill over into the peripheral blood and cause suppression of normal marrow elements. Thus, these patients present with symptoms related to lack of red cells causing anaemia, tiredness and malaise, lack of platelets leading to a bleeding tendency with petechial haemorrhages (Fig. 8.1) and lack of white cells causing an increased risk of infections, especially mouth ulcers, and fever. Leukaemias may be acute or chronic.

Acute leukaemias

In acute leukaemias, the marrow is filled with immature precursor cells (blasts). Patients typically have a rapidly progressive course with a high mortality rate without treatment. There are two main types of acute leukaemias: acute lymphoblastic leukaemia (ALL) and acute non-lymphoblastic leukaemia (ANLL), which includes myeloid, monocytic, erythroid and megakaryocytic leukaemias. These may arise de novo or may develop from pre-existing conditions such as myelodysplastic or myeloproliferative syndromes. Many of these leukaemias are associated with specific chromosomal abnormalities.

Acute lymphoblastic leukaemia. ALL is predominantly a condition affecting young children and only rarely affects adults. It presents with the symptoms described above and, when suspected, the diagnosis is made on examination of the peripheral blood, where there are increased numbers of lymphocytes and lymphoblasts, and confirmed on examination of the bone marrow, where there are increased numbers of lymphoblasts with suppression of normal marrow elements. Other organs may also be involved including the liver and spleen causing hepatosplenomegaly and there may also be infiltration of the brain and meninges and of the gonads, especially the testes. Treatment is by inducing remission through obliteration of the neoplastic cells with a combination of chemotherapy and radiotherapy, followed by maintenance therapy which may also include the use of bone marrow transplantation. Prognosis nowadays is excellent but a number of factors determine which forms of ALL respond best to different modalities.

Acute non-lymphoblastic leukaemia. ANLL is a condition most commonly seen in adults and is subcategorized into eight forms according to the French–American–British (FAB) system, from M0 to M7. The commonest types are those showing myeloblastic (M1), myelocytic (M2) and myelomonocytic (M4) differentiation. Presenting symptoms are as for ALL (Fig. 8.2) and treatment regimes are similar, although the overall prognosis is less good than for ALL.

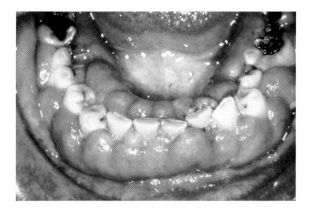

Fig. 8.2 Infiltration by acute myelomonocytic leukaemia resulting in gingival enlargement.

Chronic leukaemias

These generally present in an older age group but may occur in childhood. The two main types are chronic lymphocytic leukaemia (CLL) and chronic myeloid (granulocytic) leukaemia (CGL).

Chronic lymphocytic leukaemia. CLL is a disease of late adult life, over the age of 50 years, and is a neoplastic proliferation of small mature lymphocytes in the bone marrow, usually of B cell type although approximately 5% are of T cell type. Initially, the neoplastic lymphocytes fill up the marrow spaces without loss of normal haemopoietic elements, so that there are large numbers of peripheral blood lymphocytes and there is enlargement of lymph nodes (lymphadenopathy) and the spleen (splenomegaly). The lymph nodes show effacement of the normal architecture with features of a low-grade diffuse small cell lymphocytic lymphoma (see below). The diagnosis is made on the peripheral blood findings of marked lymphocytosis and confirmed on bone marrow aspiration or trephine biopsy. Symptoms relate to the lymph node or splenic enlargement but autoimmune haemolytic anaemia or thrombocytopenia may occur. Prognosis is related to the stage of disease, which is determined by the extent of marrow suppression and involvement of extramedullary tissues. A form of B cell leukaemia which presents with pancytopenia due to hypersplenism is characterized by small B lymphocytes with multiple cell surface projections, so-called hairy cell leukaemia.

Chronic granulocytic leukaemia. CGL is one of the myeloproliferative syndromes (see below) and is one of the first neoplastic conditions to have a consistent chromosomal abnormality. This is the Philadelphia chromosome (Ph[1]) which is a reciprocal translocation of the long arms of chromosomes 9 and 22: t(9;22)(q34;q11), which results in formation of the *bcr-abl fusion* gene which produces a protein with tyrosine kinase activity. Approximately 90% of CGL patients are Ph[1]-positive and have a reasonably good prognosis, whereas those that are Ph[1]-negative have a considerably worse survival time. CGL is a disease of adulthood (30–40 years) and presents with hepatosplenomegaly due to infiltration of liver and spleen by neoplastic cells. There is a peripheral blood leukocytosis including neutrophils and precursor cells and there is often anaemia but thrombocytopenia is relatively infrequent in the early stages. CGL, depending on its Ph[1] status, follows an indolent course before transformation ultimately into an acute leukaemia which in 75% of cases is acute myeloblastic leukaemia. The transformation is heralded by the presence of increased numbers of blasts in the marrow and in the peripheral blood, so-called blast crisis, and is often associated with rapidly developing anaemia and thrombocytopenia, as well as problems with response to infections.

Myeloproliferative syndromes

These are neoplastic proliferations of marrow stem cells which are capable of differentiating into erythroid, myeloid, megakaryocytic and fibroblastic lines. There is considerable overlap between the various manifestations which include polycythaemia rubra vera (PRV), CGL, primary thrombocythaemia and primary myelofibrosis. As the diseases progress, there is marrow replacement by the neoplastic cells which results in extramedullary haemopoiesis and hepatosplenomegaly. Most eventually transform into acute leukaemia, mainly of ANLL type.

Plasma cell tumours

These are neoplasms derived from terminally differentiated bone marrow-derived B lymphocytes. They may present as a diffuse condition, multiple myeloma; as a solitary lesion, plasmacytoma; and as an IgM-secreting tumour, Waldenström's macroglobulinaemia.

Multiple myeloma occurs in patients over the age of 50 years and can cause a number of presenting complaints. Expansion of tumour cells within the marrow leads to bone destruction which causes bone pain, pathological fractures and hypercalcaemia. The plasma cells secrete a monoclonal antibody usually of IgG type, which may be detected as a monoclonal band on electrophoresis of either serum or urine. In the urine, this is known as Bence

Jones protein. The erythrocyte sedimentation rate (ESR) is raised as a result of the increased protein (globulin) levels in the blood. The presence of increased immunoglobulins may lead to relative impairment of immune activity (immune paresis) and this may predispose to infection. The deposition of immunoglobulin light chains in the form of casts in renal tubules may precipitate renal failure. Light chains may aggregate to form amyloid of amyloid light chain (AL) type, causing the deposition of insoluble protein in various tissues which can cause, in particular, renal failure. Diagnosis is made on the finding of excess plasma cells in the bone marrow on aspiration or trephine biopsy, along with confirmation of the other findings of a paraprotein in serum or urine.

Plasmacytomas are solitary lesions of localized clusters of neoplastic plasma cells which can cause bony destruction or soft tissue masses.

Waldenström's macroglobulinaemia is a monoclonal proliferation of plasmacytoid lymphoid cells secreting IgM, which causes hyperviscosity. Occasionally, patients are found to have a monoclonal band on electrophoresis but investigations fail to reveal an underlying neoplastic process, so-called 'benign monoclonal gammopathy'. Most patients eventually develop myeloma.

Histiocytoses

These are neoplasms derived from histiocytic cells, especially Langerhans' cells which are normally found

---

SUMMARY BOX
WHITE CELL DISORDERS

- White cells are responsible for much of the body's response to injury/infection.
- Increased white cell counts occur in response to bacterial infection or necrosis (neutrophils), in allergic conditions (eosinophils) and in viral conditions (lymphocytes).
- Reduced white cell counts (leukopenia) may lead to infections, especially around the oral cavity; reduced neutrophils (neutropenia) may be associated with generalized abnormalities of bone marrow, particularly leukaemias.
- Leukaemia is a neoplastic proliferation of marrow cells which may differentiate along several lines; it may be acute or chronic and the predominant cell line may be lymphoid or non-lymphoid.
- Acute leukaemias are aggressive neoplasms which affect a younger age group; treatment is by chemotherapy and radiotherapy.
- Chronic leukaemias are more usual in an older age group and CGL is associated with the Philadelphia chromosome.

ASPECTS OF HAEMATOLOGICAL DISEASE OF PARTICULAR RELEVANCE TO DENTISTRY

- Oral manifestations of anaemia include a sore smooth tongue, angular cheilitis and recurrent oral ulceration.
- Excessive bleeding may occur following surgical dental procedures in patients with coagulation, bleeding and platelet disorders.
- Neutropenia may lead to candidal infection and recurrent oral ulceration.
- Leukaemia may present with gingival bleeding and enlargement.

in the skin and lymph nodes, where they function as antigen-presenting cells. They occur particularly in children but may also occur in adults. There are three main patterns of disease, with considerable overlap: eosinophilic granuloma (unifocal disease); Hand–Schüller–Christian disease (multifocal disease) and Letterer–Siwe disease (acute disseminated disease).

DISEASES OF LYMPH NODES

Lymph nodes are aggregates of lymphoid tissue situated at points of drainage of lymphatic vessels. They are ovoid or reniform structures ranging in size from millimetres to centimetres in diameter and are found particularly in the head and neck region, axilla, groins, hila of the lungs, mesentery of the gastrointestinal tract and in the para-aortic regions. Lymphatics drain into lymph nodes through subcapsular sinuses on the convex surface of lymph nodes (afferent lymphatics) and pass through to exit at the hilum of the lymph node (efferent lymphatics). Lymph nodes are arranged in series with each smaller node linking to the next larger node in its chain, eventually draining into the left subclavian vein via the thoracic duct. Within the node there is an internal structure with cortex containing lymphoid follicles with germinal centres of predominantly B lymphocyte lineage. In the germinal centres there are macrophage-derived cells called follicular dendritic cells which act as antigen-presenting cells. In the interfollicular paracortical zones the cells are of predominantly T cell lineage, along with sinuses containing interdigitating reticulum cells, also of macrophage origin, and high endothelial venules which permit lymphocyte trafficking.

Lymphadenopathy

Lymph node enlargement may occur for a number of reasons. There may be reactive changes when the pattern reflects the initiating stimulus and the main mode of response.

- *Follicular hyperplasia*, where the B-cell-dependent follicles and germinal centres become enlarged, may be due to non-specific forms of chronic inflammation and in response to generalized diseases such as rheumatoid disease and the early stages of HIV infection.
- *Paracortical hyperplasia*, indicating activation of the T-cell-dependent zones, may be a feature of drug hypersensitivity, e.g. due to phenytoin therapy in epilepsy, or viral infections such as infectious mononucleosis caused by the Epstein–Barr virus.
- *Sinus hyperplasia*, where there is an increase in macrophages in the medullary sinuses, may be seen in nodes draining sites of chronic inflammation, tumours, e.g. breast carcinoma, and exogenous material such as anthracotic pigment in lymph nodes at the lung hilum. A similar lesion is seen in lymph nodes draining chronic inflammatory skin conditions where macrophages containing melanin and lipid may be seen, so-called dermatopathic lymphadenopathy.
- *Acute lymphadenitis* is characterized by enlarged tender nodes in which there is follicular hyperplasia and neutrophil polymorph infiltration and is usually due to bacterial infections.
- *Granulomatous lymphadenitis* may be localized or generalized. Causes include tuberculosis where there is usually typical caseous necrosis, sarcoidosis where the granulomas are well-formed and lack surrounding lymphocytes, cat scratch disease which is caused by a microorganism transmitted by cats and contains granulomas with central necrosis including polymorphs, Crohn's disease where the granulomas are similar to those in sarcoidosis, and toxoplasmosis where there are small clusters of macrophages at the edge of germinal centres.

Neoplastic diseases

The commonest form of neoplasia involving lymph nodes is metastatic disease, particularly of carcinomas but also of melanoma and sarcomas. Biopsy of the nodes may be necessary for diagnosis and the type of tumour may be confirmed by the use of immunohistochemistry, which shows characteristic expression of markers specific for different cell types. This may be very important in deciding on the need for further surgery, radiotherapy or chemotherapy.

Malignant lymphomas

These are primary lymphoid neoplasms derived from tissue-based and nodal lymphocytes. There are two main categories of lymphoma: Hodgkin's disease (HD) and non-Hodgkin's lymphoma (NHL). It is important that the differentiation between these two forms of lymphoma is made as there are important considerations involved in deciding on appropriate treatment.

Hodgkin's disease. This is a neoplastic proliferation of an atypical lymphoid cell, the Reed–Sternberg cell, the exact origin of which is uncertain. Staging of the disease, which determines treatment regimes, is based on the extent of involvement. Stage I disease involves one node group only, Stage II disease involves several groups of nodes on the same side of the diaphragm, Stage III disease is present in node groups on either side of the diaphragm or involves the spleen, and Stage IV disease has disseminated involvement of one or more extranodal sites such as liver or bone marrow, with or without nodal involvement. Clinical subclassification of HD is made on the absence (A) or presence (B) of constitutional symptoms such as fever, night sweats or weight loss.

The histological diagnosis is based on the finding of the characteristic Reed–Sternberg (RS) cell in the appropriate cellular background. The classical RS cell is binucleate with prominent mirror-image eosinophilic nucleoli (Fig. 8.3). The different histological types of disease are related to the host immune response to the neoplastic cells. Lymphocyte-predominant (LP) HD accounts for

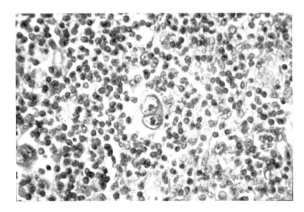

Fig. 8.3 Photomicrograph of a classical binucleate Reed–Sternberg cell in a background of lymphocytes, plasma cells and eosinophils, typical of Hodgkin's disease.

10% of the total and occurs in young males, usually in Stage I or II. Mixed cellularity (MC) HD is a disease of later life, accounting for 20% of the total, and more commonly presents in Stage III or IV. The commonest form of HD (60–70% of the total) is the nodular sclerosis (NS) type, which mainly affects young adults, especially in the mediastinum. There is a division of the involved lymph node by broad bands of fibrosis producing a nodular appearance. Two subtypes are recognized. Lymphocyte-depleted (LD) HD accounts for less than 5% of the total and is a disease of the elderly. Most present with late stage disease (Stage III or IV) and have a poor prognosis.

Prognosis in HD depends on the histological type. The best outcome is seen in LPHD and NSHD Type I while the worst is seen in LDHD and NSHD Type II. MCHD has a variable prognosis depending on the stage at presentation. Within each type, factors associated with poor prognosis are advanced stage at presentation, constitutional symptoms and an older age group. Overall, 10-year survival figures for LPHD are over 80%, for NSHD Type I 75%, for MCHD 60%, for NSHD Type II 55% and for LDHD 5%.

Non-Hodgkin's lymphoma. These are neoplasms derived from lymphoid cells which originate from either nodal or extra-nodal tissue, usually of mucosa-associated lymphoid tissue (MALT), especially in the gastrointestinal tract and bronchi but also in sites of chronic inflammation, e.g. thyroid or from skin. Lymphocytes can be of either B or T cell type and the neoplasms that originate from them reflect the stages of differentiation of the normal lymphocyte from their site of origin through their maturation in lymph nodes to their final destination. Tumour behaviour is broadly determined by the rate of proliferation of the neoplastic cells and this is to some extent reflected in the size of the cells. The larger the cell and the more hyperchromatic the nuclei the more likely the tumour is to be aggressive in clinical and biological behaviour. The classification of non-Hodgkin's lymphoma is one of the more fluid areas in diagnostic histopathology and is the subject of much debate and controversy. What is important in NHL classification is providing sufficient information to clinical oncologists to decide on the appropriate treatment regimes which will help in predicting how patients will behave clinically. Because many of the normal counterparts of lymphoid neoplasms are not easily identified, the newest classification of NHL, the revised European–American lymphoma classification (REAL), places many neoplasms into an unclassified category. In general, the previous classifications in widespread use placed tumours into low, intermediate or high grades (the American Working Formulation) or low or high grades (the European Kiel classification). This grading system suggests that high-grade tumours have high rates of cell division and rapid tumour expansion. If untreated, high-grade tumours have a poor prognosis and lead to early death. Low-grade tumours have a lower rate of cell proliferation, grow slowly and have an indolent clinical course, causing death only after many years. Intermediate-grade tumours lie somewhere between the two extremes.

B cell lymphomas. Tumours derived from B cells range from small lymphocytic lymphomas to large cell immunoblastic lymphomas. Low-grade B cell lymphomas contribute about 50% of the total of NHL, while high-grade B cell tumours are responsible for about 30% of the total. B cell lymphocytic lymphoma is the tissue counterpart of chronic lymphocytic leukaemia and is a low-grade tumour with a slow clinical course, associated with lymphadenopathy, anaemia and immune deficiency. Tumours of B cell origin may show plasmacytic differentiation and secrete immunoglobulins, especially IgM in Waldenström's macroglobulinaemia. Those derived from follicular centre cells (centrocytic or centroblastic lymphomas) often have a follicular (nodular) pattern in their early stages but may become diffuse at a later stage. Follicular lymphomas of follicle centre origin are the commonest form of NHL and tend to occur in an older age group. Diffuse centroblastic lymphoma is a high-grade tumour but responds reasonably well to aggressive chemotherapy. Immunoblastic lymphomas of B cell origin are very aggressive high-grade tumours which present early because of rapidly developing lymphadenopathy, and may arise on the basis of pre-existing low-grade lesions. Lymphoblastic lymphoma is the tissue counterpart of acute lymphoblastic leukaemia and presents with rapidly developing lymph node enlargement, especially in children. Burkitt's lymphoma is associated with Epstein–Barr virus infection and the endemic form is most commonly seen in children in Africa who present with tumours of the jaw, gut and ovaries.

T cell lymphomas. Tumours of T cell origin of low grade are responsible for about 10% of the total of NHL. They often present in the skin causing erythematous rashes (mycosis fungoides), sometimes with circulation of the characteristic convoluted 'cerebriform' neoplastic cells in the blood (Sézary's syndrome). High-grade T cell lymphomas also contribute 10% of the total and are being recognized more frequently because of the use of immunohistochemistry which allows the identification of specific T cell surface and cytoplasmic markers. One form is associated with human T-lymphotropic virus type 1 (HTLV-1) especially in Japan and the Caribbean regions.

Mucosa-associated lymphoid tissue. Tumours of MALT occur in the gut, especially in the small bowel, the tonsils, the bronchi, the salivary glands and the thyroid gland. They arise in pre-existing lymphoid tissue which may be constitutionally present or may develop in association with autoimmune disease (Graves' or Hashimoto's disease in the thyroid and Sjögren's syndrome in the salivary glands).

Treatment

This is determined by the age and clinical condition of the patient, on the histological type of the neoplasm, whether T or B cell in origin, on the grade of the tumour and on the stage (extent of spread) of disease. Low-grade tumours are difficult to cure because of their low proliferative rates and, although they have an indolent course, they will eventually cause significant morbidity and mortality in affected patients. Paradoxically, high-grade tumours are more easily induced into remission by the use of aggressive chemotherapy when this is possible in younger patients, and the mortality rates are higher in older patients and those with more widespread dissemination at the time of presentation.

SUMMARY BOX
LYMPH NODE ABNORMALITIES

- Lymph node enlargement (lymphadenopathy) may be reactive or neoplastic.
- Neoplastic lymphadenopathy may be primary or secondary; secondary carcinomas are common as are metastatic melanoma and sarcoma.
- Lymphoma is a malignant neoplasm of lymphoid tissue; the main classification is into Hodgkin's disease and non-Hodgkin's lymphoma.
- Hodgkin's disease is a neoplastic proliferation of an atypical lymphoid cell, the Reed–Sternberg cell; treatment is determined by the stage of disease reflecting the spread of tumour.
- Non-Hodgkin's lymphoma may be nodal or extra-nodal in origin and can be of B or T cell type; treatment and prognosis are determined by the grade of tumour and the histological subtype.

SPLEEN

The spleen is an organ in the left upper quadrant of the abdomen normally weighing up to 180 g. It functions as a filter for red cells reaching the end of their life span within the red pulp, which also has macrophage activity, while the white pulp (Malpighian corpuscles) is a site for antigen trapping and presentation by lymphocytes. The spleen may become enlarged (splenomegaly) which is detectable by palpation of the spleen below the left rib cage. The spleen may be increased in size from:

- infective causes – bacterial infections including infective endocarditis, viral infection especially infectious mononucleosis, protozoal infection particularly malaria and leishmaniasis (kala azar)
- vascular causes – mainly due to portal hypertension in hepatic cirrhosis
- neoplastic causes – such as Hodgkin's and non-Hodgkin's lymphoma, chronic leukaemias, extramedullary haemopoiesis in myeloproliferative syndromes and marrow replacement by tumours
- haematological causes – haemolytic anaemias, autoimmune thrombocytopenia
- immune-mediated causes – such as Felty's syndrome in rheumatoid disease
- miscellaneous causes – sarcoidosis, amyloidosis and inherited metabolic storage disorders (such as Gaucher's and Niemann–Pick diseases).

Functional hyperactivity of the spleen (hypersplenism) may or may not be associated with splenomegaly. It is a cause of morbidity because of the possibility of sequestration of red cells, white cells and platelets, leading to pancytopenia. The other major condition associated with hypersplenism is premature destruction of red cells causing haemolytic anaemia. Enlarged spleens are at increased risk of rupture in response to relatively minor trauma.

Patients with lack of splenic function (hyposplenism) are at increased risk of infection due to capsulated bacteria including *Streptococcus pneumoniae*, *Haemophilus influenzae*, *Neisseria meningitidis* and *Escherichia coli*. This may lead to septicaemia, intravascular coagulation and multi-organ failure. Characteristic abnormalities of red cells may be seen in the peripheral blood, including Howell–Jolly inclusion bodies and target cells. Hyposplenism is usually caused by surgical removal of the spleen for traumatic damage or inherent disease but may be seen in severe sickle cell disease because of multiple infarcts or in coeliac disease.

SUMMARY BOX
SPLEEN

- The spleen normally filters red cells near the end of their life span with other macrophage activity (red pulp) and antigen trapping and presentation by lymphocytes (white pulp).
- Splenomegaly is physical enlargement of the spleen, occurring in infections, portal hypertension, haematological neoplasia, Felty's syndrome, sarcoidosis, amyloidosis and inherited storage disorders.
- Hypersplenism is functional overactivity of the spleen (with or without splenomegaly) leading to a reduction in all cell types in the blood (anaemia, especially of haemolytic type, leukopenia, thrombocytopenia).
- Hyposplenism is a reduction or lack of splenic function, which causes an inability to deal with specific microorganisms, especially capsulated bacteria.

CASE STUDY 8.1
BLEEDING FROM THE GUMS

A 6-year-old boy was brought to his dentist by his mother because of recent bleeding from his gums. She also reported that he had been feeling tired and was not his usual boisterous self. The dentist noted that his gums were soft and elicited contact bleeding on gentle pressure. He also observed that the tonsils were increased in size and appeared inflamed. No intrinsic abnormality was identified in the teeth. There was no past history of note and the family otherwise were well. The dentist arranged for a blood test at the local haematology department.

This showed a haemoglobin of 6.8 g/dl, a platelet count of $26 \times 10^9/l$ and a white cell count of $14.6 \times 10^9/l$ with a differential white cell count showing 90% lymphoblasts in the peripheral blood. He was admitted to hospital where bone marrow tests including an aspirate and trephine biopsy were performed. After the results of these tests became available, he was commenced on combination chemotherapy introduced via a Hickman line into the right side of his heart.

He lost all of his hair and had several episodes of severe infection affecting his skin and lungs over the succeeding months. He received support with platelet transfusions for episodes of bleeding and intensive care admissions. He also required radiotherapy to his brain and gonads. However 6 months later he returned to school and 15 months later he was off all treatment. His hair had grown back and he was back to his old mischievous self.

1. What are the possible causes of his initial presentation to his dentist?

2. What is the most likely diagnosis from the blood count and bone marrow tests?
3. Why did he have problems with infections and bleeding?
4. What long-term problems may arise in his case?

Suggested responses

1. Bleeding from the gums has many causes. In this case bleeding is due either to a low platelet count or to infection (gingivitis). There may possibly be problems of coagulation such as factor VIII (haemophilia A) or factor IX (Christmas disease) deficiency but these are unlikely in the absence of a positive family history. Nutritional problems associated with vitamin C (ascorbic acid) deficiency may present with bleeding as also may inherited abnormalities of collagen metabolism.

2. The appearances in the peripheral blood are those of anaemia and thrombocytopenia with a raised white cell count due to lymphoblasts. This is strongly suggestive of acute lymphoblastic leukaemia (ALL) which should be confirmed on bone marrow aspirate or trephine biopsy. This is a malignant neoplasm of bone marrow stem cells in which differentiation is along the lymphoid line. It is a highly aggressive tumour which previously had a very high mortality rate, but the use of intensive regimes of chemotherapy and radiotherapy has improved the outlook considerably.

3. At the time of first presentation, the effect of the growth of malignant lymphoblasts in the marrow is to reduce the production of normal constituents such as platelets, red cells and other white cells particularly neutrophils required for defence against bacterial infections. Later on in the course of his disease, treatment with cytotoxic drugs and radiotherapy may have the same effect of reducing normal marrow-derived cells. This is to maximize the possibility of destroying the abnormal cells in the marrow and to allow the regrowth of non-neoplastic cells.

4. There is always a danger that, despite intensive chemo- and radiotherapy, the tumour may recur. This is associated with some specific genetic abnormalities which should be identified at first presentation. This may indicate a need for a different approach such as earlier bone marrow transplantation from a matched relative or perhaps an unrelated donor or possibly by an allogeneic transplant where marrow is harvested from the boy himself and treated to remove malignant cells before reinfusion. In the long term, infertility is a potential problem because of the chemotherapy and specific radiotherapy to gonads. The chemotherapy used may also damage genetic material and there is an increased risk of development of secondary malignancy especially of the lymphoid system, particularly leading to non-Hodgkin's lymphoma.

9 Respiratory disease

NORMAL DEFENCE MECHANISMS

There are several naturally occurring defence mechanisms in the respiratory tract to protect against infection, which may become altered or damaged in pathological conditions. These include:

- *Nasopharyngeal filtering systems.*
- *The mucociliary apparatus.* This may be impaired either through loss of cilia, which may be caused by cigarette smoking, inhalation of hot gases, viral diseases such as influenza or genetic defects such as Kartagener's syndrome or immotile cilia syndrome, or by changes in the composition of mucus, which may occur in dehydration, chronic bronchitis or cystic fibrosis.
- *Intra-alveolar macrophages.* Alveolar macrophage function may be impaired in cigarette smokers or in chronic alcoholics. When there is obstruction of bronchial secretions, e.g. by a tumour or a foreign body including teeth aspirated after dental extraction, there is increased risk of infection. Nosocomial infections are infections with virulent organisms acquired particularly in hospital. Patients with pulmonary oedema, most commonly due to acute left ventricular failure, are at increased risk of pulmonary infections.
- *The cough reflex.* There may be loss or suppression of the cough reflex during the use of anaesthetic agents or opiate drugs, in coma, in patients with severe chest pain, e.g. after rib fractures, or abdominal pain, e.g. after surgery, or in neurological conditions such as Guillain–Barré syndrome and motor neuron disease.

INFECTIONS

Respiratory tract infections (RTIs) may be classified as either upper RTIs, which are mainly due to viral infections and are usually of little clinical significance, and lower RTIs, which are usually due to bacterial infections and are often quite serious. Bacterial infections of the lungs include bronchopneumonia, lobar pneumonia and atypical pneumonia.

Bronchopneumonia

This is infection of the lung centred on bronchi and bronchioles with extension outwards into the adjacent lung parenchyma. It may be caused by a wide range of bacteria including microorganisms which normally reside in the respiratory tract (commensal organisms) and which in appropriate circumstances cause pathological effects. These include *Haemophilus influenzae*. It tends to occur in individuals with reduced levels of immunity (although not absolutely immunosuppressed) such as premature infants and neonates, the elderly and severely ill patients. It is also a particular problem in patients with long-standing chronic lung disease such as chronic bronchitis or emphysema, where there is progression from bronchial infection into bronchopneumonia.

Gross appearances

Grossly, the lungs show multiple areas of patchy grey-green consolidation, which tend to occur in dependent parts of the lung, the lower lobes in ambulant patients and the posterior aspects of the lungs in bed-ridden patients.

The firm areas of consolidation may become confluent but in most instances, more than one lobe is involved so that differentiation from lobar pneumonia is fairly readily accomplished (Fig. 9.1A). Occasionally, bronchopneumonia may progress to the formation of a lung abscess.

Histological appearances

Histologically, there is an exudate of polymorphonuclear leukocytes and fibrin within bronchioles and alveolar spaces, which tends to be patchy between lobes with areas of relatively normal lung parenchyma intervening

(Fig. 9.1A). Bacteria are usually difficult to identify. Bronchopneumonia may resolve completely but it may also heal by fibrosis. Occasionally pleurisy may also supervene.

Lobar pneumonia

This is infection of the lung characteristically caused by the microorganism *Streptococcus pneumoniae*, also known as the pneumococcus. It is a disease generally of young previously healthy individuals, and is more common in males than in females. It may also be associated with chronic alcoholism.

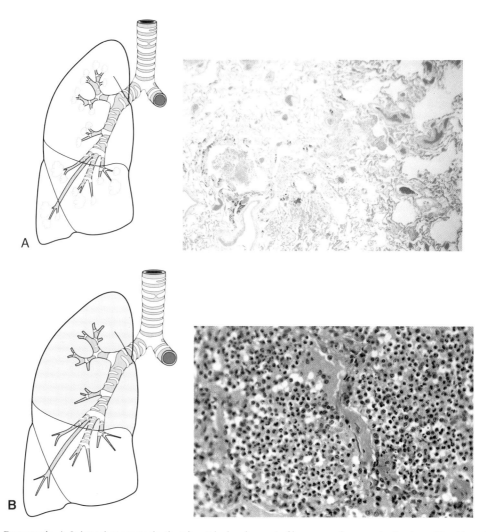

Fig. 9.1 **Pneumonia. A.** In bronchopneumonia, there is patchy involvement of lung parenchyma centred on bronchi and bronchioles, as shown in the photomicrograph. **B.** In lobar pneumonia, the whole of one lobe is involved, generally with sparing of the remainder of the lung; the photomicrograph shows filling of alveolar spaces by a dense polymorph infiltrate with admixed fibrin.

Pathology

Grossly, it affects the whole of one lobe only and typically causes confluent consolidation (Fig. 9.1B). There are four classical stages:

1. congestion – where the lung is red and boggy mainly because of congestion and oedema
2. red hepatization – where the lung is red and firm owing to the presence of abundant fibrin within alveolar spaces
3. grey hepatization – where the lung is grey and firm owing to the accumulation of large numbers of intra-alveolar polymorphs (Fig. 9.1B)
4. resolution – which is the return to complete structural and functional normality.

Complications

These may develop, including abscess formation, pleurisy, dissemination of the infection throughout the body and death. Occasionally, there may be a failure of resolution resulting in fibrosis.

Lung abscesses

These develop where there is localized suppuration and necrosis of lung tissue. They may arise in the absence of previous lung infection, such as when there is aspiration of infected material. This may occur in coma or intoxication, as a consequence of dental or pharyngeal surgery, through the movement of material from the stomach or paranasal sinuses and by the introduction of foreign bodies including teeth. Abscesses may also develop as a complication of pre-existing pneumonia, particularly lobar pneumonia (*Strep. pneumoniae*), or infection with virulent organisms such as *Staphylococcus aureus* and *Klebsiella pneumoniae*. They may also arise from septic embolism, e.g. from infective endocarditis, distal to obstructive lesions of bronchi such as tumours or foreign bodies, penetrating trauma such as stab wounds or by direct spread from liver abscesses.

Atypical pneumonia

This is pulmonary infection with varied symptoms, patchy radiological appearances and is usually due to non-bacterial causes. It may occur in a previously healthy population but more commonly in malnourished, alcoholic or immunosuppressed individuals. The commonest organisms involved include *Mycoplasma pneumoniae*,

viruses especially adenovirus, chlamydial species especially *C. psittaci*, members of the rickettsial group particularly *Coxiella burnetii*, and the bacterial agent *Legionella pneumophila*. This last mentioned organism may mimic lobar pneumonia but in most cases it exhibits the features of atypical pneumonia.

Pathology

Grossly, the lungs show patchy involvement of more than one lobe, occasionally involving a whole lobe, with areas of congestion in the absence of consolidation. Histologically, the inflammatory process affects predominantly the interstitial tissues of the lung, not the alveolar spaces as in lobar or bronchopneumonia, and the inflammatory cells are mainly lymphocytes and macrophages, rather than the polymorphs seen in the other forms. There may be intra-alveolar proteinaceous material with some hyaline membrane formation. The long-term effects are uncertain. Most patients survive but there is an undoubted mortality associated with these atypical pneumonias, probably related to the underlying immune status of the patient.

Aspiration pneumonia

This is usually associated with regurgitation of food in patients with impaired consciousness, particularly during anaesthesia, drug overdose or long-standing neuromuscular diseases such as strokes or motor neuron disease. It is a potential hazard of dental procedures using general anaesthesia. Gastric acid itself may induce a chemical pneumonitis, which may lead to adult respiratory distress syndrome. Microorganisms of mixed type may also be inhaled including anaerobes, and lung abscess is a common complication.

Tuberculosis

Primary tuberculosis (see also Ch. 3, p. 34)

In patients without immunity, the first exposure to *Mycobacterium tuberculosis* leads to the condition of primary tuberculosis. Since the usual mode of transmission of the human strain of the organism is by inhalation to the lungs, the primary focus (also known as the Ghon focus) occurs in the lung periphery in the basal segments of the upper lobes or the apical segments of the lower lobes (Fig. 9.2A). Locally, there is drainage of the organism via the lymphatics to the regional lymph nodes at the

---

SUMMARY BOX
LOWER RESPIRATORY TRACT INFECTIONS (PNEUMONIAS)

Bronchopneumonia
- Patchy inflammation.
- Centred on bronchi/bronchioles.
- Often secondary to pre-existing lung conditions.
- Common in very young or very old.

Lobar pneumonia
- All or most of a lobe involved.
- Otherwise healthy adults, males more than females.
- Caused by *Strep. pneumoniae* in 90% of cases.

Atypical pneumonia
- Interstitial inflammation.
- Lack of cellular alveolar exudate in immunosuppressed individuals especially in AIDS; common organisms include *Pneumocystis carinii*, fungi (candida and aspergillus), viruses (cytomegalovirus and measles).
- In non-suppressed individuals, organisms include *Mycoplasma pneumoniae* and other viruses (influenza and adenovirus).

lung hilum, where an identical pattern of granulomatous inflammation results. The combination of the peripheral lung lesion and the hilar lymph node involvement is the primary complex (or Ghon complex; Fig. 9.2B). The possible outcomes of primary tuberculosis include:

- healing by fibrosis often accompanied by dystrophic calcification
- erosion of blood vessels with spread of the organism

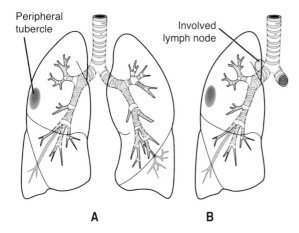

Fig. 9.2   Primary tuberculosis. A. Lungs showing typical distribution of primary lesion in peripheral aspect of lung (Ghon focus). **B.** Lung with hilar lymph node involvement (Ghon complex).

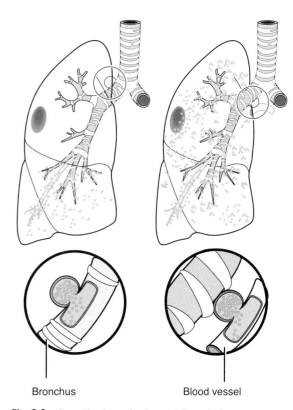

Bronchus   Blood vessel

**Fig. 9.3   Complications of primary tuberculosis.
A.** Mycobacteria spread via the bronchi to cause tuberculous bronchopneumonia. **B.** Organisms spread via the bloodstream to cause miliary involvement, here illustrated in the lung but it may also be seen in other organs, especially liver, spleen, kidneys and meninges.

either to single organs or diffusely to multiple organs with miliary involvement (Fig. 9.3)
- erosion of bronchi with spread to other parts of the lung with tuberculous bronchopneumonia (Fig. 9.3).

Secondary tuberculosis

In patients who have had previous exposure to *Mycobacterium tuberculosis* or have been immunized by BCG, the next encounter with the organism leads to secondary tuberculosis, also known as post-primary or reactivated tuberculosis. This typically involves the upper lobes/apices of the lungs (Assmann focus) where a local hypersensitivity response leads to cavitation of lung tissue (Fig. 9.4A). This heals by fibrosis and dystrophic calcification, although the organism may remain viable within the fibrotic area and later become reactivated (Fig. 9.4B). It may spread within the lung through the airways causing tuberculous bronchopneumonia. It may

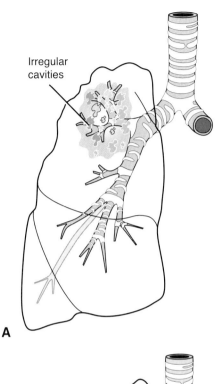

Irregular
cavities

A

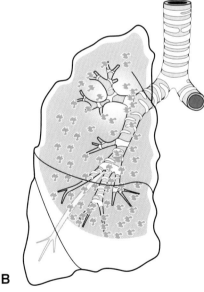

B

Fig. 9.4 Secondary (reactivated) tuberculosis. A. Secondary tuberculosis characteristically involves the apex of the lung, and **B.** may spread through the lung parenchyma by a process of fibrocaseous destruction leading to massive loss of functional lung tissue.

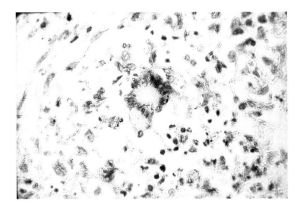

Fig. 9.5 Photomicrograph of Ziehl–Neelsen-stained section of lung showing a granuloma with central necrosis and abundant acid-fast bacilli stained red.

SUMMARY BOX
TUBERCULOSIS

- First exposure to M. *tuberculosis* occurs in the periphery of the lung and causes an inflammatory response at the site (Ghon focus).

- Local lymphatic drainage to the lung hilar nodes leads to the formation of a primary (Ghon) complex.

- The infection is usually contained within the lung and leads to immunity.

- In some individuals, the organism can spread via the bloodstream to distant sites causing miliary (disseminated) tuberculosis or to single organs such as bone, kidneys, brain and genital tract.

- Later, at times of relative immunosuppression, the disease may become reactivated, or the patient may become reinfected, causing secondary tuberculosis.

- Secondary tuberculosis occurs typically in the lung apex and causes extensive fibrocaseous destruction of lung tissue; infection may spread elsewhere in the lung causing TB bronchopneumonia or may spread to other organs throughout the body.

CHRONIC OBSTRUCTIVE AIRWAYS DISEASE (COAD)

This is a clinical syndrome which encompasses both chronic bronchitis and emphysema where patients develop progressive respiratory insufficiency accompanied by changes in blood concentration of the main respiratory gases, oxygen (O_2; reference range for arterial blood PO_2, 12–15 kPa) and carbon dioxide (CO_2; reference range for arterial blood PCO_2, 4.4–5.6 kPa). The two conditions exist at either end of a spectrum of clinical disease. Both

also spread via the bloodstream to cause single organ involvement in sites such as adrenal glands, kidneys, Fallopian tubes, epididymis, brain, meninges, spine, vertebrae and joints, especially knees (Fig. 9.5).

127

groups of patients complain of shortness of breath and on blood gas analysis of arterial blood are shown to have low O_2 levels (hypoxaemia/hypoxia). At the predominantly chronic bronchitis end of the spectrum, this is accompanied by normal CO_2 levels (normocapnia) and these patients are usually cyanotic, i.e. there are increased levels of reduced haemoglobin in the blood producing a blue appearance to the skin and mucous membranes. As the degree of pulmonary damage including pulmonary arterial disease progresses, the patients develop right ventricular strain, hypertrophy and ultimately failure, the condition referred to as cor pulmonale, which causes peripheral oedema. This combination of shortness of breath, blue skin and oedema produces the features of the 'blue bloater'. Where the pulmonary emphysema end of the spectrum of COAD predominates, there is impairment of gas exchange at the alveolar–capillary level. In general, because of the relative diffusion capacities of O_2 and CO_2, it is usually possible for carbon dioxide to be cleared from the alveoli. When there is extensive emphysematous damage, the ability to clear CO_2 is reduced and thus high levels develop in the blood (hypercapnia). Despite the patient's shortness of breath, this gives an appearance of inappropriate health with a bright pink colour to the skin and mucous membranes and bounding pulses. These patients are referred to as 'pink puffers' as they continue to breathe rapidly in an attempt to inhale greater quantities of air.

Chronic bronchitis

This is mainly a clinical entity rather than a pathological diagnosis, as there may not always be an inflammatory component within the bronchi. The clinical condition is defined by the presence of a cough productive of sputum for 3 months in 2 consecutive years. The usual exogenous causes are irritation of the airways mainly by cigarette smoking and atmospheric and industrial pollution, while endogenous causes include chronic asthma, cystic fibrosis and recurrent aspiration. The pathological changes mirror the clinical picture: there is hypersecretion of mucus with increased goblet cells in the surface epithelium, hyperplasia of submucosal glands, squamous metaplasia of the lining bronchial epithelium and variable degrees of chronic inflammatory cell infiltration of the submucosa. The smaller bronchi and bronchioles also show mucous plugging and mural fibrosis. The combination of increased mucus intermingled with normal commensal microorganisms and with impaired defence mechanisms such as loss of the normal ciliary clearing system makes these patients prone to acute exacerbations of their chronic lung disease leading to bronchopneumonia.

Emphysema (Fig. 9.6)

This is defined as abnormal permanent dilatation of the airways distal to the terminal bronchioles accompanied by destruction of their walls. Some definitions do not require destruction, merely permanence, but this may lead to confusion and the inclusion of conditions which are not truly emphysema. The pathogenesis of emphysema is thought to relate to an imbalance between the levels of protease and antiprotease activity within the alveolar spaces, based on animal experiments and on the human disease of α_1-antitrypsin deficiency. In this condition, there is a deficiency of the protease inhibitor (Pi), α_1-antitrypsin, which has more than 130 alleles producing multiple molecular variants. The normal phenotype is PiMM and the commonest variant is PiZ which may manifest as PiMZ or PiZZ. Carriers of the PiZZ phenotype, if smokers, have a 90% risk of lung damage and if non-smokers, have a 70% risk. PiMZ carriers probably have an increased risk of emphysema. The likely pathway is that cigarette smoking activates alveolar macrophages which release neutrophil chemotactic factor; polymorphs accumulate in the alveoli which release elastase and generate oxygen-derived free radicals. Normally, the actions of elastase are inhibited by α_1-antitrypsin but in significant reductions of this protease inhibitor, the unopposed action of elastase may cause damage to the lung parenchyma resulting in emphysema.

Types of emphysema

A number of clinically significant varieties of emphysema are described. Centrilobular (or centriacinar) emphysema refers to dilatation of the respiratory bronchioles particularly and tends to be more severe at the apices of the lung (Fig. 9.6B). It occurs in coal miners and cigarette smokers and often coexists with chronic bronchitis. Panacinar (or panlobular) emphysema refers to uniform dilatation of the respiratory bronchioles and acini and tends to more pronounced in the lower lobes (Fig. 9.6C, D). This form is particularly associated with α_1-antitrypsin deficiency. Other forms include paraseptal emphysema which occurs adjacent to areas of scarring and may lead to pneumothorax, bullous emphysema where there are giant air spaces (> 1 cm in diameter), often apical, which may occur in any true form of emphysema, and focal dust emphysema which is associated with centrilobular deposition of carbon.

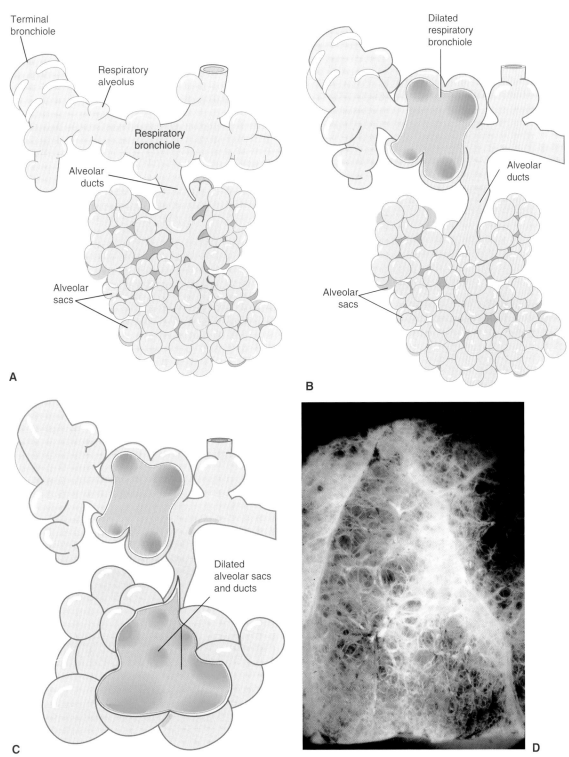

Fig. 9.6 **Emphysema. A.** Structure of normal distal airways from terminal bronchiole onwards, including respiratory alveolus, respiratory bronchiole, alveolar ducts and alveolar sacs. **B.** In centrilobular (centriacinar) emphysema, there is dilatation of the respiratory bronchiole, whereas **C.** in panacinar (panlobular) emphysema, there is dilatation of the whole of the airspace beyond the terminal bronchiole. This has implications for the pathogenesis of this condition. **D.** Photograph showing lung with well-developed panacinar emphysema.

Some conditions exist which bear the title of emphysema but do not fulfil the strict criteria defined above. They include compensatory emphysema where hyperinflation of the contralateral lung occurs in response to collapse or pneumonectomy, interstitial emphysema where there is tearing of lung tissue in response to coughing, trauma or artificial respiration, and surgical emphysema where gas accumulates in extrapulmonary tissues.

Asthma

This is a reversible form of airways obstruction caused by a hypersensitivity reaction to extrinsic allergens such as house dust mite (*Dermatophagoides pteronyssinus*) and grass pollens, principally developing in childhood or early adulthood. This often occurs in a background of atopic reactions such as infantile eczema or food intolerance. It is a common clinical problem especially in childhood and appears to be increasing in incidence, although this may be a result of increased awareness among the general public and medical practitioners rather than a genuine phenomenon. Similar reactions may occur in later adult life as a response to drugs such as aspirin and penicillin and other chemicals, and, rarely, in the absence of any known irritant.

Clinically, patients present with tightness in the chest and shortness of breath which is most pronounced on exhalation, causing loud wheezing and a non-productive cough. As the attack progresses, increased mucus production occurs in which abundant eosinophils are present. Attacks may last for minutes, hours or days and can be treated by the use of bronchodilator agents or corticosteroids. Occasionally, the attacks may become almost continuous, the condition of status asthmaticus, and such patients may require artificial ventilation to maintain respiratory function.

Pathology

Grossly, the lungs during an acute attack may become hyperinflated, so that the right and left lungs meet in the midline anteriorly, and the bronchi and bronchioles become plugged with mucus. Histologically, the airways are distended by mucus in which eosinophils and desquamated epithelial cells are visible. These cells may become twisted into shapes known as Curschmann's spirals. The bronchial basement membrane becomes thickened and hyaline and the submucosa shows congestion, oedema and eosinophil infiltration, and crystalline material known as Charcot–Leiden crystals may also be seen. In long-

standing cases, smooth muscle hypertrophy of the bronchi and bronchioles is present. Other changes such as mucous hyperplasia as in chronic bronchitis and pulmonary hypertension may be seen in severe chronic cases.

Bronchiectasis

This is an abnormal permanent and irreversible dilatation of bronchi, resulting in the formation of large spaces and cavities in the lungs, which may be either localized or generalized. There is often superimposed infection because of the presence of abundant mucus which serves as an ideal culture medium for bacteria such as *Pseudomonas aeruginosa* and *Staphylococcus aureus*. The condition develops as a result of obstruction of bronchi with collapse of the lung and added infection. Underlying causes of focal bronchiectasis include obstruction of bronchi by tumours and foreign bodies, extrinsic compression by hilar lymphadenopathy and retained viscous secretions. Causes of more generalized disease include aspiration or inhalation, e.g. of gastric contents, post-infective damage to bronchial epithelium by viral, bacterial, mycobacterial and fungal infections, abnormal host immune response and inherited disorders including cystic fibrosis and abnormalities of cilia and bronchial cartilage.

Pathology

Grossly, there is dilatation of bronchi of either saccular or cylindrical type. Histologically, there is destruction of the normal components of the bronchial wall, including bronchial glands, smooth muscle and cartilage, with replacement by chronically inflamed fibrous tissue in which lymphoid follicles are often prominent. The surface epithelium may show squamous metaplasia. A long-term complication in a minority of cases is amyloidosis of AA type.

INTERSTITIAL LUNG DISEASES

Pulmonary fibrosis

This is a condition characterized by interstitial fibrosis with progressive destruction of lung parenchyma leading to respiratory failure, and is usually classified on the basis of an aetiological factor if known. A significant proportion of these patients have no identifiable risk factor and thus fit the category of cryptogenic fibrosing

CHRONIC OBSTRUCTIVE AIRWAYS DISEASE

Chronic bronchitis
- Clinical definition of productive cough for 3 months over 2 years.
- Hypersecretion of mucus with bronchial gland hyperplasia.
- Strongly associated with smoking.

Emphysema
- Permanent dilatation of airways distal to terminal bronchioles owing to destruction of elastin in walls.
- Frequently seen with chronic bronchitis and also associated with smoking
- Caused rarely by α_1-antitrypsin deficiency.

Asthma
- Paroxysmal attacks of bronchospasm due to increased irritability of airways.
- Hyperinflated lungs with mucus plugging.
- Hyperplastic bronchial mucous glands and smooth muscle hypertrophy.

Bronchiectasis
- Permanent dilatation of bronchi owing to destruction of walls associated with obstruction and infection.
- Secondary changes lead to further airways damage.
- Clinically, patients have a productive cough with foul-smelling sputum.

alveolitis (CFA). In this condition, there is fibrosis of the alveolar walls, which contain a chronic inflammatory cell infiltrate; within the alveoli, there is an accumulation of macrophages and proliferation of type II pneumocytes and there may be progression to the formation of so-called honeycomb lung. Two common subtypes are recognized: usual interstitial pneumonia (UIP) where there is predominantly fibrosis and chronic inflammation and a relentless clinical course; and desquamative interstitial pneumonia (DIP) where the main feature is intra-alveolar accumulation of macrophages and, clinically, a response to corticosteroids is likely. The pathogenesis of this condition is uncertain but is probably related to the activation of alveolar macrophages by cytokines leading to the release of growth factors which cause proliferation of cells such as fibroblasts, myofibroblasts and smooth muscle cells in the lung interstitium and the subsequent release of collagen. The damage to type I pneumocytes, the hyperplasia of type II pneumocytes and accumulation of alveolar macrophages is probably a result of the initial insult, unknown in CFA, but similar changes occur in patients with rheumatoid arthritis, systemic lupus erythe-

matosus and ankylosing spondylitis and in response to some drugs and chemicals.

Sarcoidosis

This is a multisystem disorder which is characterized by non-caseating epithelioid granulomas. The organs most commonly affected are lungs, hilar lymph nodes, liver, spleen, heart, skin (erythema nodosum), eyes and nervous system but almost any organ or tissue may be involved. The mode of clinical presentation depends on the organ involved but pulmonary disease, either in the form of asymptomatic radiological abnormality or shortness of breath, is one of the most frequent. It is a relatively uncommon disease but is more common in people of Afro-Caribbean and Irish origin and is more frequent in Scandinavia. It is slightly more common in women and it may present at any age, although it tends to do so in the third and fourth decades.

Pathology

The characteristic pathological lesion is a granuloma composed of a central collection of epithelioid macrophages with giant cells of both Langhans' and foreign body type and a peripheral zone of lymphocytes. Necrosis is usually absent and, in particular, caseation is not seen. Occasional inclusions may be seen including Schaumann (large conchoidal basophilic bodies containing calcium and iron) and asteroid (star-shaped eosinophilic material) bodies. The granulomas may resolve or may heal by hyaline fibrosis and, in the lungs, which are involved in over 80% of cases, may contribute to interstitial pulmonary fibrosis.

Diagnosis

The diagnosis is made by the histological identification of the characteristic granulomas, but it is important to exclude other causes of granulomatous inflammation, particularly tuberculosis. In the serum, raised levels of angiotensin-converting enzyme (ACE) are found in 60% of patients with sarcoidosis. The Kveim–Siltzbach test is also used in diagnosis. It consists of an intradermal injection of material extracted from spleen or lymph nodes from patients with known sarcoidosis. The site of injection is then biopsied 6 weeks later and a positive result is indicated by the presence of sarcoid granulomas. The cause of sarcoidosis is unknown but it is thought to be a T cell-mediated delayed hypersensitivity (type IV) reaction to an inhaled antigen. A number of suggestions have been made including mycobacteria, viruses, mycoplasma, fungi, bacteria, organic and inorganic material, but no one agent has been proven.

Asbestosis

This condition exists when there is extensive pulmonary fibrosis associated with the accumulation of asbestos bodies in the lung tissues. Asbestos is a group of substances which are fibrous silicates of magnesium inhaled as dusts into the lung tissues as a result of industrial exposure, in shipyard workers, brake shoe manufacturers, boiler laggers and others, but may also cause disease in those exposed to asbestos incidentally. Two main types of asbestos fibres are identified. Serpentines are long curved flexible fibres which are resistant to air flow and impact in the upper airways where they cause fibrosis; the best example of this type is chrysotile (white asbestos). Amphiboles are short straight brittle fibres which move to the lung periphery where they are both fibrogenic and carcinogenic; the best example of this type is crocidolite (blue asbestos). Fibrosis tends to develop around respiratory bronchioles and spread into the interalveolar walls. The disease begins subpleurally and may progress into honeycomb lung. The disease can be confirmed by the finding of asbestos bodies in the lung. These are asbestos fibres coated in haemosiderin-rich proteins which have a drumstick shape.

Other effects of exposure to asbestos include hyaline pleural plaques, recurrent pleural effusions, fibrous pleural obliteration, and malignant tumours of both lung (mainly adenocarcinoma) and pleura (mesothelioma).

Silicosis

This is the disease caused by the inhalation of silica dust in individuals such as coal miners, rock and slate quarry workers, sandblasters and stone masons. The presence of silica in the lungs induces a dense fibrotic reaction which may attain quite a large size. The pathogenesis of this condition is uncertain and it may be that silica is antigenic or it may be toxic to alveolar macrophages.

Coal miner's pneumoconiosis

This can be either simple or complicated. In the simple form, coal dust is deposited in respiratory bronchioles and adjacent alveoli, particularly in macrophages. Fibrosis develops with obliteration of bronchioles and there may

be focal dust emphysema. Grossly in the lungs, there are multiple black macules up to 0.2 mm in diameter mainly in the upper lobes. The complicated form, previously called progressive massive fibrosis, is characterized by larger stellate confluent fibrotic areas which show central breakdown. As the disease progresses, patients develop respiratory failure and ultimately right ventricular failure. There is an association with pulmonary tuberculosis but it is unclear whether the onset of severe pulmonary disease is the cause of coexistent tuberculosis or an effect of it.

Extrinsic allergic alveolitis

This is an example of a type III hypersensitivity reaction where the antigen is an organic dust derived mainly from microbiological agents. Clinically, patients present

---

SUMMARY BOX
INTERSTITIAL LUNG DISEASE

Pulmonary fibrosis
- Progressive interstitial fibrosis with loss of lung parenchyma and eventual respiratory failure.
- Classified on aetiological agent if known but most fit the category of cryptogenic fibrosing alveolitis, of which there are two main subdivisions (usual and desquamative interstitial pneumonitis).

Sarcoidosis
- Multisystem disease with particular involvement of intrathoracic tissues.
- Characteristic non-caseating epithelioid granulomas with subsequent interstitial fibrosis.

Asbestosis
- Pulmonary fibrosis associated with the presence of asbestos bodies in the lung.
- Seen especially at the lung periphery.
- Also associated with pleural fibrosis and bronchial and pleural neoplasms.

Silicosis
- Caused by inhalation of silica dust, inducing intense fibrosis.

Coal miner's pneumoconiosis
- May be simple or complex.
- In simple form, fibrosis with focal dust emphysema.
- In complex form, progressive massive fibrosis, leading to respiratory failure.

Extrinsic allergic alveolitis
- Type III hypersensitivity reaction to antigens derived from organic dusts.
- Interstitial pneumonitis with progressive fibrosis.

acutely with fever, malaise and breathlessness approximately 6 hours after exposure to the antigen and symptoms persist for up to 24 hours. With chronic disease, patients develop permanent respiratory insufficiency. The characteristic histological features are the presence of interstitial pneumonitis including chronic inflammatory cells and occasional non-caseating granulomas and, with repeated exposure, progressive fibrosis up to honeycomb lung. The condition of extrinsic allergic alveolitis has a number of other names depending on the allergen, including bird-fancier's lung, farmer's lung where the allergen is derived from mouldy hay, *Micropolyspora faeni*, and air conditioner/humidifier lung.

LUNG CANCER

Cancers in the lung may be either primary or secondary with the lung being the commonest site for secondary malignancies from anywhere in the body. Primary tumours may be central, i.e. in and around the hilum of the lung and of bronchial origin (Fig. 9.7), or peripheral, i.e. away from the hilum and of bronchiolar or alveolar origin. Carcinoma of the lung is categorized on the basis of the dominant histological pattern, although with extensive sampling, it is often possible to identify more than one cell type. Squamous carcinoma is the commonest type accounting for 40% of all lung tumours, while adenocarcinoma is responsible for 20% and small cell carcinoma for 25%. The remainder fit the category of large cell carcinoma, which probably represents a mixture of undifferentiated squamous and adenocarcinomas.

Clinical features

Clinically, carcinomas of the lung present in a number of ways. Ulcerating tumours cause haemoptysis (coughing up blood) while obstructing tumours cause shortness of breath, distal pneumonia which may be resistant to antibiotic therapy, bronchiectasis, lung abscesses and lung collapse. Diagnosis is usually made on chest radiography and the histological type can be confirmed by sputum cytology or bronchial biopsy. A tissue diagnosis is important because the therapeutic options depend on the histological type.

Squamous carcinoma

This is the commonest type of primary lung carcinoma and is nearly always central in position. It is seen more

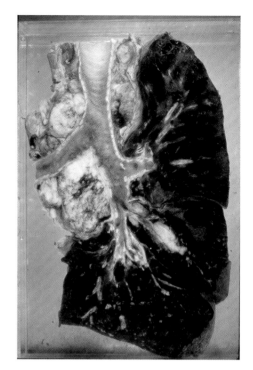

Fig. 9.7 Carcinoma of bronchus arising in lower lobe of left lung, with extensive hilar lymph node spread.

frequently in males than in females and is particularly associated with cigarette smoking. Under normal circumstances, there is no squamous epithelium in the bronchial mucosa but it develops at sites of chronic irritation, e.g. due to cigarette smoking and atmospheric pollution. It may then undergo a process of intraepithelial neoplasia (dysplasia), which at its most severe amounts to carcinoma in situ. From this stage, invasive carcinoma ensues. Most squamous carcinomas are reasonably well differentiated and show such squamous features as epithelial pearl formation, individual cell keratinization and intercellular bridge ('prickle') formation (Fig. 9.8). The majority arise in main bronchi and have a cheesy creamy-grey appearance. This tumour is relatively slow growing and is the most likely lung carcinoma to be amenable to curative surgical resection.

Adenocarcinoma

This tumour may either be central or peripheral. Central tumours may arise from bronchial epithelium or from underlying bronchial submucous glands. The sex incidence is almost equal and there is an association with

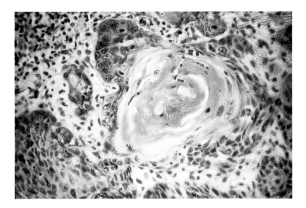

Fig. 9.8 Histological section of primary bronchial carcinoma showing keratin pearl formation typical of well-differentiated squamous carcinoma.

smoking, although this is less strong than in other lung carcinomas. The site of origin tends to be from smaller bronchi than that of squamous carcinoma. Peripheral adenocarcinomas may arise from a number of cell types including columnar bronchiolar cells, Clara cells and type II pneumocytes and are often found in areas of pre-existing scarring, with spread into the overlying pleura. It is essential that the possibility of a metastatic adenocarcinoma should also be excluded. The World Health Organization (WHO) classification gives four patterns of adenocarcinoma: acinar, papillary, solid and bronchiolo-alveolar, but only the last mentioned, which tends to grow slowly within alveoli, is commonly described.

Small cell carcinoma

This is a tumour of neuroendocrine origin, associated with cigarette smoking, which has a very high growth fraction and has often metastasized at the time of diagnosis. The original name for these tumours was oat cell carcinoma because of the nature of the predominant cell type with its oval shape, high nuclear–cytoplasmic ratio and hyperchromatic nuclei. However, variation in nuclear size and shape is seen and larger 'intermediate' cell variants are described. These tumours are almost always central in position and show extensive necrosis with a characteristic DNA deposition on blood vessel walls. These tumours, because of their widespread dissemination before diagnosis, are generally felt to be incurable by surgical resection and are often treated by aggressive chemotherapy. The prognosis, however, remains poor.

Large cell carcinoma

This is a separate category in the WHO classification but it probably represents those tumours which are so poorly differentiated that they do not show features of either glandular (adenocarcinoma) or squamous differentiation. More importantly, they are not small cell carcinomas. Histologically, the tumours tend to have sheets of large cells, sometimes including prominent multinucleated giant cells.

Spread of lung carcinomas

This may be:

- direct spread into surrounding tissues, including blood vessels in bronchial mucosa causing haemoptysis; into nerves such as the brachial plexus causing arm pain and cervical sympathetics causing Horner's syndrome (ptosis, miosis, anhidrosis and enophthalmos); into pericardium and heart; into pleura, chest wall and vertebrae; and into mediastinum and oesophagus
- via lymphatics into hilar lymph nodes, mediastinal lymph nodes, cervical lymph nodes and elsewhere; where the thoracic duct is obstructed, backpressure into pulmonary especially subpleural lymphatics causes lymphangitis carcinomatosa, although this can also occur with secondary carcinomas
- to distant organs via the bloodstream, e.g. to the adrenal glands (50% of cases), liver (30%), brain (20%) and bone (20%).

Paraneoplastic syndromes

Many carcinomas, particularly lung carcinoma, may present with features related to secretory products of the tumours rather than direct metastatic effects. These are referred to as paraneoplastic syndromes. They include:

- ectopic hormone production such as antidiuretic hormone (ADH) and adrenocorticotrophic hormone (ACTH), both from small cell carcinoma, and parathyroid hormone (PTH) causing hypercalcaemia from squamous carcinoma
- peripheral neuropathy and myopathy
- acanthosis nigricans
- finger clubbing
- hypertrophic pulmonary osteoarthropathy
- thrombophlebitis migrans (as in pancreatic carcinoma).

Staging

The TNM staging system is a useful method for determining the stage of disease and thus, for predicting prognosis. The system is based on tumour (neoplasm) parameters: T, size of the primary lesion; N, extent of nodal metastasis and M, presence or absence of distant metastasis.

T_x: only demonstrable by exfoliative cytology
T_1: ≤3 cm and beyond lobar bronchi
T_2: >3 cm or any size extending to hilum
T_3: any size within 2 cm of carina
N_0: no nodal involvement
N_1: ipsilateral lymph node involvement
N_2: mediastinal lymph node involvement
M_0: no distant metastasis
M_1: distant metastasis including scalene nodes or contralateral hilar nodes

The prognosis in lung carcinoma depends to a great extent on the histological type but because many of the tumours have metastasized widely at the time of presentation, much of the treatment available is palliative only. While small cell carcinoma is universally considered to be inoperable and thus only suitable for chemotherapy, the other main forms of lung carcinoma are also unlikely to be susceptible to any mode of potentially curative therapy. The overall 5-year survival rate in all forms of lung carcinoma is approximately 30%.

Bronchial carcinoids and other low-grade tumours

Carcinoid tumours are neoplasms derived from the neuroendocrine cells of the bronchial epithelium. They present clinically in a non-specific way with cough or shortness of breath or with an abnormal chest X-ray. They usually occur in young adults and are not related to cigarette smoking. They are embryologically of foregut origin but are typically non-secretory. Grossly, they are fleshy tumours arising in larger bronchi and often have a dumb-bell shape. Histologically, they are packeted tumours with some rosette formation and few mitotic figures They may be locally invasive but rarely metastasize.

A group of tumours known as atypical carcinoid tumours occurs in an older age-group, probably associated with cigarette smoking, which have a higher mitotic rate and are more likely to metastasize. They are intermediate between typical carcinoid tumours and small cell carcinoma in terms of histological appearance and clinical behaviour.

Another group of tumours previously known as bronchial adenomas, which are similar to tumours in salivary glands, also occur in the bronchi. They include adenoid cystic tumours, mucoepidermoid tumours, pleomorphic adenomas, cystadenomas, acinic cell tumours and oncocytomas. In general they are benign tumours or show the clinical behaviour of low-grade malignant tumours with local recurrence rather than distant metastasis.

SUMMARY BOX
CARCINOMA OF THE LUNG

- Secondary carcinomas are common.
- Primary carcinomas are among the commonest malignant tumours of the western world.
- It is strongly associated with cigarette smoking and also with occupational exposure to carcinogens.
- Histological types include squamous cell carcinoma, adenocarcinoma, small cell carcinoma and large cell undifferentiated carcinoma.
- There is generally a poor prognosis, with small cell carcinoma the worst.

Pleural mesothelioma (Fig. 9.9)

This is a malignant tumour of pleura which is strongly associated with previous asbestos exposure. There may be a long latent period from the time of exposure to asbestos, which itself may be incidental. Clinically, the patients present with recurrent pleural effusions. Grossly, the tumour encases the lung in firm grey-white tissue and infiltrates into the underlying lung and into the overlying chest wall, producing restrictive effects on lung function. Histologically, it may be difficult to differentiate mesothelioma from metastatic adenocarcinoma, but in other areas of the tumour, a sarcoma-like pattern may be identified. The prognosis is extremely poor in view of the mode of infiltration making surgical resection virtually impossible.

ASPECTS OF RESPIRATORY DISEASE OF PARTICULAR RELEVANCE TO DENTISTRY

- Aspiration pneumonia is a potential complication of a general anaesthetic.
- Patients with chronic obstructive airways diseases may have problems with dental procedures, especially general anaesthetics.
- Anti-smoking counselling and interventions given by dentists may help to prevent the development of chronic lung conditions and carcinoma.

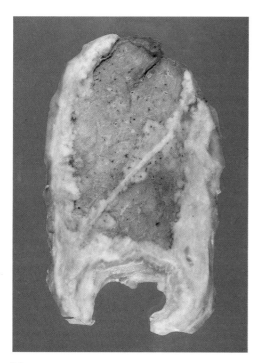

Fig. 9.9 Pleural mesothelioma: gross photograph of lung and pleura demonstrating encasement of lung by dense white tumour of pleura, typical of pleural mesothelioma.

CASE STUDY 9.1
BLOOD IN THE SPUTUM

A 57-year-old man presented to his GP with a history of a cough productive of green, tenacious sputum for the last week and on two occasions he had noticed blood within the sputum. At times, he felt hot and shivery. His GP knew this man well because he was a frequent visitor to the surgery with chest infections, particularly in the winter. He was a cigarette smoker, currently on 20/day although in the past he had smoked up to 60/day. On examination, the GP noted crackles and wheezes in the right lower lobe and prescribed an antibiotic for him.

A week later, he returned to his GP, having completed the course of antibiotics. Although the feelings of hot and cold had cleared up, he was still coughing up sputum, more frequently with blood streaks in it. The GP re-examined him and still noted crackles and wheezes. He referred him then for a chest X-ray at the local hospital. This showed an area of consolidation at the right lower lobe but there was also an opacity near the hilum. When the report arrived back at the surgery some days later, the GP immediately referred the man to the local chest physician.

A bronchoscopy revealed a lesion in the right lower lobe bronchus which was biopsied. Fragments were sent to the histopathology department and reported as 'pieces of bronchial mucosa and submucosa infiltrated by a malignant tumour composed of cells with variable amounts of cytoplasm, large nuclei, intercellular bridges ("prickles") and occasional keratin pearls. These are the appearances of ...'. As a result of this report, the patient was subjected to more investigations including a CT scan of the chest, after which he was offered surgery. A week later, a right pneumonectomy was performed. The specimen was sent to the pathology laboratory.

He made a good postoperative recovery and gave up cigarettes. No further treatment was recommended. 18 Months later, he collapsed at home and was dead on arrival at hospital. A coroner's postmortem was carried out. The pathologist reported that he had died of a myocardial infarct but also found evidence of metastases of his primary bronchial carcinoma.

1. What are the possible causes of this man's symptoms?
2. What features in the pathology report of the pneumonectomy specimen may be of value in determining the prognosis of this patient?
3. Where are the likely sites of spread of this tumour and by what routes might they arrive there?

Suggested responses

1. The cough associated with features of infection (hot and shivery) suggests pneumonia. However, the finding of blood in the sputum (haemoptysis) is more ominous. This may be associated with pneumonia but should also raise the possibility of tuberculosis, pulmonary thromboembolism/ infarction or pulmonary neoplasia. The features described in the X-ray report are of pneumonia distal to an obstructive lesion in the right lower lobe region and strongly suggest the likelihood of neoplasia. However, there are significant differences in the management of lung tumours related to the histological type so it is important to have a tissue diagnosis before considering management options. Thus, a bronchoscopy with biopsy of any lesion identified should be undertaken in the first instance. Other investigations which might be considered at this stage or later would be to stage the disease, i.e. to determine the extent of tumour – local spread, lymph node involvement, distal (haematogenous) metastases. Some lung tumours have a tendency to cause paraneoplastic syndromes, particularly small cell carcinoma producing ectopic ACTH (Cushing's syndrome), inappropriate ADH

secretion (diabetes insipidus) and myasthenia-like syndrome, and squamous carcinoma producing hypercalcaemia via ectopic PTH secretion.

2. These are the features of a reasonably well-differentiated squamous cell carcinoma. It is important to differentiate this from small cell (oat cell) carcinoma because treatment for the latter is rarely amenable to a surgical approach. The histological type is predictive of outcome (squamous or adenocarcinoma > large cell carcinoma > small cell carcinoma) as are the presence of lymph node metastases, pleural involvement and involvement of the resection margin.

3. There may have been recurrence at the surgical site, particularly if the resection margin was involved, but this is unlikely at 18 months. Lymph node metastases may have been present in the mediastinum – lung hilum or paratracheal nodes, supraclavicular or cervical nodes, rarely para-aortic nodes. Haematogenous spread may have been seen in the left lung, liver, adrenal glands, brain or bone; other sites such as spleen or kidneys are much less commonly involved.

CASE STUDY 9.2
WHEEZING

A 16-year-old female was admitted to Casualty with severe shortness of breath which developed after a row with her boyfriend. On examination, she was noted to be wheezing and investigation showed a reduced peak expiratory flow rate with a low PO_2 and a slightly reduced PCO_2.

She was treated with bronchodilator therapy and her general condition improved, and she was discharged home. 2 weeks later her condition deteriorated with repeated episodes of shortness of breath and wheezing.

She was readmitted to hospital and was treated with bronchodilator therapy and corticosteroids, given initially in high dose. A chest X-ray showed evidence of right lower lobe consolidation.

In addition to the therapy described above, she was also given an antibiotic and her condition again improved with discharge 4 days after admission.

1. What is the most likely diagnosis in this case?
2. What precipitating factors may be important in the development of her chronic condition and in the acute exacerbations causing sudden shortness of breath?
3. Of which type of hypersensitivity reaction is this an example? Describe the pathogenic mechanisms involved.
4. If a bronchial biopsy were taken during the acute attack, what histological features would be seen?

Suggested responses

1. This is a case of asthma, probably of extrinsic allergic type, which is a form of reversible obstructive airways disease.

2. In the chronic condition, the common precipitating factors in a young age group include allergy to a range of substances especially the house dust mite, viral infections, occupational exposure to allergens or direct bronchial irritants, some drugs such as aspirin or β-antagonists, psychological stress, exertion and cold air. Acute attacks may be precipitated by all of the above conditions and, in particular, may be precipitated by infections, especially bacterial super-infection following initial viral infection.

3. This is an example of type I hypersensitivity, which is the commonest predisposing condition to asthma. Initial exposure to an allergen leads to antibody production of IgE type which on subsequent exposure leads to a complex between IgE and mast cells. This leads to recruitment of T lymphocytes and eosinophils and later release of various inflammatory mediators such as leukotrienes, prostaglandins and platelet-activating factor. Locally, there is oedema and mucus hypersecretion and, along with bronchial smooth muscle contraction, this leads to the characteristic expiratory wheezing noted in this condition.

4. The walls of bronchi are usually oedematous and are infiltrated by inflammatory cells including lymphocytes, eosinophils, mast cells and macrophages. There is often epithelial necrosis and the lumen contains mucus plugs originating from hyperplastic bronchial submucous glands and including Curschmann spirals, eosinophils and Charcot–Leyden crystals derived from eosinophil granules. The smooth muscle layer is often hypertrophic and in long-standing disease, the basement membrane is thickened with increased subepithelial collagen deposition.

CASE STUDY 9.3
NIGHT SWEATS

A 24-year-old Malaysian male in the last year of a PhD course in the UK noted a lump in the left side of his neck just above the clavicle. He had first noticed it 8 weeks previously and it had gradually increased in size over that time. He was otherwise well but on direct questioning by his GP, he admitted to several episodes of drenching night sweats, such that there was a need to change the bedclothes. He denied a cough or haemoptysis (coughing up blood).

On examination, the mass was not fixed but had a lobulated

appearance. Clinically, he was suspected of having Hodgkin's disease. An open biopsy was performed at which a lymph node measuring 6.3 cm in maximum dimension was removed and submitted for histopathological examination. Histological examination revealed a lymph node whose architecture was effaced by numerous epithelioid granulomas with several Langhans'-type giant cells. Most of the granulomas were non-caseating but some showed central necrosis with caseation. A Ziehl–Neelsen (ZN) stain was positive for acid-fast bacilli.

The patient had a chest X-ray which showed an apical cavity. Several specimens of sputum and urine were collected for microbiological examination, after which he was commenced on triple antibiotic therapy appropriate to the likely organism. This man was sharing a flat with two other Asian students.

1. What possible causes of the lump in his neck should be considered?
2. What do the night sweats indicate?
3. What do these histological appearances suggest?
4. Of what type of immunological reaction is this situation characteristic? Describe the likely sequence of events in this patient.
5. What further action needs to be taken in this case?
6. What possible complications may occur?

Suggested responses

1. From the described position, this is most likely to represent a lymph node and possible causes of lymphadenopathy in this age group and ethnic background include infective diseases and neoplasia, particularly Hodgkin's disease. The infective causes should include bacterial infections but more likely are tuberculosis and fungal infections. Non-lymph-node causes of neck lumps are unusual at that site but should include thyroid lumps and extension of lesions from the anterior mediastinum.

2. Night sweats particularly of the severity described are indicative of a severe chronic infective condition such as tuberculosis or of underlying neoplastic disease such as Hodgkin's or non-Hodgkin's lymphoma, where such a symptom indicates type B (constitutional) disease.

3. The description is that of chronic granulomatous inflammation and in the absence of caseation would suggest sarcoidosis. However, the finding of caseation necrosis along with Langhans'-type giant cells and the recognition of acid-fast bacilli on ZN staining is characteristic of infection

with mycobacteria, almost certainly tuberculous. It is important to obtain samples for culture to allow sensitivity tests of the mycobacterium to be done and to ensure correct antimicrobial therapy.

4. The lesion described is a typical example of a type IV hypersensitivity reaction which is a T-cell-mediated delayed hypersensitivity response to the presence of mycobacterial infection (see Chs 3 and 4). This man probably had infection with *Mycobacterium tuberculosis* as a child in Malaysia, following which he would have had immunity to infection. On first exposure to the organism, there is little or no acute inflammatory response but the mycobacteria are recognized by T cells, which release cytokines which attract bone-marrow-derived macrophages to the site of the infection, most commonly by the inhaled route in the lungs. These macrophages may change shape to become epithelioid in character, so-called because of their resemblance to squamous epithelial cells of the skin or buccal mucosa. They aggregate together to form a granuloma and the fusion of several macrophages leads to the formation of a Langhans'-type giant cell, which has a horseshoe-shaped ring of nuclei around enlarged cytoplasm. The effect of lysosomal enzymes on the mycobacterial cell wall leads to necrosis of caseation type, characteristic of tuberculous infection. The inflammatory process may spread to the regional and distant nodes, as in this case involving the supraclavicular nodes. It is likely that this man had a dormant primary infection with tuberculosis and on moving to a foreign country and living in relatively impoverished conditions that the infection became reactivated.

5. Tuberculosis is an infectious condition and should be reported to the appropriate authorities responsible for public health. Those people in close contact with the patient should also be contacted and offered screening for TB in the form of a chest X-ray and a tuberculin skin test such as Heaf or Mantoux, which uses the principles of delayed hypersensitivity to assess whether an individual is immune to the disease. If the chest X-ray is clear and the skin test is negative, they should then be offered vaccination with BCG (bacille Calmette–Guérin).

6. The disease may spread to other body sites either as single organ involvement, particularly to the kidneys, bones including spine, joints especially knees, and reproductive organs such as epididymis in males and ovaries and Fallopian tubes in females, or by blood-borne spread to several organs at once (miliary spread) when kidneys, liver, spleen and meninges are particularly at risk.

10 Diseases of the gastrointestinal tract

LIPS, TEETH AND GINGIVAE, ORAL MUCOSA, SALIVARY GLANDS AND PHARYNX

LIPS

The vermilion border of the lips, particularly the lower lip, may be exposed to ultraviolet radiation in outdoor workers and in those living in tropical latitudes. The affected lip appears pale owing to damage to the underlying connective tissue, referred to as solar elastosis. Of greater clinical significance is the occurrence of solar keratosis which is a premalignant lesion characterized by microscopic dysplasia. Squamous cell carcinoma typically presents as a painless, non-healing ulcer or raised area on the lower vermilion border which can be easily overlooked. Transplant recipients are particularly prone to developing lip cancer due to immunosuppression, thought to result from loss of a mechanism which destroys UV-damaged cells.

Angular cheilitis is a relatively common disorder characterized by sore crusting areas at the angles of the mouth. Often it results from saliva tracking from the mouth onto the skin as a result of habitual licking, worn dentures or neurological disorders. Infection by *Candida albicans* and *Staphylococcus aureus* is frequently present. Iron-deficiency anaemia is a common predisposing factor.

Melanotic macules involving the lips and circumoral skin may be a feature of Peutz–Jeghers syndrome, a hereditary disorder which includes intestinal polyps.

Squamous papillomas present as small solitary or multiple white cauliflower-like growths and are common on the lips. They are caused by human papilloma viruses and in children are frequently acquired by chewing warts on the fingers.

The lower labial mucosa is a common site for small relapsing cysts arising from the minor salivary glands known as mucoceles. In contrast, cystic or solid swellings involving the upper labial mucosa are more likely to be salivary neoplasms.

SUMMARY BOX
LIPS

- Chronic UV exposure damages the lower lip.
- The lower lip is a common site for squamous carcinoma.
- *Candida albicans* and *Staphylococcus aureus* infection is common in angular cheilitis.
- Mucoceles are a common cause of swelling in the lower lip.
- Salivary tumours are more likely to occur in the upper lip.

TEETH AND GINGIVAE

The most common disorder of the teeth is dental caries (see also Ch. 5 on microbiological aspects). This is an acquired disorder which involves progressive demineralization of the dental enamel resulting in porosity and ultimately cavitation. Bacterial invasion of the dentine may then follow, leading to demineralization, discoloration and destruction of the dentine matrix. Eventually, the bacteria can reach the dental pulp and infection can lead to acute or chronic pulpitis. The inflammatory process may then spread to the periapical bone and can lead to

139

acute alveolar abscess, apical granuloma or radicular cyst formation.

Other acquired forms of disease leading to loss of dental hard tissue include erosion, abrasion and attrition. Rarely, genetic disorders lead to defective tooth formation, the best-known example being amelogenesis imperfecta where the enamel may be hypomineralized or hypoplastic. Systemic disease, excessive fluoride ingestion and drugs taken during the period of tooth formation may affect tooth development.

Gingivitis is the generic term used to describe chronic inflammation of the gingival tissue characterized by redness and swelling. It is very common and is related to accumulation of dental plaque which releases toxins and other irritants into the marginal tissue. Destruction of the supporting tissues of the teeth by chronic inflammation is referred to as periodontal disease, though this term includes a variety of related disorders.

Drug-induced gingival overgrowth is most often caused by continuous therapy with either phenytoin, cyclosporin or nifedipine and is characterized by generalized enlargement of the gingivae which can be so extensive that the crowns are covered. Such gingival enlargement can also be a feature of leukaemia, particularly acute lymphoblastic and myelomonocytic types.

A localized swelling of the gingivae is referred to as an epulis. Local irritation is the most common cause of an epulis, though systemic factors such as pregnancy may predispose to some forms of epulis. Almost all of the disorders referred to in the next section on oral mucosa may arise on the gingivae.

SUMMARY BOX
TEETH AND GINGIVAE

- Dental caries, gingivitis and periodontal disease have an extremely high prevalence in humans.
- Gingival overgrowth can be caused by drugs, leukaemia, inflammatory diseases, genetic and other disorders.
- Epulis is a term used to describe a localized swelling of the gum.

ORAL MUCOSA

Inflammatory

Recurrent oral ulceration

Also known as recurrent aphthous stomatitis, this is an extremely common disorder of the oral mucosa, estimated to affect 25% of the population. The most common type is minor recurrent oral ulceration where shallow ulcers up to 10 mm in diameter appear singly or in crops on the non-keratinizing areas of the oral cavity. The ulcers have a flat yellowish base and are surrounded by erythematous mucosa. They typically heal without scarring after 10–14 days. Clinically more severe types are known; major recurrent oral ulceration causes larger, more persistent ulcers which tend to affect the posterior part of the oral cavity and pharynx, and herpetiform recurrent oral ulceration is characterized by crops of pinhead-size ulcers which persist and become confluent with time.

The pathogenesis of recurrent oral ulceration is not fully understood but it is thought to involve a T cell event occurring in relation to small vessels. Recurrent oral ulceration can be a feature of Behçet's syndrome where the pathogenesis involves circulating immune complexes. Most cases of recurrent oral ulceration are idiopathic and may have a genetic basis. Gastrointestinal disease, particularly coeliac disease and inflammatory bowel disease, anaemia and stress may predispose to recurrent oral ulceration.

Lichen planus

This is a chronic mucocutaneous disorder which involves the mouth in around 65% of cases. On the skin it presents as an itchy macular–papular rash typically involving the flexor surfaces of the limbs and sometimes other sites. The prevalence is estimated at 0.5–1.9% in the population. The papules are violaceous and show distinctive white lines known as Wickham's striae (Fig. 10.1). In the oral cavity, the buccal mucosa and lateral tongue are most frequently involved but the palate, gingivae, labial mucosa and floor of mouth may be affected. The lesions

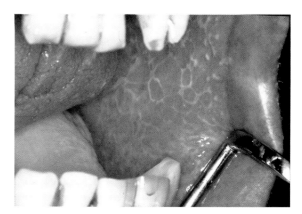

Fig. 10.1 **Buccal mucosa showing the characteristic Wickham's striae of oral lichen planus.**

are typically bilateral. Various oral lesions may occur including white lace-like lines forming networks (reticular lesions), white plaques and small white papular lesions which frequently coalesce. In the atrophic form of lichen planus, the epithelium is thinned and appears intensely erythematous. This lesion is one cause of desquamative gingivitis, a clinical term used for any red, atrophic disorder affecting the gingival tissue. Superficial ulceration may occur in lichen planus, leading to pain.

The pathological processes in lichen planus involve destruction of the epithelial basal cells, often by apoptosis. A discrete subepithelial band of T lymphocytes and histiocytes is typically seen in biopsies of lichen planus. The apoptotic basal cells appear as condensed hyaline bodies with nuclear fragmentation and are known as Civatte bodies. The epithelium may show keratosis or atrophy and it often exhibits irregular elongation and widening of the rete processes. The 'saw tooth' pattern which is typical of skin lesions is not always seen in oral biopsies.

The pathogenesis of lichen planus is poorly understood but it is thought to involve modification of the antigenic structure of the epithelial cells. Interleukins may upregulate intercellular adhesion molecules to which T lymphocytes bind. Destruction of the basal epithelium is thought to be mediated by CD8 cytotoxic lymphocytes.

The atrophic form of lichen planus is recognized as a possible premalignant condition, i.e. where there may be a slightly increased susceptibility to carcinogens. The frequency of malignant change is, however, very small.

Lupus erythematosus, drug reactions and graft-versus-host disease can also cause lichenoid mucositis.

ognized: type 1 HSV is typically associated with oral infections and type 2 HSV with genital infection. Both are DNA viruses. Primary infection with HSV can be subclinical, manifest as pharyngitis or present as primary herpetic gingivostomatitis. Infection is acquired by droplet spread or contact and typically young children and young adults are affected. There is malaise and fever followed by an outbreak of vesicles on the oral mucosa (Fig. 10.2). The gingivae are frequently involved and the vesicles break down to form ulcers rapidly. Bilateral tender cervical lymphadenopathy is characteristic also. Finger sucking may spread the infection to the hands resulting in painful herpetic whitlows and the eyes may also be involved. HSV infects the oral epithelial cells causing cytopathic changes, degeneration and formation of intraepithelial vesicles. The infection resolves in 14–21 days but the virus may remain latent in the trigeminal ganglion. Reactivation may result in virus travelling down the axoplasm to the lips and face. Depression of immunity, either local or general, can then trigger recurrent herpetic infection. This is known as herpes labialis (cold sores) and attacks are not accompanied by systemic illness.

Varicella zoster virus. This may also lie dormant in the trigeminal ganglion following chickenpox. Reactivation can lead to shingles involving one or more branches of the trigeminal nerve. Recurrent infection is often painful and may lead to toothache-like symptoms.

Coxsackievirus A, measles virus, Epstein–Barr virus and cytomegalovirus can also cause oral infections.

SUMMARY BOX
INFLAMMATORY CONDITIONS OF THE ORAL MUCOSA

- Recurrent oral ulceration affects 25% of the population and may be related to gastrointestinal disease and anaemia.
- Lichen planus is a mucocutaneous disorder affecting around 1% of the population.
- Desquamative gingivitis may be caused by lichen planus, vesiculobullous disorders, allergy, hormonal factors and other diseases.

Infections

Viral infections

Herpes simplex viruses (HSV). These are a common cause of infection in the mouth. Two types are rec-

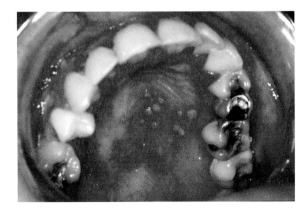

Fig. 10.2 Clinical photograph demonstrating typical vesicles of oral herpes simplex virus infection.

Bacterial infections

Infections of the oral mucosa include acute ulcerative gingivitis, which is characterized by gingival necrosis resulting in pain, bleeding and halitosis. The infection is polymicrobial and there is overgrowth of fusiform and spirochaetal organisms. Local factors and suppression of immunity, for example in HIV infection, may predispose to the condition. In African countries, severe gangrenous destruction of the orofacial region known as noma (cancrum oris) may follow acute ulcerative gingivitis. Cervicofacial actinomycosis is a chronic infection typified by foci of suppuration with discharge through multiple sinuses. It is a mixed infection which includes various *Actinomyces* species. Syphilis, tuberculosis and leprosy can cause oral infections.

Fungal infection

This is a common condition and is most often due to *Candida albicans*. Other *Candida* species which can produce infection include *C. glabrata*, *C. tropicalis*, *C. krusei* and *C. parapsilosis*. *Candida* is a commensal organism with carriage rates of 20–40%. They are opportunistic pathogens and a variety of local and systemic factors may predispose to infection in the mouth. Acute pseudomembranous candidiasis (thrush) is characterized by white loose plaques which can be scraped off the oral mucosa leaving a red bleeding surface (Fig. 10.3). Erythematous and atrophic lesions can also form. In chronic hyperplastic candidosis the yeast invades the superficial layers of the oral epithelium. Rare immunodeficiency syndromes can result in chronic infection involving the mucosal surfaces and skin, particularly the nails (hereditary mucocutaneous candidiasis syndromes).

HIV infection in the mouth

Human immunodeficiency virus (HIV) is transmitted by blood or body fluids. Transmission of the virus generally does not produce symptoms, but there may be diarrhoea, rash, fever and an oral erythematous eruption. This is self-limiting and following seroconversion most patients remain symptom free for many years. Oral candidosis is a frequent feature of infection and occurs in approximately 25% of HIV symptomless carriers and over 90% of those who have developed acquired immune deficiency syndrome (AIDS). Other characteristic HIV-related oral lesions include linear gingival erythema, periodontitis (Fig. 10.4) and necrotizing stomatitis. Hairy leukoplakia is the term applied to a lesion which typically involves the lateral aspects of the tongue. It presents as white plaques which may be smooth, ridged or papillary. The plaques contain swollen cells in the prickle cell layer which contain large numbers of Epstein–Barr virus particles. Hairy leukoplakia is frequently seen in HIV patients with low CD4 counts indicating severe depression of immunity and it has also been found in renal transplant recipients. Kaposi's sarcoma is seen in around 25% of AIDS patients and it presents on the skin or oral mucosa, most often the palate (Fig. 10.5). Early lesions are seen as pigmented spots but these soon progress to dark red or purple raised swellings. Kaposi's sarcoma is considered to be a multicentric vascular proliferation in response to persistent infection with human herpesvirus 8 (HHV8). Non-Hodgkin's lymphoma, atypical oral ulceration,

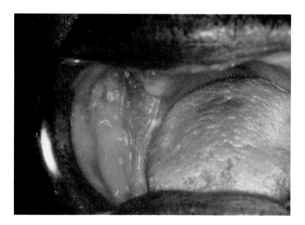

Fig. 10.3 Tongue and buccal mucosa showing the typical yellow-white coating of oral candidiasis (thrush).

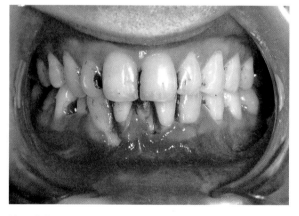

Fig. 10.4 Clinical photograph from a patient with HIV infection showing a very florid pattern of acute periodontitis.

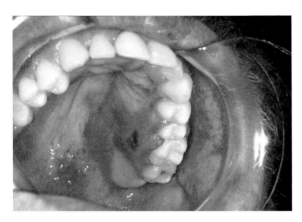

Fig. 10.5 Clinical photograph from a patient with HIV infection demonstrating the characteristic purple-red lesion of Kaposi's sarcoma.

thrombocytopenic purpura and salivary gland disease are also associated with HIV infection.

SUMMARY BOX
INFECTIONS OF THE ORAL MUCOSA

- HSV is a common cause of acute stomatitis in children and young adults.

- Oral lesions strongly associated with HIV include erythematous candidiasis, hairy leukoplakia, Kaposi's sarcoma, linear gingival erythema, HIV-related periodontitis and stomatitis, non-Hodgkin's lymphoma.

- Acute *Candida albicans* infection presents in pseudomembranous (thrush) form and atrophic (erythematous) form.

- Chronic *Candida albicans* infection presents in atrophic, hyperplastic and mucocutaneous forms.

Squamous cell carcinoma

Squamous cell carcinoma accounts for over 90% of primary cancer in the oral cavity. It is estimated that there are over 350 000 new cases per annum globally, with over 2500 in the UK. The disease has a high morbidity and there is around 50% 5-year survival overall. Epidemiological evidence suggests that the incidence of oral squamous cell carcinoma is increasing, particularly in the younger age groups. The major aetiological factors are tobacco and alcohol for intra-oral carcinoma and ultraviolet light for lip carcinoma. When alcohol and tobacco are taken together, their effects are synergistic in terms of risk. Chronic iron deficiency, particularly in primary sideropenic anaemia with oesophageal web

(Patterson–Kelly or Plummer–Vinson syndrome) and diets deficient in antioxidant vitamins A, C and E are also significant risk factors for oral cancer. The prevalence of oral squamous cell carcinoma is high in the Indian subcontinent and Southeast Asia owing to the use of betel quid (pan). Pan is held habitually in the mouth for several hours. It may include tobacco but other constituents of pan such as areca nut may also be carcinogenic. Pan is also thought to be the major aetiological factor for submucous fibrosis, which is a recognized precancerous condition.

Gross pathology

Oral squamous cell carcinoma can present in many forms and is often painless until advanced. Classically, oral carcinoma is described as a persistent non-healing ulcer with raised rolled margins (Fig. 10.6). However, it can also present as a white patch, red patch, proliferating mass or with fixation of tissues. The latter feature is due to the excessive fibrosis often stimulated by the invading squamous cells and it may result in, for example, tongue deviation on protrusion. Clinically, the fibrosis is often palpable and is referred to as induration. Invasion of bone, muscle and adjacent anatomical structures is common. Metastatic spread to regional lymph nodes in the neck is frequent and may be the presenting sign. Blood-borne distant metastases tend to occur late in the course of the disease. They are rarely important clinically because most incurable patients experience problems with local destruction of vital tissues in the neck.

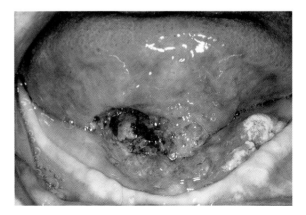

Fig. 10.6 Clinical photograph of elderly edentulous patient with an ulcerating tumour of the floor of the mouth, typical of squamous carcinoma. Note the white plaques in the adjacent mucosa, characteristic of leukoplakia.

Histopathology

Oral squamous cell carcinomas are variable but all show invasion of the underlying connective tissue by malignant squamous cells. Well-differentiated tumours show intercellular bridges (desmosomes) and tend to form characteristic whorls of keratin, known as keratin pearls. In moderately differentiated carcinomas, keratin pearls may be less conspicuous and there is usually nuclear and cellular pleomorphism, nuclear hyperchromatism, increased and atypical mitosis and individual cell keratinization. Apoptosis may also be seen to a variable degree. Some examples are poorly differentiated or anaplastic and cytokeratin markers may be required to establish the diagnosis. The carcinoma cells are supported by vascular fibrous stroma which often contains large numbers of reactive chronic inflammatory cells. Necrosis may be present and is thought to be due to failure of the vascular stroma to keep pace with growth of the carcinoma cells. Invasion pattern is a key feature in oral squamous cell carcinoma. Invasion on a broad, cohesive front is generally regarded as a good prognostic sign while single cell diffuse invasion is associated with a poor prognosis. Sarcolemmal, perineural, lymphatic, vascular and bone invasion are also regarded as poor prognostic indicators. Metastatic spread to regional lymph nodes in the neck adversely affects prognosis, particularly when the nodal deposit extends through the lymph node capsule resulting in clinical fixation of the node.

Prognosis depends strongly on clinical stage, and detection of small (early) neoplasms is critical to outcome both in terms of survival and morbidity. The TNM system (see Ch. 9, p. 135) is used to determine clinical stage, which acts as an important guide to planning therapy. It should be noted that gross invasion of adjacent structures indicates a T4 carcinoma and hence Stage 4 disease, even in the absence of nodal metastasis. A simplified TNM system used for oral carcinoma as follows:

- Tumour:
  T_1: primary tumour <2 cm diameter
  T_2: primary tumour 2–4 cm diameter
  T_3: primary tumour >4 cm diameter
  T_4: large tumour >4 cm with invasion of adjacent structures.
- Nodes:
  N_0: no enlarged nodes
  N_1: single ipsilateral node <3 cm diameter
  N_2:
    a. single ipsilateral node 3–6 cm diameter

  b. multiple ipsilateral nodes <6 cm diameter
  c. bilateral or contralateral nodes <6 cm diameter
  N_3: any node >6 cm diameter.
- Metastasis:
  M_0: no distant metastasis
  M_1: distant metastasis.

The clinical stage is derived from the TNM findings using the combinations below. Note that the system can also be used by the pathologist to determine the pathological stage (pTMN stage) in cases where the carcinoma is resected.

• Stage 1	T_1	N_0	M_0
• Stage 2	T_2	N_0	M_0
• Stage 3	T_3	N_0	M_0
or	$T_1, T_2,$ or T_3	N_1	M_0
• Stage 4	T_4	N_0 or N_1	M_0
or	any T	N_2 or N_3	M_0
or	any T	any N	M_1

Survival is usually measured at 5 years and varies from around 70–80% for Stage 1 disease to 15–20% for Stage 4 disease.

SUMMARY BOX
ORAL CANCER

- Oral cancer globally causes over 350 000 new cases per annum.
- Over 2500 cases of oral cancer occur in the UK per annum.
- There is a wide geographic variation in oral incidence.
- Mortality of oral cancer is around 50% at 5 years.
- Tobacco and alcohol are principal risk factors for oral cancer.
- Intercellular bridges and keratin pearls are key histological features.
- Survival depends on TMN stage and invasion pattern.
- Clinical presentation is variable; any suspicious lesion should be biopsied.

Other neoplasms

As mentioned previously, oral squamous cell carcinoma accounts for over 90% of primary oral cancers. Other causes of primary malignant disease are malignant melanoma, non-Hodgkin's lymphoma, minor salivary gland carcinomas, Kaposi's sarcoma and, rarely, soft tissue, bone and odontogenic malignancies.

Odontogenic tumours arise from the tooth-forming epithelium and mesenchyme and most often occur within the jaw bone, although some are located in the gingivae. Almost all are benign and range from hamartomas to locally invasive behaviour. The best-known example is ameloblastoma, which tends to expand the jaw and undergo cystic change. It is locally infiltrative but does not metastasize and can be cured by resection with a small margin of normal tissue.

Leukoplakia and erythroplakia

Numerous lesions can present in the mouth as white or red patches and their differential diagnosis is beyond the scope of this text. Leukoplakia is defined as a predominantly white lesion that cannot be clinically or pathologically categorized as being due to any other condition. Erythroplakia is similarly defined, except that it is a red patch. Diagnosis is therefore made by exclusion and both lesions have variable clinical and histopathological appearances. Tobacco use is recognized as a major aetiological factor. A significant proportion of lesions show evidence of epithelial dysplasia and a number transform into oral squamous cell carcinomas (see Fig. 10.6). The risk is greater in erythroplakia and in lesions showing dysplasia microscopically. Malignant transformation may occur rapidly or after many years of follow-up in a small proportion of cases, at a rate of approximately 1.5% per year.

SUMMARY BOX
PREMALIGNANT CONDITIONS

- Leukoplakia and erythroplakia are premalignant lesions.
- Tobacco use is a major aetiological factor for both conditions.
- Epithelial dysplasia is a risk factor for malignant change.
- Transformation is more likely in the floor of the mouth and the ventral tongue.
- Diagnosis is clinical and no specific histological features are present.
- Non-homogeneous lesions are more likely to transform than simple plaques.
- Erythroplakia carries a higher risk than leukoplakia.

Fibrous hyperplasia

Chronic irritation of the oral mucosa from habitual biting, ill-fitting dentures and irregular teeth often results in benign swellings in the mouth. There is hyperplasia of the fibrous tissue of the lamina propria and the overlying epithelium often shows hyperkeratosis. These lesions are referred to as fibroepithelial polyps and are treated by excision with elimination of the causative irritative factor.

SALIVARY GLANDS

The salivary glands comprise three paired major glands, the parotid, submandibular and sublingual, together with intraoral minor salivary glands.

Sialadenitis

This is an inflammatory group of disorders which may relate to bacterial or viral infection, obstruction, trauma, irradiation and autoimmune disease.

Acute bacterial sialadenitis mainly involves the parotid gland and is related to ascending infection by *Streptococcus pyogenes*, *Staphylococcus aureus* and *Haemophilus* species. There is swelling, pain, redness of overlying skin and sometimes exudation of pus from the parotid duct. Chronic bacterial sialadenitis affects the submandibular gland more commonly than the parotid and is often related to obstruction by salivary calculus (stone) or low-grade ascending infection. Typically, the patient experiences pain and swelling at meal times and the gland becomes progressively enlarged and fibrotic. Viral infection of the major glands is quite common in childhood and the major cause is the mumps paramyxovirus. After resolution immunity is long-lasting.

Sjögren's syndrome is an autoimmune disorder characterized by lymphocytic infiltration of the salivary and lacrimal glands and the presenting signs are often dry eyes or dry mouth. Primary Sjögren's syndrome involves only the salivary and lacrimal glands. Secondary Sjögren's syndrome includes a connective tissue disorder, most often rheumatoid arthritis. Autoantibodies to extractable nuclear antigens are commonly detectable in Sjögren's syndrome and are important in diagnosis. Malignant non-Hodgkin's lymphoma may arise in the salivary glands in Sjögren's syndrome, usually of mucosa-associated lymphoid tissue (MALT) type.

HIV-associated salivary disease usually involves the parotid gland and is due to the formation of multicystic lesions, intraparotid lymph node swelling or Sjögren's syndrome-like disease.

Salivary gland tumours

Tumours of the salivary glands are uncommon and account for around 3% of all tumours. Most occur in the major salivary glands and over 90% are found in the parotid.

Pleomorphic adenoma

The most common type of salivary gland tumour is the pleomorphic salivary adenoma and this accounts for around 65% of parotid tumours and 45% of minor and submandibular gland tumours. Pleomorphic adenomas are benign and are generally slow growing and painless, presenting as a rubbery nodule (Fig. 10.7). Histopathologically they show a variety of appearances and contain epithelial and myoepithelial cellular elements as well as a characteristic myxoid or chondroid stroma. An important feature is that the connective tissue capsule does not envelope the neoplasm completely. This results in extracapsular extension and, despite the benign nature of the neoplasm, multifocal recurrence can follow enucleation. For this reason the pleomorphic adenoma is normally excised with a small margin of surrounding normal tissue. Malignant transformation of pleomorphic adenoma after many years is well recognized.

Warthin's tumour

This is also a benign lesion which is slow growing and occurs almost exclusively in the parotid gland. Up to 10% of cases have bilateral tumours. The tumours are thought to arise from salivary gland epithelial inclusions in lymph nodes.

Malignant tumours

Malignant tumours of the salivary glands account for around 1% of all cancers and, although rare, there is a relatively high proportion of malignant tumours in the minor glands compared to the parotid gland.

Adenoid cystic carcinoma. This is a relatively slow-growing tumour which arises mostly in middle-aged or elderly patients. Histopathologically it shows a characteristic cribriform (Swiss cheese) pattern. It tends to extend along peripheral nerve branches and has a poor long-term prognosis.

Mucoepidermoid carcinoma. Mucoepidermoid carcinoma is characterized by squamous and mucus-secreting cellular differentiation. Some examples occur in a younger age group and it shows a spectrum of behaviour from low-grade to highly aggressive malignancy.

Acinic cell carcinoma. This is rarer and the cells resemble serous acini or other epithelial elements. Generally acinic cell carcinoma is regarded as low grade but it is difficult to predict its biological behaviour.

Other forms of salivary carcinoma are recognized.

Most malignant lymphomas arising in the salivary glands do so on the basis of pre-existing autoimmune disease in mucosa-associated lymphoid tissue and are typically of low grade.

SUMMARY BOX
SALIVARY GLANDS

- Causes of sialadenitis include infection, irradiation and autoimmune disease.
- Obstructive sialadenitis is most common in the submandibular gland.
- Over 90% of salivary tumours occur in the parotid gland.
- Pleomorphic adenoma is the most common salivary tumour.

PHARYNX

Pharyngitis and tonsillitis are common. Most frequently, acute pharyngitis is caused by virus infection. Streptococcal pharyngitis is important because of its association with important hypersensitivity disorders such as rheumatic fever and Henoch–Schönlein purpura.

Malignant tumours arising in the pharynx include squamous cell carcinoma and non-Hodgkin's lymphoma. Many carcinomas in this site are anaplastic. Nasopharyngeal carcinoma is of particular interest because its epidemiology contrasts with that of oral and oropharyngeal squamous cell carcinoma. Nasopharyngeal carcinoma is rare in the West (under 1%), but in parts of China

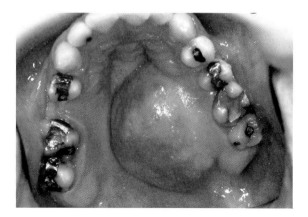

Fig. 10.7 Nodular mass typical of a pleomorphic adenoma of minor salivary gland.

it accounts for almost 50% of all cancers. Epstein–Barr virus infection and genetic susceptibility (HLA-A2 and -BW46) have been implicated in accounting for the high incidence of the disease in China.

OESOPHAGUS, STOMACH AND INTESTINES

OESOPHAGUS

Non-neoplastic diseases

A number of congenital disorders may affect the oesophagus including agenesis, stenosis and atresia which may be associated with a tracheo-oesophageal fistula.

Inflammatory conditions include reflux of gastric contents causing oesophagitis and in severe cases, peptic ulcer disease (see below). Long-term inflammation may lead to metaplastic changes in the oesophagus with a change from the normal squamous lining to gastric columnar type; subsequent intestinal metaplasia may occur in this condition known as Barrett's oesophagus. This is a risk factor for the development of oesophageal neoplasia, especially adenocarcinoma.

The oesophagus may be the site of specific infections, particularly fungal infection with candida, and viral infections with herpes simplex. The features are similar to those seen elsewhere and are especially important in immunosuppressed patients. Less common infections are tuberculosis and Chagas' disease, while the oesophagus may also become inflamed in uraemia and following ingestion of corrosive chemicals.

Mechanical disorders of the oesophagus are relatively common especially hiatus hernia where there is an abnormality of the sphincter mechanism of the lower oesophagus, mainly in the diaphragm, which allows the stomach to move upwards into the thoracic cavity. This predisposes to inflammation such as reflux oesophagitis and peptic ulcer disease.

The oesophagus may become obstructed from tumours (see below), strictures from inflammatory conditions and rare conditions such as achalasia and scleroderma. Rupture of the oesophagus may arise from prolonged vomiting inducing tears in the wall (Mallory–Weiss syndrome), from infiltrating tumours or as a result of medical or surgical procedures such as endoscopy and injection of varices.

Varices are dilated veins, seen especially in the lower one-third of the oesophagus, arising from portal–systemic anastomoses in portal hypertension. They have a tendency to bleed, particularly in patients with chronic liver disease who also have abnormalities of blood clotting.

Carcinoma (Fig. 10.8)

Risk factors for the development of oesophageal carcinomas include excess alcohol consumption, cigarette smoking and the ingestion of nitrosamines or aflatoxins in foods, which may explain the increased incidence in China, Iran and parts of Africa. The Plummer–Vinson syndrome is associated with iron-deficiency anaemia and oesophageal webs and the early development of squamous carcinoma. Barrett's columnar-lined oesophagus is associated with adenocarcinoma in the lower oesophagus. Tumours may be identified in the upper (20%), middle (50%) or lower (20%) oesophagus, while squamous carcinoma accounts for approximately 90% of cancers, with Barrett's oesophagus-associated adeno-

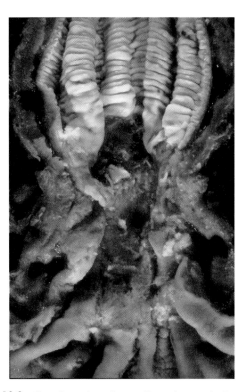

Fig. 10.8 Oesophageal carcinoma. Gross photograph of an oesophagogastrectomy in which there is an infiltrating stenosing tumour in the lower oesophagus. Note the shiny oesophageal squamous epithelium above and the dull gastric columnar epithelium below.

carcinoma accounting for 10% of cases. Patients may present with dysphagia, weight loss or recurrent episodes of aspiration pneumonia. Spread occurs by direct local infiltration into surrounding structures, by lymphatic spread to regional lymph nodes or by haematogenous spread to liver or lung. The prognosis is very poor, with 70% of patients dead within 1 year and a 5-year survival rate of less than 10%.

STOMACH

Peptic ulcer disease

Aetiology/pathogenesis

Peptic ulcers occur as a result of an imbalance between gastric acid production and resistance of the mucosa to this acid by the bicarbonate buffer in the mucous layer. In gastric ulcers, gastric acid levels are mainly normal or even reduced and, thus, impaired cytoprotection is the most likely cause. This is often associated with *Helicobacter pylori* infection of the gastric body region. Patients with autoimmune chronic gastritis (pernicious anaemia) also have an increased risk of gastric ulcer disease. In duodenal ulcers, gastric acid levels are usually high, possibly with an impaired feedback mechanism. The majority (>90%) of duodenal ulcers are associated with chronic antral gastritis due to *H. pylori* infection and in many of these cases it is possible to identify foci of gastric metaplasia in the duodenum, which *H. pylori* may colonize, inducing similar active chronic inflammation. Non-steroidal anti-inflammatory drugs (NSAIDs) are associated with peptic ulcer disease especially in the elderly, probably through their effect on mucosal prostaglandin metabolism.

Helicobacter pylori *and NSAIDs in peptic ulceration*

It is now widely accepted that *H. pylori* plays a causal role in chronic active antral gastritis. Unfortunately the relationship between gastritis and the symptoms of non-ulcer dyspepsia is unclear and eradication of *H. pylori* in this condition is of unpredictable clinical benefit. The best evidence that *H. pylori* plays a causal role in duodenal ulceration (DU) stems from the very substantial protection against ulcer relapse that its eradication affords. Acid and *H. pylori* infection are probably both of crucial importance in duodenal ulcer disease. Ulcers can be kept healed by suppressing either, but in the case of acid this requires long-term drug treatment or surgery, whereas

H. pylori can be eradicated in a large proportion of people by a 1- to 2-week course of two or three drugs, including one or two antibiotics, in combination.

The prevalence of *H. pylori* infection in gastric ulceration (GU) (70–80%) is somewhat lower than in chronic active gastritis and DU (90–100%) and fewer data are available on the effects of eradication, though there is limited evidence that these cases too may gain some protection from relapse. Nevertheless there is a substantial proportion of GU cases (20–30%) that are independent of *H. pylori* infection. Non-steroidal anti-inflammatory drugs (NSAIDs) may be important in these.

For the moment, attempts to eradicate *H. pylori* infection in routine clinical practice are probably best made with a combination of acid suppression therapy and antibiotics active against *H. pylori*. Combinations of a proton pump inhibitor (e.g. omeprazole) with an antibiotic (e.g. amoxycillin or clarithromycin) are effective, although reported eradication rates vary widely (30–95%).

NSAIDs are very widely used and the majority of patients can take them without problems. They are potent inhibitors of prostaglandin synthesis in the gastric mucosa and in a small proportion of cases they may induce or exacerbate peptic ulceration. There is also evidence that they can induce intestinal ulceration and stricture formation and exacerbate inflammatory bowel disease. It is likely that their use in the elderly is contributing to the increase in complicated peptic ulceration seen in this group at a time when complications are on the decline in younger subjects. NSAIDs should not be given lightly to patients with dyspepsia or a history of peptic ulceration, but neither is it good medicine to withhold NSAIDs indiscriminately from these patients if they are severely afflicted with joint disease or other causes of severe pain. The risks and benefits should be discussed with individual patients and consideration given to the co-prescription of an H_2-receptor antagonist or a prostaglandin analogue.

Other general factors may also be implicated in peptic ulceration. Psychological stress (type A individuals) and cigarette smoking increase the risk and various genetic factors including blood group O may predispose to the development of disease. Hypergastrinaemia, most graphically seen in Zollinger–Ellison syndrome (ZES), also increases the risk of ulceration.

Acute peptic ulcers

These may occur at any age and are usually associated with stress, e.g. severe burns (Curling's ulcer), brain damage

(Cushing's ulcer), or drugs, e.g. aspirin, NSAIDs, and possibly alcohol. They present with bleeding, are often multiple, measure up to 1–2 cm in diameter and are seen in the first part of the duodenum or any part of the stomach. They are differentiated from chronic peptic ulcers in the lack of muscularis propria involvement.

Chronic peptic ulcers (Fig. 10.9)

These are decreasing in incidence particularly in the younger age groups, although the incidence of gastric ulcers is increasing in the elderly population, possibly associated with NSAID use. Duodenal ulcer is still predominantly a disease of young males. Chronic ulcers occur in the stomach on the lesser curve, in the first part of the duodenum, at the cardio-oesophageal junction, in Meckel's diverticula or at multiple sites in patients with ZES. Most are solitary and measure between 1 and 3 cm in diameter, although occasionally they are much larger. They have sharply punched out edges with the gastric rugae running right up to the edge. There are distinct layers in the base of the ulcer – a surface layer of poly-

morphs and amorphous debris, a layer of fibrinoid necrosis with underlying granulation tissue, and deep scar tissue involving the muscularis propria (Fig. 10.9B). This may also extend more deeply into serosa or surrounding structures, e.g. pancreas, transverse colon, liver. There is a variable inflammatory infiltrate and blood vessels often show endarteritis obliterans. The immediately adjacent epithelium shows regenerative features occasionally mimicking dysplasia. The epithelium away from the ulcer may show features of *H. pylori*-associated chronic gastritis or gastric metaplasia in the duodenum.

Complications

The complications of peptic ulceration may be predicted from knowledge of the first principles of general pathology. All chronic inflammation will eventually lead to fibrosis and so pyloric stenosis or an 'hourglass' deformity may result. Haemorrhage is almost inevitable from chronic ulcers, either as a slow trickle from granulation tissue leading to positive faecal occult bloods and iron-deficiency anaemia, or more active bleeding from a larger

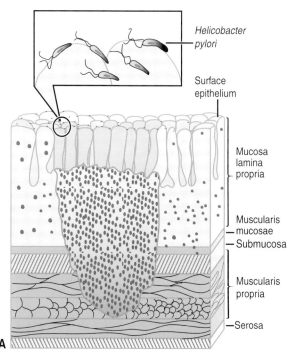
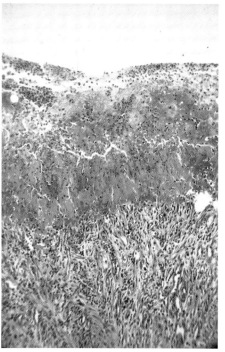

Fig. 10.9   Peptic ulcer. A. In this chronic gastric (peptic) ulcer, there is loss of the superficial epithelium and replacement by necrotic debris on the surface, fibrinopurulent inflammation and granulation tissue below this and a deeper layer of fibrous tissue which extends through the muscularis propria. The adjacent epithelium shows chronic gastritis with *Helicobacter pylori* infection. **B.** Photomicrograph of a typical chronic peptic ulcer showing necrotic debris on the surface with an underlying layer of fibrinopurulent inflammation and a deeper layer of granulation tissue.

artery causing haematemesis or melaena. Occasionally a large artery may become eroded leading to catastrophic, life-threatening bleeding. Fibrous tissue developing gradually is protective but rapidly developing chronic ulcers do not produce much fibrosis and rupture easily, especially anteriorly from the duodenal bulb. The release of gastric acidic contents is extremely irritant to the peritoneum and potentially infective, causing severe peritonitis. If an ulcer perforates into the lesser sac posteriorly it may track upwards into the subphrenic region with abscess formation. As Robbins states: 'cancers often ulcerate, ulcers rarely cancerate.' When carcinoma of the stomach develops in a patient with a proven benign chronic gastric ulcer, it is likely that the original gastric ulcer has not been sampled widely enough and was probably malignant from the beginning. However, evidence is accumulating that risk factors for peptic ulcer disease, particularly *H. pylori*-associated chronic gastritis, may by a process of atrophy and intestinal metaplasia also predispose to gastric carcinoma. While this is an attractive and plausible hypothesis, direct evidence is still lacking.

SUMMARY BOX
PEPTIC ULCER DISEASE

- Imbalance between acid production and mucosal cytoprotection.
- In gastric ulcers, acid levels are low or normal, while in duodenal ulcers acid levels are usually high.
- There is a strong association with *Helicobacter pylori* gastritis in >90% of duodenal ulcers and >70% of gastric ulcers.
- Acute ulcers are associated with stress, burns, raised intracranial pressure, drugs such as aspirin and non-steroidal anti-inflammatories, and alcohol.
- Chronic peptic ulcers are usually solitary and penetrate the muscularis propria.
- Characteristically there are four layers: necrotic debris, fibrinopurulent material, granulation tissue and fibrosis.
- Complications include acute bleeding causing haematemesis or melaena, chronic bleeding causing iron-deficiency anaemia, fibrosis causing obstruction, and very rarely carcinoma.

Chronic gastritis

This is defined as inflammation of the stomach where the main inflammatory cell type is mononuclear (lymphocyte or plasma cell). It may occur predominantly in the gastric body (corpus) region or the gastric antrum, occasionally affecting both in equal measure (pangastritis).

Autoimmune-type chronic gastritis. Body gastritis alone is often associated with atrophy and intestinal metaplasia and is seen in patients with autoantibodies directed against gastric parietal cells or intrinsic factor (pernicious anaemia).

Bacterial gastritis. Antral-predominant gastritis or pangastritis (both body and antrum) is most commonly seen in *H. pylori* infection, the former especially in duodenal ulcer patients and the latter in gastric ulcer disease. There may also be more active (neutrophilic) inflammation and also atrophy or metaplasia.

Chemical gastritis. This is often seen in stomachs where there is reflux of duodenal (biliary and alkaline) contents through a damaged or surgically absent pylorus; rarer forms include lymphocytic, eosinophilic and granulomatous gastritis.

SUMMARY BOX
CHRONIC GASTRITIS

- Autoimmune: type A chronic gastritis, associated with autoantibodies against parietal cells and intrinsic factor; leads to pernicious anaemia, glandular atrophy and intestinal metaplasia; increased risk of gastric carcinoma.
- Bacterial: type B gastritis, associated with *Helicobacter pylori* infection; causes active chronic inflammation and later atrophy and intestinal metaplasia; strong association with peptic ulceration, duodenal > gastric.
- Chemical: type C gastritis; associated with chemical injury such as bile reflux and non-steroidal anti-inflammatory drugs.

Gastric carcinoma

This has been decreasing in incidence over the last 50 years for reasons which are not clear. The tumour is particularly common in Japan, Chile and Iceland, where the ingestion of smoked foods is high. The effects of environmental influences are further supported by the decreased incidence in Japanese migrants to the USA, compared with native Japanese and the intermediate group of Hawaii-based Japanese. Nitrosamines are thought to be the most important factor. It is a tumour of late middle-aged and elderly people and is more common in males. A number of precancerous lesions are recognized, including pernicious anaemia (chronic atrophic gastritis), neoplastic polyps and possibly intestinal metaplasia, which may be linked with *H. pylori* infection, although evidence for this suggestion is still lacking.

Morphology

The tumour may present in an early phase – early gastric cancer – when the tumour is confined to the mucosa and submucosa of the stomach, without evidence of lymph node spread. This is seen particularly in countries such as Japan, where population screening is performed and thus identifies earlier cases. This is reflected in the excellent 5-year survival figures of 85%. In contrast, the tumour in low-prevalence countries such as the UK usually presents at a more advanced stage. There are a number of appearances possible:

- a fungating exophytic growth projecting into the gastric lumen
- a malignant ulcer with raised rolled edges with loss of the normal rugal pattern at the margins (Fig. 10.10)
- a diffusely infiltrating lesion with thickening and contraction of the stomach giving the so-called leather bottle appearance (linitis plastica).

Ulcerating lesions may be difficult to differentiate clinically and multiple biopsies are required to separate benign from malignant pathologies.

Histopathology

Microscopically, the vast majority of gastric tumours are adenocarcinomas of varying differentiation. Well-formed glands may be seen, but particularly in the diffusely infiltrative type, individual signet ring cells may be seen with an intense stromal desmoplastic fibrotic response.

Spread

The spread of gastric carcinoma is one of the best exam-ples of spread of malignant tumours in general. There may be direct local spread into surrounding structures such as pancreas, transverse colon, spleen and liver. Lymphatic spread into local and regional groups occurs early and when the thoracic duct is involved, there may be back pressure into the left supraclavicular node group (Virchow's node) which is one of the classical modes of presentation. Haematogenous spread to liver and lungs also may be noted early in the course of disease. As the tumour spreads through the gastric wall, individual tumour cells and clusters may seed in the omentum and mesentery, and with peritoneal fluid involvement, meta-stasis may be seen in the ovary (Krukenberg tumour) and rectovesical pouch.

Prognosis

This depends on the stage of the tumour, i.e. the depth of invasion of the primary tumour and its consequent risk of metastasis. Early gastric cancer, as seen in Japan, has a 5-year survival of 85%, but it must be remembered that in the UK only 5–10% of tumours will be identified at this stage. Tumours with full-thickness wall involvement without lymph node spread have a 30% 5-year survival but similar full-thickness tumours with positive lymph nodes have a 5% 5-year survival.

SUMMARY BOX
GASTRIC CARCINOMA

- Geographical variations suggest that environmental factors are important.
- Predisposing conditions include pernicious anaemia and intestinal metaplasia; the role of *Helicobacter pylori* infection is less clear.
- Most cases present at an advanced stage and have a poor prognosis.
- Early gastric cancers have a good prognosis but are identified infrequently in western populations.
- Gastric carcinomas may spread locally into surrounding tissues, via lymphatics to regional and distal lymph nodes, via the bloodstream to liver and lungs and transcoelomically to the peritoneum and ovaries.

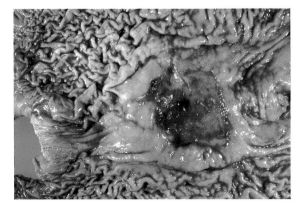

Fig. 10.10 Gross photograph of an ulcerating tumour of the stomach with raised rolled edges and loss of the adjacent rugae, typical of adenocarcinoma.

SMALL INTESTINE

Malabsorption

This is a clinical syndrome characterized by increased faecal fat excretion (steatorrhoea) and the systemic effects of deficiency of vitamins, minerals, proteins and carbohydrates; not all of these features need necessarily be present in all patients and some patients may have malabsorption of specific dietary contents.

Inadequate digestion

The normal digestion of food requires the interaction of gastric, pancreatic and biliary secretions, even before absorption across the bowel wall can take place. Thus, post-gastrectomy patients lacking gastric digestive action may malabsorb, and various pancreatic conditions such as chronic pancreatitis, cystic fibrosis and previous surgical resection cause a lack of pancreatic enzymes such as lipase, amylase and trypsin with resulting impaired absorption of fats, carbohydrates and proteins. Bile salts secreted by the liver via gall bladder bile are important for fat emulsification and absorption of fat-soluble vitamins (A, D, E and K); normally bile salts are reabsorbed in the terminal ileum and thus diseases affecting this region such as Crohn's disease may impair upper small bowel function. Obstructive jaundice for whatever reason and bacterial overgrowth syndromes (jejunal diverticulosis, post-surgical blind loops) may cause a lack of functional bile salts, and some drugs, e.g. cholestyramine and neomycin, may precipitate bile salts. Some endocrine disorders, e.g. carcinoid syndrome, VIPoma (Verner–Morrison syndrome) and Zollinger–Ellison syndrome, may also cause malabsorption by impairing the digestive phase.

Primary mucosal disease

When the preabsorption digestive phase has taken place, an adequate amount of functioning mucosa is required for the uptake of the broken-down fats, carbohydrates and proteins in their constituent fatty acid, saccharide and amino acid forms. The most important disease causing malabsorption in the western world is coeliac disease (see below) while tropical sprue and post-infective malabsorption are more common on a global basis. A less common condition affecting the mucosa is Whipple's disease (intestinal lipodystrophy) which is a multisystem disorder, involving lymph nodes, joints, heart, lungs and brain, with a characteristic histiocytic infiltrate in the lamina propria of the upper small intestine in which periodic acid–Schiff (PAS)-positive bacillary bodies are seen; this condition responds to antibiotic therapy. Biochemical abnormalities such as abetalipoproteinaemia, disaccharidase deficiencies and malabsorption of specific

amino acids, e.g. Hartnup disease, are examples of selective malabsorption syndromes. Radiation enteritis may reduce the functional mass of cells available for absorption, while amyloid deposition in vessels and lamina propria may have a similar effect. An inadequate quantity of functionally normal small intestine, e.g. after surgical resection, jejunoileal bypass for obesity and mesenteric vascular disease with infarction, will also lead to malabsorption. Reduction or complete obstruction of lymphatic drainage from the lamina propria and submucosa may cause malabsorption particularly of fats. This occurs secondary to disease of intra-abdominal lymph nodes, such as lymphoma or tuberculosis, or as a primary, usually congenital, abnormality of lymph drainage. Microscopically, there is dilatation of lymphatic channels in the mucosa and submucosa (intestinal lymphangiectasia).

Coeliac disease

This is also known as non-tropical sprue or gluten-sensitive enteropathy and is caused by a T-lymphocyte-mediated hypersensitivity reaction to the α-gliadin fraction of the wheat protein gluten. This is a rare condition which is seen more often in people of Irish and Scottish extraction and has a strong familial tendency with specific HLA associations (HLA-B8/DW3). Patients may present with recurrent oral ulceration and serologically there may be antibodies against gliadin and endomyseum. The diagnosis is suggested on small intestinal biopsy (either by Crosby capsule or by direct endoscopic biopsy). The normal small intestinal architecture shows a basal proliferative crypt zone and a taller villous component, the normal ratio of which is 1:3 or 4. It is the villous component with its surface microvilli which provides the surface area for normal absorption in the small bowel, and in coeliac disease there are variable degrees of villous atrophy with crypt hyperplasia. There are also increased numbers of T lymphocytes in the surface epithelium and of plasma cells in the lamina propria. The dissecting microscopic appearances reflect the severity of disease, showing the variation from the normal 'finger-like' pattern to partial atrophy through subtotal atrophy to total atrophy patterns. The diagnosis is confirmed by the response clinically and pathologically to withdrawal of gluten from the diet. Complications include splenic atrophy in adults, dermatitis herpetiformis, and an increased risk of small intestinal lymphoma (enteropathy-associated T cell lymphoma, previously known as malignant histiocytosis of the intestine) and of extracolonic epithelial malignancy.

- Clinically, malabsorption may present with diarrhoea and the effects of lack of vitamins, minerals, proteins and carbohydrates.

- Malabsorption may be due to inadequate digestion from pancreatic or gastric disease, a lack of enzymes such as sucrase or lactase, or from small intestinal disease.

- The commonest cause is coeliac disease (gluten-sensitive enteropathy); it is diagnosed on small intestinal biopsy where villous atrophy and crypt hyperplasia are seen; long-term complications include enteropathy-associated T cell lymphoma.

Small bowel neoplasia

Adenocarcinoma of the small intestine is extremely rare, except in the region of the ampulla of Vater where it may be associated with colonic polyposis syndromes and in cases of Crohn's disease where there is a slightly increased incidence. The commonest neoplasm of the small intestine is lymphoma. The small bowel is a very active immunological site, where there is a well-developed 'homing' system for circulating B cells, mainly of IgA type. Thus, most lymphomas are of non-Hodgkin's type of B cell origin and have a reasonably good prognosis when confined to the bowel. In the Mediterranean basin, there is a form of lymphoma known as α-chain disease associated with immunoproliferative small intestinal disease (IPSID), possibly precipitated by infection. There is also an increased risk of lymphoma in gluten-sensitive enteropathy (coeliac disease) but in this case, the neoplastic cell is of T cell type, as would be predicted from the immunopathological basis of this condition. Burkitt's type lymphoma may be seen particularly in Africans.

Carcinoid tumours are the second commonest neoplasm occurring in the small intestine (see 'Appendix' below).

Tumours of mesenchymal origin are also relatively common in the gastrointestinal tract, particularly in the small intestine. The commonest of these is of smooth muscle type, which may achieve a large size. Modes of presentation include ulceration with bleeding and anaemia, intestinal obstruction or intussusception. The differentiation of benign from malignant is difficult and relies on a number of features including size, mitotic rate and presence or absence of necrosis. Again, the only reliable feature is the development of metastasis. Other mesenchymal tissues may produce intestinal tumours, especially adipose tissue (lipomas/liposarcomas), nerves

(neurofibromas/neurofibrosarcomas) and blood vessels (haemangiomas/angiosarcomas).

APPENDIX

The commonest condition affecting the appendix is acute appendicitis. This is a disease of western populations, probably associated with a low-fibre diet, which affects children and adolescents mainly. It occurs because of obstruction of the appendiceal lumen by faecoliths (concretions of faeces), lymphoid hyperplasia, parasites such as *Oxyuris vermicularis*, Crohn's disease and rarely carcinoid tumours (see below). The disease starts with mucosal ulceration and then is followed by a transmural polymorph infiltrate. There is a risk of perforation with development of peritonitis or, if contained locally within the right iliac fossa, an appendix abscess. Rarely, inflammation will spread via the portal venous system (portal pylephlebitis) to the liver, causing abscess formation. Clinically, patients present first with periumbilical pain and vomiting. The pain later spreads to the right iliac fossa where there may be tenderness and guarding. Treatment is by surgical removal (appendicectomy), sooner rather than later to avoid the complications of peritonitis and abscess formation.

Carcinoid tumours

These are tumours derived from the neuroendocrine cells normally present in the gut, which secrete a variety of amines and hormones, especially serotonin (5-hydroxytryptamine). The commonest site of origin is the appendix but may also be found in the ileum, rectum, stomach and colon. Grossly, these tumours are yellow and arise in the submucosa; from there they may ulcerate the overlying mucosa or infiltrate into the muscularis or serosa. Histologically, the cells are small, round and relatively uniform, and grow in nests and cords. The secretory products can be demonstrated by histochemical, immunohistochemical and electron microscopic means. Most of these tumours are asymptomatic and are found incidentally at appendicectomy for example. The vast majority are benign and do not metastasize; it is not possible to predict clinical behaviour on histological grounds. However, a proportion of carcinoid tumours (5% of appendiceal, 15% of rectal and 60% of ileal tumours) may become malignant. This can only be reliably recognized when metastasis, predominantly to the liver, has occurred. The liver normally inactivates serotonin to

5-hydroxyindoleacetic acid (5HIAA; the basis of bio-chemical diagnosis) but when metastases overwhelm the liver's capacity, then the carcinoid syndrome may ensue. This is characterized by smooth muscle stimulation, causing cramps, diarrhoea and bronchospasm, by vaso-dilatation causing episodic flushing in the skin, and by cardiac valve (pulmonary and tricuspid) fibrosis.

COLON AND RECTUM

Inflammatory bowel disease

Idiopathic inflammatory bowel disease includes Crohn's disease and ulcerative colitis. Other conditions which can mimic the presentation of these two entities include ischaemic colitis, radiation colitis, antibiotic-associated (pseudomembranous) colitis and other rarer conditions for which underlying causes can usually be recognized.

Crohn's disease

This is a chronic inflammatory condition which may affect any part of the whole gastrointestinal tract, from mouth to anus. Most commonly it affects the terminal ileum and the colon. In the oral cavity, patients may present with lip swelling, granulomatous gingivitis, mucosal tags, cobblestone mucosa and deep fissured oral ulcers. The disease appears to be increasing in incidence and is seen most frequently in northwestern Europe and the USA. Both sexes are affected equally and the disease may occur at any age, although it has its highest incidence in young adults. There is not uncommonly (20–30%) a positive family history, although this may include either Crohn's disease or ulcerative colitis. The cause is un-known. A similar disease in cattle (Johne's disease) is caused by mycobacteria, although the evidence in humans for an infectious cause is lacking. Immuno-logical injury is also postulated as an aetiological mecha-nism, particularly as the granulomas characteristically seen in Crohn's disease are reminiscent of a type IV hypersensitivity reaction. Occasionally antibodies against colonic epithelial components are seen and T lymphocyte dysfunction may be apparent.

Gross appearances (Fig. 10.11A). Ileal disease alone (30%) or in combination with colonic disease (50%) is the most common site of involvement, while colonic disease alone (20%) is less frequent. Many patients with Crohn's disease (75%) have perianal lesions such as abscesses, fistulas and skin tags, regardless of rectal

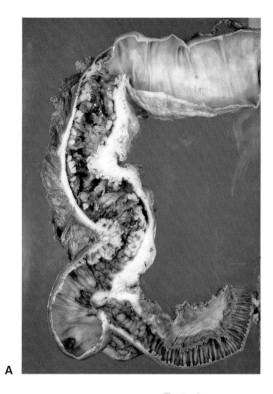

A

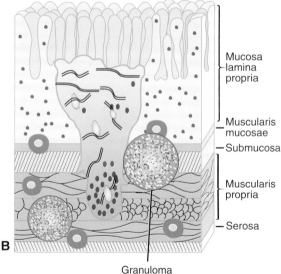

B

Mucosa
lamina propria

Muscularis mucosae

Submucosa

Muscularis propria

Serosa

Granuloma

Fig. 10.11 Crohn's disease. A. Part of a right hemicolectomy specimen in which there is involvement of the terminal ileum and part of the ascending colon, with sparing of the caecum and transverse colon. The mucosa in the involved areas shows ulceration and cobblestoning, with thickening and fibrosis of the wall. The appearances are typical of Crohn's disease. **B.** Transmural inflammation affecting all layers of the bowel wall (mucosa, submucosa, muscularis and serosa). There is fissuring ulceration extending from mucosa into muscularis propria and in places non-caseating epithelioid granulomas are present, along with lymphoid follicles.

involvement. The disease is typically segmental in distribution with large areas of uninvolved bowel intervening between abnormal areas ('skip lesions'). In the acute phase, the bowel is swollen, reddened and ulcerated. More chronically, there is thickening and rigidity ('hosepipe thickening') with fibrosis causing luminal narrowing and obstruction. The serosa is dull and granular and there may be 'fat-wrapping' in the involved segment, where the mesenteric fat surrounds the anti-mesenteric serosa. As in the oral cavity, the mucosa may have areas of serpiginous ulceration with adjacent oedematous, hyperplastic mucosa, creating a 'cobblestoned' appearance. The ulcers may be superficial and shallow or deep and fissuring, the latter penetrating into the wall causing adhesions or fistulas between the bowel and adjacent structures.

Microscopic appearances (Fig. 10.11B). There is typically transmural inflammation with mucosal crypt distortion, fissuring ulcers, neuronal hyperplasia, lymphoid follicles and fibrosis. The most characteristic feature is the presence of non-caseating epithelioid granulomas in any of the bowel layers but this feature is seen only in 60–70% of patients. The diagnosis is made on the basis of a combination of clinical, radiological and pathological features and it is important to remember that overlap may occur with ulcerative colitis and other conditions.

Complications. These relate mainly to fibrosis causing obstruction, and to fistula formation between small bowel and small bowel, small and large bowel, bowel and vagina, bowel and bladder, and bowel and skin. There may be malabsorption, particularly if there is terminal ileal disease, of vitamin B_{12} and bile salts leading to megaloblastic anaemia and fat malabsorption respectively, the latter because bile salts are required for the emulsification of fats and fat-soluble vitamins in the upper small bowel. Chronic iron-deficiency anaemia may result from blood loss, and protein-losing enteropathy may also occur. Extracolonic manifestations include arthritis, ankylosing spondylitis if the patient is HLA-B27-positive, and uveitis. There is a small increased risk of colonic carcinoma.

Ulcerative colitis (UC)

This is a chronic inflammatory condition of the large bowel of unknown aetiology with a tendency to relapses and remissions. The disease commonly presents in the third decade, but may occur at any age, and is slightly more frequent in females. It is seen most often in western Europe and North America. No infectious agent has been identified but antibodies cross-reacting between intesti-

nal epithelial cells and certain *Escherichia coli* serotypes may be found in the serum of some patients with the disease. An allergy to food proteins has been speculated as a cause and the disease may be precipitated by psychological stress. A positive family history may be recognized in up to 30% of cases, but the history may be of either UC or Crohn's disease.

Gross appearances (Fig. 10.12A). This condition primarily involves the rectum (in almost all cases) and spreads proximally in a continuous manner, sometimes to involve the whole colon – 'pancolitis'. The appendix may

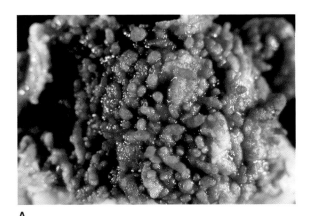

A

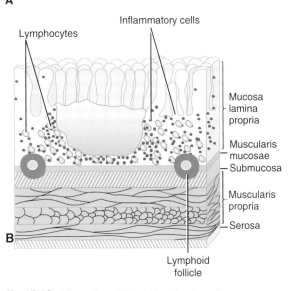

B

Fig. 10.12 Ulcerative colitis. A. Pseudopolyps. Gross photograph of a colon showing extensive involvement with ulcerative colitis. There is regenerative activity in the epithelium adjacent to areas of ulceration, producing a pseudopolypoid appearance. **B.** In ulcerative colitis, all of the inflammatory process is present above the muscularis mucosae in the mucosa, involving the epithelium and lamina propria. There is a shallow ulcer with surrounding inflammation composed of polymorphs and mononuclear cells, mainly lymphocytes.

be affected and the ileum for a few centimetres may show non-specific inflammatory changes known as 'backwash ileitis'. UC is a disease almost exclusively of the mucosa, except in the rare instance where there is severe acute disease, including involvement of all bowel layers with dilatation, thinning and possible rupture – so-called 'toxic megacolon'. The mucosa is diffusely hyperaemic in the acute phase with superficial ulcers. In the recovery and chronic phases, there is regeneration of the epithelium, producing inflammatory 'pseudopolyps', while elsewhere the mucosa may be atrophic.

Microscopic appearances (Fig. 10.12B). Histologically, the inflammatory infiltrate which involves the lamina propria comprises neutrophil polymorphs, lymphocytes and plasma cells. Neutrophils may be seen in crypt epithelium and lumina – 'crypt abscesses' – and there may be depletion of goblet cells. In the chronic disease, there is crypt loss and distortion with abnormal architecture and branching. Metaplastic features including a change to gastric pyloric glands and to Paneth cells may also be seen. Usually, the inflammation is confined by the muscularis mucosae although, occasionally, the submucosa is involved; the muscularis propria is not affected.

Diagnosis depends on a combination of clinical, radiological and pathological features. Differentiation from Crohn's disease on endoscopic biopsy material may be difficult since superficial ulceration, crypt abscesses and mucosal distortion may be seen in either condition. Multiple biopsies showing a mixture of normal and abnormal features are more likely to be from Crohn's disease and the finding of a non-caseating epithelioid granuloma is only seen in Crohn's disease. However, food granulomas and disrupted crypts with mucus granulomas may be seen in both diseases.

Complications. The complications of UC include anaemia and electrolyte imbalances due to ulceration and bleeding. This may be particularly marked in toxic megacolon which may cause perforation and has a high mortality rate. Extracolonic disease is especially seen in UC and includes arthritis, ankylosing spondylitis, uveitis, a necrotic skin condition of the extremities known as pyoderma gangrenosum, oral pyostomatitis vegetans and sclerosing cholangitis, which causes fibrosis around bile ducts leading to obstructive jaundice. Chronic ulcerative colitis carries an overall increased risk of carcinoma of about 10%, which is related to severity and extent of disease and its duration. The risk is greater in severe pancolitis of greater than 20 years' standing but many patients now have elective panproctocolectomies for severe symptomatic disease or where dysplasia is recognized on surveillance biopsies. The most common procedure now is the formation of an ileoanal reservoir ('pouch') rather than an ileostomy. These pouches may develop a peculiar form of inflammation known as 'pouchitis' which may represent recurrence of the original disease in the neorectum.

Ischaemic colitis

The left side of the colon is supplied with blood via the inferior mesenteric artery, which is often involved in aortic atheroma or aneurysm formation particularly in the elderly. Although collateral supplies develop, the circulation to the splenic flexure region may be compromised by episodes of hypotension. This may lead to foci of mucosal necrosis and superficial ulceration with rectal bleeding. Most episodes resolve but occasionally healing by fibrosis with stricture formation may occur.

More widespread ischaemia, involving small and large bowel ('ischaemic enterocolitis'), may occur in shock, congestive cardiac failure or uraemia, possibly accompanied by hypotension and/or disseminated intravascular coagulation. Frank infarction of the bowel develops when there is complete occlusion of a major vessel, such as the superior mesenteric artery. This may be either by thrombosis superimposed on severe atheroma or by embolism from the chambers of the heart, i.e. from the left ventricle in post-myocardial infarction mural thrombosis or from the left atrium in mitral valve disease and/or atrial fibrillation.

Angiodysplasia

This condition is increasingly being recognized as a cause of rectal bleeding in an elderly population, where other causes such as inflammatory bowel disease, ischaemia, carcinoma and diverticular disease have been excluded. Although it may occur in any part of the gut, angiodysplasia is most commonly seen in the caecum and ascending colon where numerous thin-walled, dilated, tortuous blood vessels can be demonstrated in the mucosa and submucosa. Rupture of these vessels causes painless bleeding and the diagnosis is made by selective mesenteric angiography. Treatment is by local resection.

Pseudomembranous colitis

This condition complicates treatment with certain antibiotics, particularly lincomycin, clindamycin, ampicillin and tetracycline (all of which may routinely be prescribed by dentists). This alters the intestinal bacterial flora allowing an overgrowth of *Clostridium difficile*, whose exotoxin binds to epithelial cells and exerts a cytotoxic effect resulting in superficial necrosis and ulceration and acute inflammation. The necrotic debris attaches to the mucosa as yellow plaques or pseudomembranes. This may occur diffusely throughout the colon. The microscopic appearance is of a volcano-like fibrinopurulent exudate overlying necrotic epithelium and acutely inflamed lamina propria. The disease presents with severe diarrhoea including blood and mucus and may be rapidly fatal; it is treatable with vancomycin.

Radiation colitis

Exposure of the bowel to ionizing radiation may occur in the treatment of Hodgkin's disease, intra-abdominal malignancy and cervical carcinoma. The initial damage is usually mild leading to diarrhoea and, if the small bowel is affected, to malabsorption. Delayed effects may be seen many years later owing to progressive occlusion of blood vessels, leading to essentially ischaemia-mediated damage. This leads to ulceration and stricture formation. Microscopically there may be mucosal atrophy, vascular hyalinization and atypical mesenchymal cells ('radiation fibroblasts').

SUMMARY BOX
INFLAMMATORY BOWEL DISEASE

- Crohn's disease and ulcerative colitis are the two commonest forms, although other conditions such as ischaemic colitis, radiation colitis and pseudomembranous colitis can mimic them.
- Crohn's disease:
  - may affect any part of the gastrointestinal tract from mouth to anus
  - inflammation is typically transmural
  - in 60–70% of cases non-caseating epithelioid granulomas may be found
  - complications include fistula formation, fibrosis and obstruction.
- Ulcerative colitis:
  - affects only the large bowel
  - typically starts in the rectum and spreads proximally but may affect the whole of the colon
  - inflammation is superficial involving only the mucosa
  - complications include acute toxic megacolon, perforation and haemorrhage
  - chronic disease may cause anaemia and increased risk of colonic carcinoma.
- Both conditions are associated with extraintestinal manifestations including liver disease, skin conditions, arthritis and inflammation of the eyes.

Neoplasms
Colonic polyps

Polyps are simply projections above an epithelial surface and may be composed of a number of tissue types. The type of polyp is usually qualified on its aetiological basis and thus there are:

- inflammatory polyps
- hamartomatous polyps (juvenile and Peutz–Jeghers types)
- metaplastic (hyperplastic) polyps
- neoplastic polyps.

Inflammatory polyps are associated with inflammatory bowel disease and have no neoplastic potential. Hamartomas are tumour-like conditions composed of variable amounts of tissues indigenous to a particular anatomical region arranged in a haphazard manner. In the large bowel, the two commonest types are (a) juvenile polyps composed of cystically dilated glands set in an inflamed stroma lacking smooth muscle and (b) Peutz–Jeghers polyps composed of proliferating glands set in a stroma rich in smooth muscle. Both may occur singly or in association with polyposis syndromes; occurring alone they have little increased risk of malignancy. Metaplastic (hyperplastic) polyps are common lesions which are seen mainly in the sigmoid colon and rectum and are composed of stellate glands with serrated surface epithelium. They do not have any intrinsic malignant potential but are often seen in bowels containing neoplastic polyps and are said to be a marker of at-risk populations.

Neoplastic polyps are of three main types histologically: (a) tubular adenomas, (b) tubulovillous adenomas and (c) villous adenomas, depending on the relative composition of small tubular glands and taller villous glands (Fig. 10.13). They are now generally accepted to be the main precursor lesions for colorectal carcinoma and the risk of progression of these polyps, although low, depends on the size of the polyp (< 1 cm: < 10%; 1–2 cm: 10–30%; > 2 cm: > 50%), the histological type (villous > tubulovillous > tubular) and the degree of epithelial dysplasia (severe > moderate > mild); the more polyps a patient has the greater the risk of malignancy.

Colonic polyposis syndromes

Familial adenomatous polyposis (FAP) is a genetically inherited syndrome, associated with a mutation of the APC gene on chromosome 5. Patients suspected of having FAP are screened from their mid-teens onwards

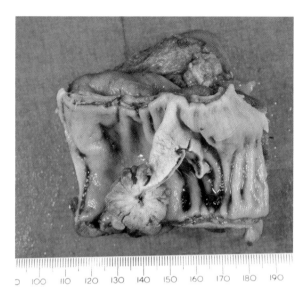

Fig. 10.13 **Gross photograph of a solitary neoplastic polyp of colon.** Note the pedunculated stalk.

for signs of colonic polyps and there is a latent period of approximately 15 years before the inevitable development of colorectal carcinoma which may be multiple. The extent of disease may be so great as to produce a 'shag pile carpet' appearance of the colon. Most patients now have an elective panproctocolectomy with pouch formation before carcinoma develops; there is also a need for genetic counselling in these patients since FAP has an autosomal dominant pattern of inheritance. FAP may present with extracolonic manifestations including jaw osteomas, odontomes, other dento-osseous abnormalities, desmoid tumours and congenital hypertrophy of the retinal pigment epithelium, some of which are part of Gardner's syndrome. Turcot syndrome is FAP associated with malignant tumours of the central nervous system. Hereditary non-polyposis colorectal cancer (HNPCC) is another inherited condition with specific chromosomal abnormalities, which may also have extracolonic neoplasms as part of the presentation.

Hamartomatous polyps may also form part of a polyposis syndrome. Juvenile polyps occur mainly in the large bowel and present with rectal bleeding or prolapse of a polyp. There is a slight increase in the risk of malignancy. The polyps in Peutz–Jeghers syndrome are most commonly found in the small bowel. There is an association with perioral pigmentation and theca/granulosa cell tumours in the ovary. There is also a slight increased risk of malignancy.

Carcinoma of the colon and rectum (Fig. 10.14)

Most of these (75%) occur in the left side of colon within 25–30 cm of the anal canal, although the incidence of right-sided tumours (caecum and ascending colon) is increasing, particularly in women. Predisposing lesions include neoplastic polyps, most of which are sporadic but may be inherited (see above), and long-standing chronic inflammatory bowel disease, especially ulcerative colitis. Right-sided colonic tumours tend to be large, polypoid, non-circumferential lesions which present with occult bleeding and anaemia whereas left-sided tumours tend to be smaller, circumferential, stenosing lesions ('napkin ring') which present with frank bleeding, altered bowel habit, alternating diarrhoea and constipation, or obstruction. Either form may present with constitutional symptoms of weight loss, pain or evidence of distal metastases. Rectal tumours may present as malignant ulcers with raised rolled edges. Histologically, most colorectal tumours are moderately well-differentiated adenocarcinomas, although mucinous (colloid) forms may also be seen. These tumours are staged by the Dukes' system on the basis of the extent of invasion through the wall and

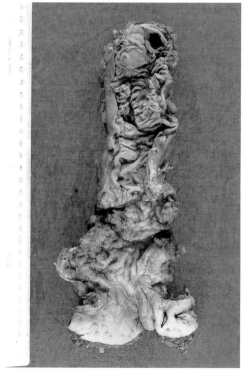

Fig. 10.14 **Gross photograph of an abdominoperineal resection of a low rectal carcinoma showing stenosis of the lumen by a polypoid tumour.**

the presence or absence of lymph node spread; this staging system has prognostic significance.

- Dukes' A tumours are confined to mucosa and sub-mucosa and have a greater than 90% 5-year survival.
- Dukes' B tumours have spread through the muscularis propria without lymph node involvement and have a 60% 5-year survival rate.
- Dukes' C tumours have extended through the full thickness of the bowel wall with lymph node spread and have approximately 25% survival at 5-years.
- These tumours may also spread haematogenously via the portal venous system, producing liver metastases, so-called Dukes' D tumours, which are associated with a poor prognosis (less than 10% survival at 5 years).

SUMMARY BOX
COLORECTAL NEOPLASIA

- Most carcinomas of the colon and rectum arise from pre-existing neoplastic polyps.
- The adenoma–carcinoma sequence is well established in morphological and molecular terms, with much of the information derived from the rare inherited conditions of familial adenomatous polyposis and hereditary non-polyposis colorectal cancer.
- Adenomas may be tubular, tubulovillous or villous in type.
- The risk of developing malignancy is related to the size of the polyp, the histological type and the degree of epithelial dysplasia.
- Most colorectal carcinomas arise on the left side of the colon and present with obstruction or a change in bowel habit, although right-sided tumours are increasing in incidence, especially in women, and present with iron-deficiency anaemia.
- Prognosis is related to the extent of spread of tumour through the bowel wall and to adjacent lymph nodes, as described in the Dukes staging system.

LIVER, GALL BLADDER AND PANCREAS

LIVER

Hepatitis

This literally means any inflammation of the liver. However, the term is usually reserved for inflammation with diffuse involvement of the liver, and thus excludes focal lesions such as abscesses, which may spread from other sources, e.g. pylephlebitis in acute appendicitis.

Other infections which may affect the liver include tuberculosis (discussed in detail elsewhere), leptospirosis, protozoal infections such as amoebiasis, rickettsial infections such as Q fever, fungal infections such as histoplasmosis, and parasitic infections such as hydatid cysts and infection with the flatworm *Clonorchis sinensis*.

Acute viral hepatitis

Most cases of acute viral hepatitis show a similar histological and clinical pattern with some minor differences allowing separation of the various types.

Hepatitis A virus (HAV). This is a DNA virus with a short incubation period (usually 4 weeks, range 2–6 weeks) which causes an acute hepatitis only, which always resolves, although about 50% are asymptomatic. There is no chronic hepatitis and there is no chronic viral carriage. It is transmitted by the faecal–oral route, and may be shed in the stools during the incubation period and for a short time after the onset of hepatitis. There may be water-borne, community (e.g. prisons, boarding schools, long-term mental institutions) and nosocomial outbreaks. Recent infection can be identified serologically by an IgM antibody response, and previous infection by a positive IgG antibody titre.

Hepatitis B virus (HBV). This is a DNA virus transmitted by parenteral/mucocutaneous exposure to infected blood or secretions. It has a long incubation period, usually 2–3 months with a range of 1–6 months. The virus can be transmitted by both acutely or chronically infected patients, including those who are asymptomatic carriers. It was particularly common after blood transfusion, although the introduction of blood donor screening has greatly reduced this mode of transmission, but is nowadays seen especially in intravenous drug abusers and may also be transmitted in the perinatal period from mother to child. It is an uncommon disease in the UK (virus carriage about 1:1000) but it is found in about 5% of the population of the Asian subcontinent and in 20% or more of the Far Eastern population. It can be prevented by screening of infected blood or blood products and those exposed occupationally to needlestick injury can be given HBV immune globulin. A vaccine is available, nowadays usually of recombinant type, which provides protection for up to 10 years and is offered to individuals at risk of exposure, such as health care workers including dentists and dental students. Three doses are given at 0, 1 and 6 months and seroconversion is confirmed by blood testing; a significant minority of those vaccinated require a booster dose. A minority of patients are asymptomatic and approximately 20% progress to chronic liver disease. It is a known cause in the longer term of hepatocellular carcinoma.

Serological diagnosis. This includes the identification of hepatitis B surface antigen (the Australia antigen; indicating acute or chronic infection or the carrier state), hepatitis B surface antibody (indicating past, resolved HBV infection), hepatitis B e antigen positivity (indicating active viral replication), hepatitis B e antibody positivity (indicating lower infectivity), hepatitis B core IgM antibody reactivity indicating recent infection and hepatitis B core antibody positivity (indicating either recent or old HBV infection). Accurate diagnosis requires a combination of tests and the detection of serum HBV DNA may also be needed.

Hepatitis C virus (HCV). This virus was previously known as the main cause of non-A non-B hepatitis. It is an RNA virus of relatively short incubation, up to 40 days. It may cause an acute hepatitis like the other viruses, but in a high proportion of cases it may be asymptomatic but nonetheless progress to chronic hepatitis in up to 80% of cases. Transmission is by blood transfusion (although screening is now available), organ transplantation, intravenous drug abuse and parenteral/mucocutaneous exposure to blood or secretions, but it is much less contagious than HBV. No vaccines or immunoglobulin are currently available and therefore care with sterilization techniques and blood donor screening is required to reduce transmission. Like HBV, it is thought to be associated with the development of hepatocellular carcinoma, although the link is less clear cut than with HBV. Diagnosis is initially suggested by positive antibody responses, although seroconversion may occur late. The current gold standard for diagnosis is the use of the polymerase chain reaction (PCR) test in serum.

Hepatitis D virus (delta agent). This is an incomplete virus which requires HBV for its replication, but otherwise its mode of transmission and incubation are as for HBV. It makes the clinical presentation of HBV more severe and is seen particularly in intravenous drug abusers and in the Mediterranean region. Diagnosis is by detection of the appropriate antigen or antibody in the serum.

Hepatitis E virus (HEV). This is a new virus, previously part of the non-A non-B group, which is particularly common in the Third World especially India, where it is associated with high morbidity and mortality in pregnant women. In other respects, it is similar to HAV infection and is seen especially in water-borne infection, suggesting a faecal–oral method of spread. No vaccine is currently available, and diagnosis is by antibody detection in serum.

Histology

Morphologically, there is diffuse involvement of the liver with the most severe changes being seen in acinar zone 3 (perivenular region). There is focal 'spotty' necrosis of hepatocytes and some cells undergo apoptosis, such cells being referred to as acidophil or Councilman bodies. Along with necrosis, there is a heavy mononuclear cell infiltrate, predominantly lymphocytes, both in the lobules and portal tracts, and the resident liver macrophages, Kupffer cells, become hyperplastic. Cholestasis may also be seen. The mechanisms of damage are unclear but are probably immunologically mediated although direct viral cytotoxicity is also a possibility. As the liver recovers, the degree of necrosis and inflammation reduces while Kupffer cell hyperplasia continues for some time. Regenerative changes occur in the hepatocytes, while in more severe cases, there may be more extensive loss of liver cells with collapse of the reticulin framework. This leads to bridging necrosis with linkage between perivenular and portal areas. Survival is related to the regenerative power of the remaining parenchyma. The most severe form of acute viral hepatitis is where there is confluent necrosis of nearly all of the hepatocytes in large areas of the liver – acute massive necrosis. This is a cause of fulminant hepatic failure and death may occur in the acute phase. If the patient survives, there is often some degree of scarring and nodule formation.

Sequelae of acute viral hepatitis

This depends on the virus involved, the degree of initial injury and the regenerative capacity of the liver. Some cases may be asymptomatic ('subclinical') and only come to light on subsequent serology or when chronic hepatitis supervenes. Most have an acute illness which then resolves. A small minority develop acute massive necrosis which may be fatal. A significant minority progress to chronic hepatitis.

SUMMARY BOX
ACUTE HEPATITIS

- Usually presents with jaundice.
- Causes include the hepatotropic viruses (A, B, C, E and delta agent), alcohol, drugs and bile duct damage.
- Very rarely, it causes massive liver necrosis and death; most commonly patients recover completely; occasionally it goes into a chronic phase which varies depending on the underlying cause.

Chronic hepatitis

This is a clinical syndrome characterized by persistent liver function abnormality without improvement for more than 6 months. It includes chronic viral hepatitis, mainly hepatitis B and C, autoimmune chronic hepatitis and drug-induced disease, but a similar morphological pattern may be seen in alcohol-induced liver injury, long-standing biliary obstruction (primary or secondary), Wilson's disease and other metabolic disorders.

Classification. Chronic hepatitis is nowadays classified on the basis of an aetiological agent, such as a virus or autoimmunity, where this is possible on clinical or serological grounds.

- *Grade.* Classification is also made on the degree of necroinflammatory activity, corresponding to the grade of disease. Necroinflammation may be portal or lobular and there may be inflammation at the interface between liver parenchyma and either portal areas or fibrous septa (so-called interface hepatitis, a phenomenon previously referred to as 'piecemeal necrosis').
- *Stage.* The extent of fibrosis corresponds to the stage of disease and is an important predictor of outcome.

The older classification of chronic hepatitis into chronic persistent hepatitis (CPH), chronic active hepatitis (CAH) and chronic lobular hepatitis (CLH) is no longer used, since it is now accepted that all forms of chronic hepatitis may progress over variable and prolonged periods.

Autoimmune-type chronic hepatitis is seen in young women who often have autoantibodies in their serum to nucleus, microsome and smooth muscle; this form of chronic hepatitis was previously referred to as lupoid hepatitis and responds well to corticosteroids. Chronic hepatitis occurs in about 5–10% of hepatitis B patients (Fig. 10.15) and rather more hepatitis C patients (70–80%); antiviral agents such as interferon-α may be used in treatment.

The significance of chronic hepatitis lies in its propensity to progress to the irreversible stage of cirrhosis with its associated problems of hepatocellular failure, portal hypertension and increased risk of primary hepatocellular carcinoma (hepatoma). However, there may be significant liver function impairment in the absence of established cirrhosis.

Alcoholic liver disease

High alcohol consumption causes a number of changes in the liver of susceptible individuals, including fatty change

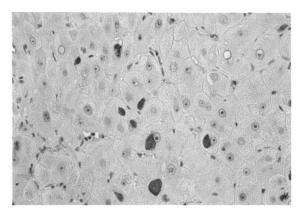

Fig. 10.15   Liver HBV (HBsAg). Immunohistochemical stain of liver demonstrating the presence of hepatitis B surface antigen as shown by the brown reaction product within the cytoplasm of hepatocytes.

SUMMARY BOX
CHRONIC HEPATITIS

- Liver disease which persists for at least 6 months.
- The common causes include viral hepatitis (especially B and C), autoimmune hepatitis, drugs and alcohol.
- It is characterized by inflammatory cell infiltration on liver biopsy which determines grade of disease; inflammation may involve portal tracts, periportal areas and hepatic lobules.
- Stage of disease reflects extent of fibrosis and determines the likelihood of cirrhosis.

(steatosis), alcoholic hepatitis, hepatic fibrosis and cirrhosis, the first three of which are thought to be reversible on withdrawal of alcohol. The exact mechanism of alcoholic liver disease is unclear but may include direct toxicity, damage by metabolites, immunologically mediated damage, free radical production and lipid peroxidation and the effect of alcohol may be aggravated by dietary imbalance and nutritional deficiencies especially of proteins and vitamins.

Steatosis.   This is the first morphological manifestation of excess alcohol consumption in the liver. This is a predictable effect and is associated with alterations in redox potential with changes in the ratio of metabolism via the alcohol dehydrogenase (ADH) and microsomal ethanol oxidative system (MEOS) enzyme systems. In the early stages, the fatty acids which accumulate in the hepatocytes are derived from body fat stores, while later they are predominantly of dietary origin. The fatty acids are esterified in the endoplasmic reticulum to triglycerides, while cholesterol esters may also accumulate. Cessation of alcohol leads to rapid reversal of this change. Occasionally massive fatty change may precipitate liver failure.

Alcoholic hepatitis (Fig. 10.16). Whereas fatty change is a predictable event, alcoholic hepatitis is much less well understood and many host factors play a part in pathogenesis. Normally, there is also fatty change on which there is superimposed ballooning and necrosis of hepatocytes associated with neutrophil polymorph infiltration, particularly in acinar zone 3. Within the damaged hepatocytes, there is accumulation of amorphous, irregular, eosinophilic aggregates composed of clumped intermediate (cytokeratin) filaments – so-called Mallory's hyaline or Mallory bodies. Giant mitochondria may also be seen. This change is thought to be reversible but continued alcohol consumption leads to persistent necrosis, fibrosis and ultimately cirrhosis.

Hepatic fibrosis. This is often seen with alcoholic hepatitis but may occur in patients who consume excessive amounts of alcohol, without hepatitis. The initial site of deposition of new fibrous tissue (rather than collapsed reticulin) is in the perivenular region (acinar zone 3) and is usually in a pericellular distribution, creating a 'chicken-wire' pattern. The cell of origin of this fibrous tissue is currently a cause of controversy and research; the present favoured explanation is the hepatic stellate (fat-storing, perisinusoidal, Ito) cell. As the degree of fibrosis progresses, fibrous septa extend from perivenular areas to other perivenular areas and to portal tracts, eventually leading to nodule formation, distortion of liver architecture and cirrhosis.

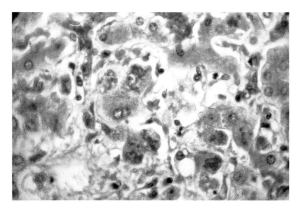

Fig. 10.16 Liver alcoholic hepatitis. Histological section of a liver in which there is swelling of hepatocytes with accumulation of bright red intracytoplasmic material (Mallory's hyaline) with some pericellular fibrosis of hepatocytes. These are typical appearances of alcoholic hepatitis.

Alcoholic cirrhosis. The end-stage of alcoholic liver disease is cirrhosis (see below) which is initially micronodular but may eventually become macronodular. In established cirrhosis, when a patient has abstained from alcohol for some time, it may not be possible to decide on an aetiological agent on histological grounds. This probably explains the variability in different series of the finding of so-called 'cryptogenic' cirrhosis.

SUMMARY BOX
ALCOHOLIC LIVER DISEASE

- Very common cause of acute and chronic liver disease.
- Mechanisms of damage include direct toxicity of ethanol or its metabolites, free radical production, immunological injury and stimulation of fibrosis.
- A range of features is seen including fatty change, alcoholic hepatitis, alcoholic fibrosis and cirrhosis, often in combination.

Cirrhosis

Cirrhosis is a condition involving the whole liver characterized by the formation of parenchymal nodules separated by fibrous tissue. It is irreversible and liver cell damage may persist on withdrawal of the toxic agent because of continuing vascular disturbance. This condition leads to progressive hepatocellular failure and/or portal hypertension; a rare complication is the development of primary hepatocellular carcinoma.

Aetiology

In western populations, alcohol is the commonest cause of cirrhosis (35%) while post-viral infection (hepatitis B and C) accounts for about 15–20%. There are a very large number of less common causes of cirrhosis which must be considered ($<5–10\%$) while the remainder are considered cryptogenic, for which no definite cause can be established on clinical, serological or pathological grounds. Biliary cirrhosis may be either primary (PBC) or secondary to some abnormality of bile flow (biliary atresia or gallstones). PBC is a disease of middle-aged women, with a strong autoimmune background, which results in progressive destruction of intrahepatic bile ducts. Primary sclerosing cholangitis causes a similar pattern of disease but is often (70%) associated with inflammatory bowel disease, especially ulcerative colitis.

There are a very large group of metabolic disorders capable of causing cirrhosis. The commonest is haemo-

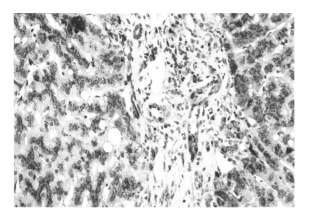

Fig. 10.17 Histological section of liver stained with the Perls' Prussian blue reaction demonstrating the presence of abundant haemosiderin within hepatocytes, typical of genetic haemochromatosis.

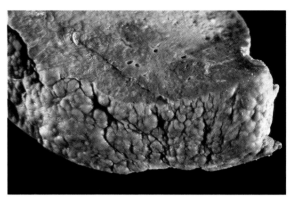

Fig. 10.18 Gross photograph of a liver slice showing nodularity of the surface typical of established micronodular cirrhosis.

chromatosis, a so-called pigment cirrhosis and part of the iron overload syndrome. In this condition, it is possible to demonstrate excess iron in the form of haemosiderin in the liver using the Perls' Prussian blue reaction (Fig. 10.17). Wilson's disease is another form of pigment cirrhosis, in this case the pigment being copper which is accumulated in excess in the liver and other sites including the basal ganglia, kidney and eyes. In susceptible individuals, the protease inhibitor α_1-antitrypsin is synthesized but not secreted by liver cells leading to the accumulation of characteristic α_1-antitrypsin deficiency globules in hepatocytes detected by the PAS stain. Rarer causes include glycogen storage diseases and an unusual form of Indian childhood cirrhosis.

Pathogenesis

Cirrhosis is a consequence of persistent loss of liver cells, for a variety of reasons (see above), accompanied by compensatory liver cell hyperplasia and nodule formation; there is chronic inflammation with the usual result of fibrosis. The irregular pattern of hyperplasia and fibrosis results in disturbance of the liver blood flow, particularly of the portal circulation. This causes further ischaemic damage to the hepatic parenchyma, regardless of the initial cause of injury, and thus there is continuing hepatocellular failure and portal hypertension.

Morphology

Grossly, in the early stages of cirrhosis, the liver may be enlarged. However, with disease progression, the liver shrinks and terminally may weigh less than 1000 g. The surface is diffusely nodular (Fig. 10.18) and on sectioning there may be evidence of fatty change (pale, yellow) or cholestasis (yellow/green). Classification on nodule size is often performed but is of little value in determining the aetiology: micronodular cirrhosis is where the nodules are all roughly the same size up to 3 mm in diameter; macronodular where the nodules are irregularly sized up to 1 cm in diameter; and a mixed type where both are present. The mixed and macronodular forms are often seen at a later stage of disease.

Histologically, there is a loss of the normal architecture (Fig. 10.19). The fibrous septa separating nodules link portal tracts to each other, to terminal hepatic venules (central veins) and terminal hepatic venules to each other, with loss of the normal relationships of these structures. They enclose nodules of hepatic parenchyma which may show variable degrees of hypertrophy

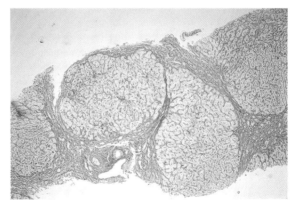

Fig. 10.19 Histological section of liver using a reticulin stain demonstrating established micronodular cirrhosis.

(increased cell size) and hyperplasia (increased cell number), and also atrophy. There may be an inflammatory infiltrate in the fibrous septa, or bile duct proliferation, both reflecting activity of disease. In the nodules there may be cholestasis, although this is often a terminal feature of hepatocellular failure, or there may be clues to the aetiology of the cirrhosis.

Complications of cirrhosis

Portal hypertension. This arises from increased portal blood flow and increased resistance and arterio-venous shunting within the liver. It leads to anastomoses between the portal and systemic circulations, especially in the lower oesophagus causing oesophageal varices which are prone to rupture. Other sites include the anorectal region, causing haemorrhoids, the periumbilical region, causing *caput medusae*, and through the splenic vein, causing splenomegaly. It may also contribute to the development of ascites.

Hepatocellular failure. The liver is the most important metabolic site in the body and its failure leads to:

- inadequate synthesis of proteins, including albumin and blood clotting factors, and
- reduced capacity to detoxify endogenous material, including breakdown products of protein metabolism and hormones, and exogenous substances, such as drugs.

Clinical consequences include ascites and oedema from hypoalbuminaemia, easy bruising and a bleeding tendency from lack of clotting factors, encephalopathy from failure to remove nitrogenous waste products, features of excess sex hormones such as gonadal atrophy, gynaecomastia, liver palms, Dupuytren's contracture and spider naevi, and increased tendency to infection from defective macrophage (Kupffer cell) activity.

Hepatocellular carcinoma. Cirrhosis is an important premalignant condition, with a greatly increased risk of hepatocellular carcinoma. This is particularly the case in HBV infection but is associated with all aetiological types of cirrhosis, especially long-standing macronodular forms.

Neoplasms

The commonest malignant tumours occurring in the liver are metastases from a variety of primary sites, particularly from within the gastrointestinal tract. Primary liver tumours are rare, although hepatocellular carcinoma is common

---

SUMMARY BOX
CIRRHOSIS

- End stage of chronic liver disease characterized by diffuse nodule formation.
- Irreversible disease associated with portal hypertension and hepatocellular failure.
- Causes include alcoholic liver disease, HBV and HCV, autoimmune diseases, and iron and copper pigment overload.
- Hepatocellular carcinoma is a long-term complication especially in HBV infection.

---

where hepatitis B virus infection is endemic, especially in sub-Saharan Africa and Southeast Asia. It may also be associated with aflatoxin ingestion. Most cases arise on the basis of pre-existing cirrhosis and should be suspected clinically when patients with long-standing chronic liver disease show rapid clinical deterioration. A useful serological marker is the detection of high levels of the onco-fetal antigen, α-fetoprotein, which may also be seen in the neoplastic hepatocytes. Prognosis is extremely poor, with most patients dead within 6 months. Cholangio-carcinoma, a malignant tumour of bile duct origin, is relatively uncommon but in Southeast Asia is often associated with infection with the liver fluke *Clonorchis sinensis* and there is also an association with chronic inflammatory bowel disease and sclerosing cholangitis. Clinically, it may present with symptoms indistinguishable from hepatocellular carcinoma but it is not associated with either cirrhosis or raised α-fetoprotein levels. Histologically, it is a mucin-secreting adenocarcinoma which produces a marked desmoplastic reaction. There is slow relentless progression with eventual haematogenous spread.

ASPECTS OF GASTROINTESTINAL DISEASE OF PARTICULAR RELEVANCE TO DENTISTRY

- Malabsorption syndromes may present as recurrent oral ulceration.
- Both major forms of inflammatory bowel disease, ulcerative colitis and Crohn's disease, may present with oral manifestations.
- Patients with familial adenomatous polyposis may present with dento-osseous lesions visible on panoramic radiographs.
- Chronic liver disease patients may have bleeding problems and difficulties with metabolism of prescribed drugs.

GALL BLADDER

Cholelithiasis

Most gall bladder diseases are associated with the formation of gallstones (cholelithiasis), which are usually found in the gall bladder and only rarely in extrahepatic bile ducts. The normal homeostasis of the gall bladder is maintained by the balance between cholesterol and bile salts/phospholipids. Stones are formed when there is supersaturation of bile, followed by initiation of stone formation, 'nucleation' (possibly related to excess mucus or infection), and further enlargement by accretion.

Pure bilirubin stones are rare (about 5% of the total) but cholesterol is present in over 90% of stones (pure, mixed or combined). Excess bile cholesterol is seen in a variety of conditions including pregnancy, diabetes, nephrotic syndrome, obesity, starvation, hyperthyroidism and treatment with clofibrate, a lipid-lowering agent. Reduced levels of bile salts/phospholipids are usually a consequence of failure of the normal enterohepatic circulation where conjugated bile acids are reabsorbed in the terminal ileum as bile salts. Conditions such as Crohn's disease or ileal surgery are the most common causes. Gallstones are found in 10–20% of autopsies and are more common in women than in men. The disease is particularly common in Native American and South American Indians. The aphorism 'fair–fat–female–fertile–forty' is a useful reminder of risk factors but it is important to remember that many people outside these groups may have gallstones.

A common incidental finding in the gall bladder is cholesterolosis, producing the appearance of 'strawberry gall bladder'. It occurs where bile cholesterol levels are high and histologically consists of macrophages filled with foam cells rich in cholesterol esters in the tips of villi.

Effects of cholelithiasis

- Many patients with gallstones are asymptomatic but if stones are found incidentally, it is suggested that up to 50% will develop symptoms eventually and this is the basis for elective cholecystectomy, nowadays commonly performed laparoscopically – so-called 'keyhole surgery'.
- Acute cholecystitis is probably due to chemical irritation of gall bladder mucosa damaged by stones. Primary infection of the gall bladder is extremely rare and, although bacteria are identified occasionally, they are probably of little significance.
- Chronic cholecystitis encompasses a wide range of clinical and pathological features. Functionally the gall bladder retains little or no absorptive capacity. Continuing inflammation at the same time as attempts at healing, owing to persistence of stones, leads to a number of features. These include a variable degree of inflammatory cell infiltration, fibrosis of the wall often with muscle layer hypertrophy, metaplastic changes in the surface epithelium, the development of tracts lined by epithelium within the wall – so-called 'Rokitansky–Aschoff' sinuses, and possibly dystrophic calcification of the wall causing a 'porcelain' appearance.
- Mucocele of the gall bladder occurs when there is complete obstruction of the cystic duct by stones producing a tense, shiny gall bladder containing clear bile.
- Empyema develops when there is intermittent blockage of the cystic duct with ascending infection leading to the formation of a ragged inflamed gall bladder with a thickened wall. This is particularly liable to rupture and may cause a biliary fistula to surrounding structures or may lead to generalized peritonitis.
- Biliary colic develops if a stone leaves the gall bladder and enters the common bile duct. The passage of the stone may cause intense pain.
- If the stone impacts in the lower bile duct it may lead to painful obstructive jaundice.
- If the sphincter of Oddi is damaged allowing reflux of intestinal contents and bacteria, then ascending cholangitis may develop.
- If there is a common channel for both pancreatic and bile duct, which occurs in 60–70% of the population, pancreatitis may ensue.
- If a large stone finds its way into the bowel, usually via a fistula, then gallstone ileus may occur.
- Persistent or intermittent obstruction of the bile ducts may induce chronic inflammation and fibrosis leading to stricture formation, and in the long term, may cause secondary biliary cirrhosis of the liver.

Neoplasms

Primary tumours of the gall bladder are rare and they are most commonly seen in elderly patients, particularly women, because of the association with cholelithiasis. Many cases are found incidentally in cholecystectomy specimens. However, in advanced disease, tumours which have spread beyond the gall bladder have a very poor prognosis.

PANCREAS

Pancreatitis

Acute pancreatitis and chronic pancreatitis are inflammatory diseases of the exocrine pancreas, which usually manifest as an attack of severe epigastric pain accompanied by elevated levels of pancreatic enzymes such as amylase in blood and/or urine. It is not known at the time of the first attack whether the pancreas was previously normal and will return to normal upon full clinical recovery (acute pancreatitis), or whether the attack merely unmasked established disease (chronic pancreatitis): this distinction ideally requires pancreatic histology but in most cases that is not feasible and pancreatic functional and morphological tests, applied 8 weeks after an attack, facilitate a retrospective diagnosis. Acute pancreatitis should not recur if the cause is removable and complications have been adequately dealt with; by contrast, recurrent attacks with progressive destruction of exocrine tissue, and eventually pancreatic islets, is the expected course in chronic pancreatitis.

Aetiological factors for acute pancreatitis may be divided into three main categories:

- those which obstruct ductal drainage and promote reflux: these include gall stones (by far the commonest cause), duodenal diverticula, pancreas divisum and ampullary stenosis or carcinoma
- those which compromise the microcirculation: these include shock, hypothermia and hypertriglyceridaemia
- those associated with deranged pancreatic acinar cell metabolism: these include trauma, infection especially viral, drugs, chemicals and toxins, hypercalcaemia, fasting followed by excess food, chronic renal failure and inflammatory bowel disease.

In up to 50% of cases, no specific aetiological factor or association can be identified, the so-called idiopathic group. Alcohol is often included as a cause of acute pancreatitis but it is likely that in chronic alcoholics, the first attack probably represents the onset of chronic pancreatitis.

By far the commonest identifiable risk factor for chronic pancreatitis is alcohol, although in tropical countries, an endemic form exists. Again, in up to 50% of cases, no identifiable factor is apparent. The first attack resolves spontaneously in the majority of cases, with blood amylase levels returning to normal by 72 hours.

The pathological features in this situation are those of acute oedematous pancreatitis with oedema, leukocyte infiltration and fat necrosis of pancreatic interstitium. In approximately 20% of cases, the gland develops the features of acute haemorrhagic, necrotizing pancreatitis where there are haemorrhages, coagulative acinar necrosis and extensive membrane necrosis; there is widespread fat necrosis in the peritoneum and bloody peritoneal exudate. Death from multisystem organ failure is the usual outcome. Of those who recover, up to 25% of patients may develop a pancreatic pseudocyst and/or abscess. The pathological hallmarks of chronic pancreatitis are patchy acinar loss, inter- and intra-acinar fibrosis, ductal distortion, and intraductal protein plugs that tend to calcify with the passage of time: the features of inflammation are superimposed during painful exacerbations.

Neoplasms

There are rare benign tumours of the exocrine pancreas including serous and mucinous cystadenomas, analogous to their ovarian counterparts. Carcinoma of the exocrine pancreas is a relatively common tumour which occurs mainly after the age of 50 and is slightly more common in men. A number of dietary factors have been postulated including coffee consumption and high-fat diets; no conclusive evidence is available. Cigarette smoking is also a risk factor. Most tumours are of ductal origin and are unequally distributed throughout the gland: 70% in the head, 20% in the body and 10% in the tail region. They present with obstructive jaundice, characteristically painless, because of the infiltration of the common bile/pancreatic duct. They are usually well-differentiated adenocarcinomas and may be difficult to distinguish histologically from chronic pancreatitis. Perineural infiltration is common and spread into surrounding structures is a frequent early finding. Lymphatic and haematogenous metastases are also early events. A well-recognized paraneoplastic manifestation is Trousseau's sign, migratory superficial thrombophlebitis, probably due to release of thromboplastins by the tumour, which may also explain the development of more severe thrombosis and disseminated intravascular coagulation sometimes seen with these tumours. Surgery (Whipple's procedure) may be effective in early stage tumours but most tumours present too late for surgical intervention and prognosis is correspondingly poor.

Tumours of the endocrine pancreas are also relatively common and are dealt with later in the endocrine diseases section (see Ch. 14).

SUMMARY BOX
EXOCRINE PANCREATIC DISEASE

- The main cause of acute pancreatitis is gallstones but many other causes may be seen; it has a high morbidity and mortality rate, and is diagnosed clinically by finding raised amylase levels in the serum.

- Chronic pancreatitis is associated with alcohol excess and gallstones; there is marked fibrosis with acinar cell loss, leading to intestinal malabsorption and later diabetes.

- Pancreatic carcinoma usually presents with painless obstructive jaundice and is associated with a very poor prognosis.

CASE STUDY 10.1
EFFECTS OF STEROIDS

A 21-year-old student who suffered from asthma experienced increasing frequent asthmatic attacks which could not be controlled by his usual medication. A corticosteroid inhaler was added to his regime and was effective in preventing attacks when used daily. After 6 weeks he began to experience a sore throat and metallic taste in the back of the mouth. He attended his dentist who found white and red areas on the soft palate, fauces and posterior tongue. Referral to the local hospital's oral and maxillofacial surgery unit was arranged.

At the hospital, the house officer found a thick, irregular, white coating involving the entire soft palate, fauces, retromolar areas and posterior tongue. The material resembled milk curds and could be wiped away to leave a red, raw, bleeding mucosal surface. The house officer took swabs and prepared smears on microscope slides of the white plaques. These were submitted to the microbiology department. The microbiology report stated that there was heavy growth of *Candida albicans* in culture and that both yeast forms and pseudohyphae were abundant in the smear.

1. What is the relationship between the use of the corticosteroid inhaler and the development of the *Candida* infection?
2. What other patterns of *Candida* infection are seen in the oral cavity?
3. Which *Candida* species may act as oral pathogens?
4. Why did the house officer submit both swabs and smears?
5. How can inhaler-related candidosis be prevented?

Suggested responses

1. *Candida* species are opportunistic pathogens and oral candidiasis (candidosis) is sometimes referred to as the 'disease of the diseased'. Local and general factors may underlie *Candida* infection; important local factors include tobacco smoking, continuous denture wearing and poor denture fit and hygiene. Numerous general factors may predispose and examples include immunosuppression in HIV infection, antibiotics, corticosteroids, debilitated patients, genetic susceptibility and diabetes. In this case, the corticosteroid inhaler has suppressed local immunity in the oropharynyx and this has resulted in acute pseudomembranous candidiasis. *Candida* is carried, principally in the dorsal tongue in approximately 40% of subjects with a medical condition and infection results from overgrowth of the organism.

2. In addition to acute pseudomembranous candidiasis (thrush) the following patterns are recognized: acute atrophic (erythematous) candidiasis (antibiotic sore mouth, HIV), chronic atrophic candidiasis (denture sore mouth), candida-associated angular cheilitis, chronic hyperplastic candidiasis and chronic mucocutaneous candidiasis (see also Chs 5 and 15).

3. *C. glabrata*, *C. tropicalis*, *C. krusei* and *C. parapsilosis*.

4. Swabs are taken in suspected *Candida* infection to enable speciation; heavy growth also indicates infection. Direct smears can be stained by the periodic acid–Schiff or Gram's methods to demonstrate yeast and pseudohyphae forms. Whilst yeast forms may be seen in carriers, the presence of thread-like pseudohyphae is indicative of infection.

5. Inhaler-related candidiasis may be prevented by use of a nebulizer and by mouth rinsing after use.

CASE STUDY 10.2
A LUMP IN THE NECK

A 55-year-old man presented to his general medical practitioner with a recent history of a lump in the left side of his neck just below the angle of the mandible. He had first noticed the lump 2 months previously but it had grown in size in the meantime. It was non-tender to the touch and was not painful.

On questioning, the man reported that he was a heavy cigarette smoker (40/day for nearly 40 years) and that he drank 3–4 pints of beer each night and spirits at the weekend. His diet was poor, consisting of pies and snacks with no fresh fruit and vegetables. On one occasion some 6 years previously, he had attended his general dental practitioner because of toothache and had been told that he had a white patch on the oral mucosa. He was offered an appointment at the oral medicine department of his local dental school but failed to attend on three occasions.

On examination, a firm mass 2.5 cm in diameter was noted in the left submandibular region which felt hard and was fixed to the underlying tissues. Within the oral cavity, an ulcerated area 2.3 cm in diameter with a raised rolled margin was identified on the left lateral border of the tongue. On protruding the tongue, it deviated towards the left side.

An incisional biopsy was taken from the intraoral mass and a needle biopsy of the neck lump was performed. The report to the surgeon described the biopsy as showing a moderately differentiated squamous cell carcinoma. The fine needle aspirate contained keratinizing squamous cells with cytological features of malignancy.

After further evaluation, no blood-borne distant metastases were apparent but because of his long history of cigarette smoking resulting in chronic lung problems and ischaemic heart disease, he was considered unfit for general anaesthesia and possible curative surgery.

1. What are the possible causes of a such a lump in the neck?
2. What points from this man's history are relevant to his presentation with a neck lump?
3. Which additional investigations should be performed to allow a management plan to be formulated?
4. What features allow the pathologist to describe the degree of differentiation?
5. From the information available to you, what stage has the carcinoma reached?
6. Which other treatment options are potentially available?

Suggested responses

1. In this case the neck lump is due to metastatic squamous cell carcinoma which has spread from the primary oral cancer to infiltrate a cervical lymph node. Other possible causes of enlargement of cervical lymph nodes are bacterial infection (unlikely in the absence of mobility, tenderness and pain), granulomatous conditions such as sarcoidosis and tuberculosis and neoplasia. The latter may be due to primary malignant lymphoma or metastatic neoplasm from more distant sites. The position of the lump is also consistent with a lesion arising in the submandibular salivary gland itself, such as chronic sialadenitis, a benign neoplasm or salivary carcinoma. Lesions arising from the thyroid gland, branchial cleft cysts, vascular malformations and soft tissue tumours also occur in this site.

2. Cigarette smoking and alcohol are common risk factors for oral cancer and the disease is still more common in males than females. The white patch seen previously by the dentist probably represented an area of leukoplakia, which in around 5–10% of cases progresses to oral squamous cell carcinoma. Both oral leukoplakia and carcinoma are typically painless until advanced and this tends to lead to late presentation with metastasis. Fixation of the lymph node to the underlying neck tissue suggests that the metastatic carcinoma has spread beyond the capsule of the node, which is an indicator of poor outcome.

3. Imaging, including radiography of the jaw to exclude bone invasion and scanning to exclude possible second primary sites in the upper aerodigestive tract are useful investigations in treatment planning.

4. Differentiation refers to the extent that the neoplasm resembles the tissue of origin, in this case the squamous epithelium of the oral mucosa. In the biopsy, the pathologist will have noted the presence or absence of intercellular bridges ('prickles') and whether or not the tumour is producing the normal product of squamous epithelium, i.e. keratin. In well-differentiated areas of squamous cell carcinomas, both features are usually present and whorls of keratin (keratin pearls) are often seen. The pattern of invasion is a particularly important feature in determining prognosis. At one extreme, invasion in a broad pushing front indicates a better prognosis, whilst at the other, diffuse, single cell infiltration and perineural spread are associated with poor outcomes.

5. Stage refers to the extent of local and distant spread that has occurred at the time of diagnosis and is normally determined clinically. Oral squamous cell carcinomas generally invade locally in the first instance and then spread to regional lymph nodes. Distant blood-borne metastasis is uncommon and usually a late event in these carcinomas. The TNM classification for this neoplasm can be summarized as T_2, N_2, M_0, i.e. primary carcinoma 2.1–4 cm, fixed unilateral node and no distant metastases. A more detailed staging classification is provided and updated by the Union Internationale Contre le Cancer.

6. Oral squamous cell carcinoma is not usually treated by chemotherapy except as an adjuvant. Radiotherapy can be provided by external beam or implant methods and the outcome is similar to surgical treatment. Often a combination of radiotherapy and surgery are used. Although overall survival for oral squamous cell carcinoma is just less than 50%, the prognosis in the case described is poor with 5-year survival rates in the region of 15–20%.

CASE STUDY 10.3
UPPER ABDOMINAL PAIN

A 41-year-old dentist presented to her GP complaining of upper abdominal pain and generally feeling tired and unwell. She is a general dental practitioner and had been under considerable stress recently, in relation to both her professional and home life. On questioning, she described pain which came on in the evening and was relieved by food or sometimes antacids, and occasionally by vomiting. There was no history of weight loss or haematemesis (vomiting blood). Her menstrual periods had been somewhat irregular recently but blood loss was not particularly heavy. On examining the patient, the GP noticed that she was pale with angular cheilitis and a reddened tongue. Abdominal examination was normal. Her GP took a blood test.

The test results came back from the laboratory and confirmed the GP's initial clinical impression. The GP then referred the patient to a gastroenterologist who performed an endoscopy under sedation. The endoscopy report described a normal oesophagus, reddened, inflamed antral mucosa and a sharp punched-out ulcer in the anterior wall of the first part of duodenum. Biopsies were taken from both duodenum and gastric antrum.

Pending the results, she was started on ferrous sulphate tablets orally and omeprazole 40 mg/day. A week later, she returned to the gastroenterologist who had the results of her biopsies. They confirmed the chronic peptic ulcer and the antral biopsy showed active chronic inflammation with *Helicobacter pylori* infection.

6 weeks later, she completed all treatments prescribed. She felt much better and a repeat blood test revealed a haemoglobin of 11.2 g/dl.

1. What are the possible causes of this woman's symptoms?
2. What blood test will the GP have requested and what are the likely results?
3. What are the histological features of a benign chronic peptic ulcer involving the duodenum?
4. What further measures should the gastroenterologist take?
5. What long-term complications may possibly arise in this woman's case?

Suggested responses

1. The usual causes of upper gastrointestinal tract symptoms include non-ulcer dyspepsia, peptic ulcer disease, gastric carcinoma (although she is a little young), hiatus hernia with reflux oesophagitis, gall bladder disease and pancreatic pain, and the possibility of myocardial ischaemic pain should be considered. The tiredness and unwell feeling are non-specific symptoms but should suggest anaemia, especially given the oral manifestations and observation of pallor. The other major cause of anaemia in a woman in this age group is excessive menstrual loss but this seems to be excluded by the history.

2. The GP should request a full blood count with examination of a blood film for red cell morphology. This is likely to show anaemia, i.e. haemoglobin less than 11.0 g/dl, probably with a low mean corpuscular volume; the blood film should show hypochromic microcytic cells, typical of iron-deficiency anaemia.

3. There are four main layers in any chronic peptic ulcer: superficial necrotic material, a layer of fibrinopurulent material (polymorphs, fibrin), a layer of granulation tissue (capillaries and fibroblasts) and a deeper layer of new collagen. The epithelium at the edge will show regenerative features and in the duodenum, there may be gastric metaplasia infected with *H. pylori*. In the vast majority of chronic duodenal peptic ulcers (>90%), there is an associated chronic antral gastritis due to *H. pylori* infection. Other features such as metaplasia may also be present.

4. Treatment initially concentrated on reduction of acid levels by the use of the proton pump inhibitor, omeprazole. However, ulcers are likely to recur after cessation of drug therapy unless the underlying cause of hyperacidity, in this case *H. pylori* infection through its ability to induce hypergastrinaemia, is eradicated. Thus, the gastroenterologist should add in at least one and probably two antibiotics such as ampicillin, clarithromycin and metronidazole for a further 2 weeks. In some cases, a repeat endoscopy may be needed to ensure complete eradication but this is usually assessed on clinical response in the first instance.

5. *H. pylori*-associated gastritis may be associated with the development of intestinal metaplasia, from which gastric carcinoma may arise. So far, this association is not definitely proven but is one of the arguments in favour of eradication therapy.

CASE STUDY 10.4
DIARRHOEA

A 30-year-old female presents to her GP with a history of 4 days of diarrhoea. On questioning, she states that mixed with the diarrhoea were small amounts of blood and mucus.

She was treated with oral fluid replacement. Investigations failed to reveal an infective cause for her condition. Her temperature, which had been slightly raised initially, returned to normal. She was referred to the local gastro-enterology clinic where a number of investigations were performed.

When she returned to the outpatient clinic 2 weeks later, the gastroenterologist read to her the histopathology report of her rectal biopsies which showed 'fragments of rectal mucosa in which there is a moderate degree of active chronic inflammation with crypt abscess formation and focal superficial ulceration. No granulomas are present and there is no evidence of dysplasia or neoplasia.'

She was commenced on mesalazine by mouth and the frequency of diarrhoea was greatly reduced. Occasionally she developed more profound symptoms requiring oral corticosteroids.

1. What are the possible causes of diarrhoea in this woman's case?
2. What initial investigations should be performed to elicit the underlying cause?
3. What further investigations are likely to be undertaken by the gastroenterologist?
4. What is the most likely diagnosis in this woman's case? Justify your diagnosis.
5. What extracolonic manifestations may occur in this condition?
6. What long-term complication of this disease may occur?

Suggested responses

1. Diarrhoea may be infectious or non-infectious in origin. Infectious causes include viruses and bacteria in which food poisoning must be considered. Non-infectious causes include exposure to drugs, e.g. antibiotics, irritable bowel syndrome, inflammatory bowel disease, diverticular disease, colonic carcinoma and thyrotoxicosis. The presence of blood and mucus raises the possibility of ulcerative colitis, dysentery, ischaemic colitis and colorectal carcinoma, although many of these conditions are unlikely in a 30-year-old woman.

2. Stools should be submitted for culture and sensitivity to exclude an infectious cause. A full blood count may show

features of infection with a raised white cell count, and urea and electrolytes tests may show features of dehydration.

3. The gastroenterologist is likely to perform a full abdominal examination including rectal examination and to perform a sigmoidoscopy (which allows direct visual examination of the distal 25 cm of rectum and sigmoid colon). He is likely to take biopsies of any abnormal area for histological examination. He may also request a barium enema radiological examination and later a colonoscopy to examine the whole of the large bowel.

4. This woman is most likely to have ulcerative colitis on the basis of disease involving the rectum which is superficial in nature and lacking granulomas. However, other investigations including radiology and colonoscopy are needed to confirm the diagnosis. Crohn's disease may have similar features on a single biopsy but more detailed examination in Crohn's disease may show the patchy nature of inflammation with uninvolved areas in between and the presence of deeper transmural inflammation and granulomas, although typical non-caseating epithelioid granulomas are found in only 60–70% of cases.

5. Patients with either ulcerative colitis or Crohn's disease have a range of extracolonic manifestations including skin lesions such as pyoderma gangrenosum and erythema nodosum, joint problems including large joint arthropathy and ankylosing spondylitis (in HLA-B27-positive individuals), eye problems such as iritis and uveitis, and liver disease such as sclerosing cholangitis.

6. There is a small but significant increased risk of colorectal carcinoma in long-standing ulcerative colitis, which is associated with severe disease of the whole colon (pancolitis) for more than 10 years. In practice this occurs very rarely because increased surveillance of these patients should recognize the pre-malignant changes of dysplasia before carcinoma develops, at which time elective surgery such as panproctocolectomy should be performed.

CASE STUDY 10.5
ABNORMAL LIVER FUNCTION TESTS

A 45-year-old male general dental practitioner went to see his general medical practitioner who was a family friend. He complained of feeling generally unwell with excessive tiredness and a dragging sensation in the right upper quadrant of his abdomen. His GP examined him and noticed that he was slightly tender in the right upper quadrant on palpation but no other specific findings were identified. On closer questioning, there was no history of nausea, vomiting or pain relieved by antacids. The GP requested a number of investigations.

2 weeks later the dentist returned to get the results of the investigations and was told that some of the liver enzymes were raised, including aspartate aminotransferase (AST) and alanine aminotransferase (ALT), which were both two to three times the upper limit of normal, and the bilirubin level which was just above normal. He was not anaemic and his white cell count was normal. The GP decided to refer his dental colleague to the local hospital where there was a special liver clinic. When seen there, he was asked more questions and had further investigations performed.

He was seen again at the clinic 1 month later when all of the results of these investigations were available. He was advised to have a liver biopsy. This was performed in hospital after checking that his bleeding status was normal. It was reported by the pathologist as showing features of alcoholic liver disease which were potentially reversible.

1. What are the possible causes of these presenting symptoms?
2. What questions relevant to liver disease in a dentist should be asked after the receipt of the original blood tests?
3. What features of alcoholic liver disease are likely to be present on biopsy?
4. What are the possible long-term complications of this condition?

Suggested responses

1. The symptoms of tiredness raise the possibility of anaemia. The dragging sensation in the right upper quadrant suggests problems related to the liver and gall bladder although it may also be related to gastric, oesophageal or pancreatic disease. In addition to upper gastrointestinal disease, the possibility of musculoskeletal problems also need to be considered.

2. The commonest cause of liver function abnormalities in the western population is excess alcohol consumption, so a detailed alcohol history should be taken. Dentists along with medical practitioners have a high risk of alcoholism. The number of units consumed per week (1 unit = 10 g alcohol) should be estimated and if he exceeds the recommended safe limits of 21–28 units he should be advised that he may be damaging his liver (the level for females is lower at 14–21 units per week). Dentists are at risk of blood-borne transmission of infections and although he should have had hepatitis B immunization, there is currently no vaccine available for hepatitis C virus infection. Therefore he should be asked about needlestick injuries or contact with jaundice. Foreign travel should be questioned because of the risk of exposure to hepatitis A virus infection from contaminated water or foods. Blood transfusion in the UK should carry very little risk of hepatitis. Exposure to drugs can sometimes cause liver disease, including prescribed drugs such as antibiotics and psychotropic agents, over-the-counter medicines and even herbal remedies. Obesity can cause fatty change in the liver and this may lead to minor abnormalities of liver function biochemically.

3. The features of alcoholic liver disease histologically include:
   a. fatty change
   b. alcoholic hepatitis characterized by ballooning of hepatocytes, accumulation of Mallory's hyaline and polymorph infiltration
   c. pericellular fibrosis in perivenular (acinar zone 3) hepatocytes, and
   d. cirrhosis where there is diffuse fibrosis with nodule formation.

The first three of these changes are potentially reversible on withdrawal of alcohol.

4. The long-term complications which may develop include cirrhosis and ultimately hepatocellular carcinoma, especially if there is another risk factor present such as viral infection or iron overload syndrome.

Diseases of the kidneys, urinary tract and reproductive organs

KIDNEY

Normal renal function

The function of the kidney is to filter approximately 170 litres of fluid per day through the glomeruli and reabsorb 168 litres of fluid through the tubules, resulting in approximately 2 litres of urine. In doing so, the kidney:

- maintains a very strict acid–base balance producing a pH range between 7.36 and 7.42
- gets rid of waste products mainly of protein metabolism
- produces strict electrolyte (Na^+, K^+, Cl^-, HCO_3^-) and water balance.

These are essential functions, derangement of which may be fatal. Other functions which are mainly hormonal in nature are also provided by the kidney including erythropoietin secretion leading to stimulation of red blood cell production by the bone marrow, vitamin D and calcium metabolism which may cause bone disease, and the renin–angiotensin system which maintains sodium homeostasis and may cause systemic hypertension.

The presenting features of renal impairment are very varied and reflect the many functions of the normal kidney, including blood in the urine (haematuria), significant amounts of protein especially albumin in the urine (proteinuria), oedema (due to hypoalbuminaemia) and systemic hypertension. Certain combinations of such symptoms and signs produce well-recognized clinical syndromes, including acute nephritis (hypertension and haematuria) and the nephrotic syndrome (oedema, proteinuria and hypertension).

Urinary tract infection

This is defined as the presence of microorganisms in the urine, and implies involvement of either the bladder (cystitis) or the kidney, collecting system and renal pelvis (pyelonephritis) or both. The diagnosis is made by the identification of 'significant' numbers of microorganisms on culture of the urine (i.e. more than 100 000 (10^5) per ml) and this is accompanied by the finding of pyuria or white blood cells in the urine (i.e. more than 10 per high power microscopic field). This is one of the commonest infections occurring in the general population and may arise at any age, depending particularly on gender.

Predisposing/risk factors

These may be considered either as general or local:

- *General.* Patients with diabetes mellitus are at increased risk, because of glycosuria; immunosuppressed patients are at risk of all types of infection; women in pregnancy also have an increased incidence of urinary infections for a number of reasons.
- *Local.* Patients who have stasis of urine may develop urinary infections and this is associated especially with obstruction due to anatomical abnormalities (more common in children) or pathological conditions such as stones, prostatic enlargement, urothelial tumours, strictures or valves; sexual intercourse increases the risk of infection in females particularly; instrumentation of the urinary tract, especially catheterization, is associated with increased incidence of urinary tract infections; reflux of urine is also a risk factor for infections and this is especially the case in children (males more than females) where there may be abnormalities

of the sphincter mechanisms between bladder and lower ureter (vesicoureteric reflux) or between upper ureter and renal pelvis (pelviureteric reflux).

Clinical features

The clinical presentation varies with age as infants and young children may not manifest the classical symptoms. Cystitis causes suprapubic pain, pain on micturition (dysuria), blood in the urine (haematuria), severe frequency of micturition and the passage of offensive urine. Pyelonephritis causes loin pain and tenderness may be elicited on examination; the other features of lower urinary infection may also be noted, but not infrequently, acute pyelonephritis may be silent and this has a danger of progressing to chronic pyelonephritis and eventually chronic renal failure.

Pathogenesis

The pathogenesis of most urinary infections is through an ascending route of infection. Commensal colonic bacteria reach the perineum and then ascend the urethra into the bladder, and if reflux of urine occurs, may further ascend into the upper urinary tract. Predisposing physical factors for this form of infection include the shorter urethra in females, infection following sexual intercourse and instrumentation of the urinary tract, and predisposing bacterial factors are their ability to adhere to the urothelium. The other less common route of infection is through the bloodstream which may occur in systemic *Staphylococcus aureus* infections.

Microbiology

The microbiology of urinary tract infections depends on whether the infection is community or hospital acquired and whether the urinary tract is anatomically normal or not. The commonest organism in all groups of patients is *Escherichia coli*, while *Proteus mirabilis*, which has a urease capability and is associated with stone formation, *Staphylococcus saprophyticus*, which is typically community acquired in young females, and *Enterococcus faecalis*, which may also be associated with infective endocarditis, are the next most frequently detected organisms. *Klebsiella* species and *Pseudomonas aeruginosa* are usually hospital acquired, while rarer causes of urinary tract infections are tuberculosis and candidiasis.

The laboratory diagnosis of urinary infections requires the collection of a midstream specimen of urine before commencing antibiotics. In the laboratory, the urine should be examined for pus cells, red cells and casts with semi-quantitative culture to confirm 'significant' (i.e. at least $> 10^4$ and probably $> 10^5$) numbers of organisms, followed by antibiotic sensitivity. Antibiotics used in the treatment of urinary infections need to be excreted in the urine and should be active against the likely pathogens. Preferably, they should be oral, safe and cheap and in pregnant women, they should not cause any problems to the developing fetus.

Pathology

Pathologically, cystitis shows non-specific features of acute inflammation only (i.e. oedema, congestion and polymorph infiltration). Acute pyelonephritis shows suppurative inflammation with microabscess formation. Polymorphs are the predominant inflammatory cell within the tubules and in the interstitium (Fig. 11.1). Complications may arise from acute pyelonephritis, including papillary necrosis where the tips of the papillae may slough off into the pelvis and ureters, pyonephrosis where there is a cavity filled with pus because of obstruction of the pelvis or upper ureter, perinephric abscess where the inflammatory process spreads across the renal capsule into the perinephric space, septicaemia where the microorganisms spread via the bloodstream, and recurrent episodes of acute infection, which develops into chronic pyelonephritis.

Chronic pyelonephritis usually occurs because of a mechanical (reflux) or obstructive lesion. Grossly, the kidney develops coarse irregular scarring in relation to distortion of the calyceal system and, with progression of disease, the kidney becomes shrunken and contracted,

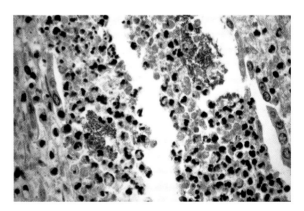

Fig. 11.1   Kidney: acute pyelonephritis. Histological picture of kidney showing acute polymorph infiltration of renal tubular epithelium with bacterial colonies within the lumen. These are the features of acute pyelonephritis.

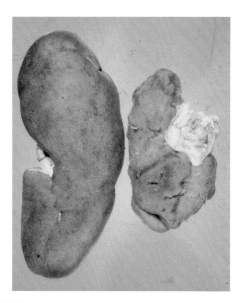

Fig. 11.2 Kidney: chronic pyelonephritis. Gross photographs showing a normal kidney on the left and a small contracted scarred kidney on the right, typical of the effects of chronic pyelonephritis.

with pitted scars on the cortical surface (Fig. 11.2). Microscopically, there is prominent tubulointerstitial inflammation, tubular atrophy and dilatation in which proteinaceous material accumulates producing an appearance resembling normal thyroid (so-called 'thyroidization'), interstitial fibrosis, periglomerular fibrosis and variable degrees of active inflammation especially in the pelvicalyceal systems. Long-term complications associated with chronic pyelonephritis include chronic renal failure, which is one of the commonest indications for dialysis and renal transplantation, systemic hypertension and occasionally septicaemia.

SUMMARY BOX
URINARY TRACT INFECTIONS

- These include infections of the bladder (cystitis) or of the kidney (pyelonephritis) by pyogenic organisms.

- Infection may be precipitated by general factors (diabetes mellitus, immunosuppression and pregnancy) and local factors (stasis, obstruction, stones, tumours, instrumentation, prostatic enlargement and some congenital anomalies of urinary anatomy); in general, UTIs are more common in women.

- Clinically, patients present with pain on micturition (dysuria) or blood in the urine (haematuria).

- Common organisms in ascending infection are derived from the perineal region and gastrointestinal.

- The major complication is chronic pyelonephritis leading to chronic renal failure.

Glomerulonephritis

This is one of the major causes of chronic renal failure. The glomerulus has a very limited range of responses to injury despite its complexity in functional terms. The three main sites of potential damage are the glomerular capillary basement membrane which is the main site of filtration, the mesangial matrix and cells which provide the structural support for glomeruli, and the glomerular capsule which is related to the surrounding connective tissue (Fig. 11.3). Clinically, glomerulonephritis tends to cause haematuria, proteinuria and hypertension. Aetiologically, immunological mechanisms account for the vast majority of cases of glomerulonephritis either in the form of circulating immune complexes which deposit in the glomeruli or, less commonly, where circulating antibodies react with the glomerular basement membrane directly. Circulating immune complexes are cleared from the body partly via the kidneys (also via the reticuloendothelial system) and because the glomeruli filter such a large volume of blood, they are particularly vulnerable to injury, while the risk is related to the size and charge of the complexes. Less frequently, the antigen is an intrinsic component of the glomerular basement membrane and this condition is known as Goodpasture's syndrome, which is a combination of pulmonary haemorrhages and glomerulonephritis.

The classification of glomerulonephritis is quite complex in clinicopathological terms and relates to aetiological factors, morphological features, and the rate of progression of clinical disease, which may be an isolated phenomenon or part of a systemic disease. Some of the

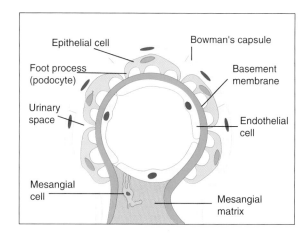

Fig. 11.3 Structure of normal glomerulus showing relations of Bowman's capsule to urinary space, the glomerular capillary basement membrane and mesangium.

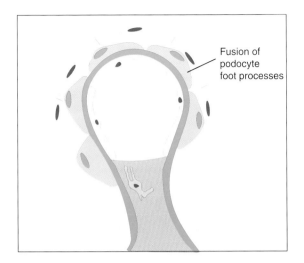

Fig. 11.4 In minimal change disease (a common cause of nephrotic syndrome in children), the main abnormality is fusion of foot processes of epithelial cells.

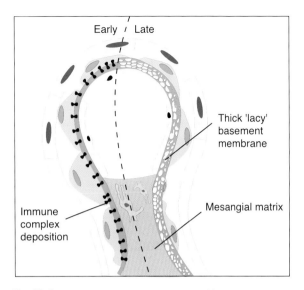

Fig. 11.5 In membranous glomerulonephritis, early stage disease is associated with immune complex deposition on the epithelium in a 'spiky' distribution, while later disease is characterized by a thickened basement membrane with a 'lacy' pattern.

commoner and clinically significant forms are outlined below.

Minimal change disease (Fig. 11.4)

In this condition, the glomeruli appear normal on light microscopy, but on electron microscopy, there is widespread fusion of epithelial cell foot processes. It is the commonest cause of the nephrotic syndrome in young children but may occur at any age. In most cases, recovery occurs but there may be relapses requiring corticosteroid or other immunosuppressive therapy.

Membranous glomerulonephritis (Fig. 11.5)

In this condition, there is diffuse capillary wall thickening with little or no mesangial involvement and with subepithelial spikes in the basement membrane, which on electron microscopy are composed of mainly IgG immune complexes. In most cases, there is no apparent cause but it may be associated with infection (hepatitis B virus, syphilis, malaria), malignant neoplasms (especially in older patients), systemic lupus erythematosus (SLE) and drug toxicity (e.g. penicillamine, gold). It characteristically causes the nephrotic syndrome or persistent proteinuria and the course is either stationary or slowly progressive to chronic renal failure, except where underlying causes such as drugs or infections are treated.

Acute diffuse proliferative glomerulonephritis (Fig. 11.6)

Histologically, this condition is characterized by an increase in mesangial cells and matrix, swollen endothelial cells and an excess of polymorphs; occasionally epithelial crescents may be present. The clinical onset is

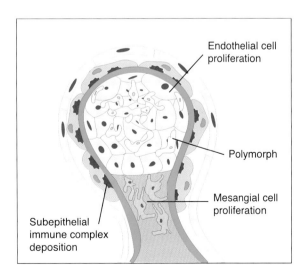

Fig. 11.6 In diffuse acute proliferative glomerulonephritis, often due to preceding streptococcal infection, there is subepithelial immune complex deposition, endothelial and mesangial cell proliferation and polymorph infiltration.

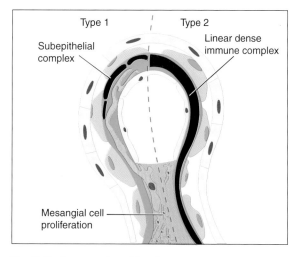

Fig. 11.7 In mesangioproliferative glomerulonephritis, there is expansion of the mesangial matrix in which immune complexes are deposited, typically of IgA type, along with proliferation of mesangial cells.

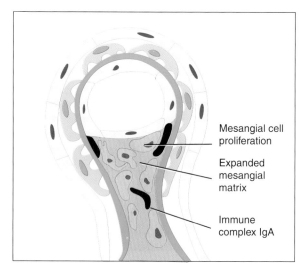

Fig. 11.8 In membranoproliferative glomerulonephritis, there is mesangial cell proliferation along with either subepithelial immune complex deposition (type I) or dense basement membrane immune complexes (type II).

typically 3 weeks after a group A β-haemolytic streptococcal throat infection with the development of the nephritic syndrome (haematuria, hypertension). Most patients recover completely but some have persistent or latent disease with a minority progressing to renal failure. Similar lesions occur in infective endocarditis and in systemic vasculitis.

Diffuse mesangioproliferative glomerulonephritis (Fig. 11.7)

Microscopically, there is an increase in mesangial cells and matrix, with ultrastructural deposits of immune complex, mainly of IgA type but occasionally of IgM type. Various clinical presentations may occur including haematuria, proteinuria or the nephrotic syndrome. Many progress slowly to glomerulosclerosis and renal failure.

Membranoproliferative glomerulonephritis (Fig. 11.8)

In this condition, there is an increase both in mesangial cells and matrix and in thickening of the capillary basement membrane, due to deposition of immune complexes and complement. Patients usually present with the nephrotic syndrome or persistent proteinuria but less frequently with acute nephritis or haematuria. There is often slow progression to renal failure.

Crescentic (rapidly progressive) glomerulonephritis (Fig. 11.9)

In this condition, cellular crescents occlude 50–100% of glomeruli with fibrin in the urinary space; the underlying glomeruli show severe damage, which may be idiopathic or associated with other forms of glomerulonephritis such as Goodpasture's syndrome or in vasculitic condi-

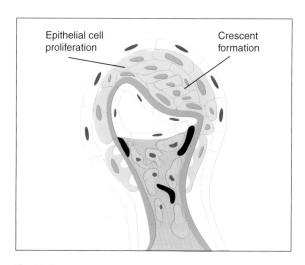

Fig. 11.9 Crescent formation may occur with many different types of glomerulonephritis; it represents a response of the epithelial cells of Bowman's capsule to injury and is often associated with a poor outcome for renal function.

tions such as polyarteritis nodosa or Wegener's granulomatosis. Most patients present with severe progressive acute renal failure which leads to a need for dialysis or transplantation. A small minority recover.

Secondary causes of glomerular disease

Many systemic conditions can result in glomerular damage and the clinical features of glomerulonephritis.

- These can be due to circulating immune complexes, in conditions such as systemic lupus erythematosus, Henoch–Schönlein purpura and infective endocarditis, or due to vascular diseases such as polyarteritis nodosa and Wegener's granulomatosis.
- Diabetes mellitus can cause a number of morphological changes in the kidney including diffuse glomerulosclerosis, nodular glomerulosclerosis (Kimmelstiel–Wilson lesions), fibrin caps and capsular drops, while the afferent and efferent arterioles show marked hyalinization. This is a late complication of diabetes, especially in the juvenile-onset insulin-dependent type where it occurs in about one-third of cases, and it tends to present with proteinuria which persists for years but may cause the nephrotic syndrome and renal failure.
- Amyloidosis refers to the deposition of an amorphous eosinophilic hyaline material in various organs of the body including the kidney. The material is of heterogeneous origin (including serum amyloid A (SAA) protein and light-chain-derived amyloid (AL) type) but has a common histological appearance and histochemical staining reaction with the Congo Red stain, which produces characteristic apple-green birefringence when viewed under cross-polarized light. Amyloid may be deposited in the mesangium, capillary basement membranes, blood vessels, tubular basement membranes and renal interstitium. The clinical presentation is usually with proteinuria which later progresses to the nephrotic syndrome and ultimately renal failure.

Acute renal failure

The kidneys may go into acute failure for a number of reasons:

- pre-renal failure, as a response to severe volume loss, e.g. in burns, severe trauma or massive haemorrhage, or circulatory failure, e.g. after myocardial infarction
- renal causes, such as acute tubular necrosis, severe glomerulonephritis, acute interstitial nephritis and vasculitis

SUMMARY BOX
GLOMERULAR DISEASES

- Most primary glomerular diseases are immunologically mediated.
- The antigenic stimulus may be part of the glomerulus itself or more commonly be formed elsewhere in the circulation.
- Antigens include infective agents, drugs, tumours and self-antigens such as the nucleus in systemic lupus erythematosus (SLE).
- Secondary glomerular damage is associated with systemic diseases such as diabetes, vasculitis including that complicating infective endocarditis, autoimmune diseases, hypertension and amyloidosis.
- Patients may present clinically with haematuria, proteinuria, hypertension, the nephritic syndrome, the nephrotic syndrome or chronic renal failure.

- post-renal causes, including obstruction, such as hydronephrosis, ureteric blockage from tumours and prostatic enlargement, and major vessel occlusion.

Clinically, patients in acute renal failure present with a reduction or complete absence of urinary output, associated with oedema, hypertension and general uraemic symptoms such as tiredness and pallor. The diagnosis is confirmed biochemically by the finding of raised blood urea and creatinine and reduced glomerular filtration rate (GFR) as shown by reduced creatinine clearance. There is often marked disturbance of electrolytes in the serum, the most worrying of which is elevation of the potassium above 6.0–6.5 mmol/l which may cause cardiac conduction abnormalities including sudden death.

SUMMARY BOX
ACUTE RENAL FAILURE

- Acute renal failure may be due to:
  - pre-renal factors such as severe volume loss
  - renal causes such as acute tubular necrosis, glomerulonephritis, vasculitis and interstitial nephritis
  - post-renal causes such as obstruction.
- Patients present with reduction or lack of urinary output, oedema, hypertension and electrolyte imbalances.
- Unless renal function is supported by, for example, haemodialysis, death rapidly ensues.

Chronic renal failure

This is end-stage renal failure for which there is no single cause. Glomerulonephritis of whatever aetiology is responsible for approximately 30% of all cases, diabetes mellitus contributes another 15–20% of cases, while vascular diseases including hypertension are the cause of about 15% of cases, and polycystic disease of the kidneys is the underlying factor in 10% of cases. There are then a large number of other causes including chronic pyelonephritis, urinary obstruction, interstitial nephritis, analgesic nephropathy, amyloidosis, multiple myeloma, hereditary factors and occasionally no apparent cause can be identified.

Clinically, these patients have reduced urinary output, sometimes with nocturia, associated with hypertension, oedema and uraemic symptoms including tiredness, pallor and anaemia. There may be bone disease including osteomalacia, because of impaired vitamin D metabolism, osteitis fibrosa cystica and a spectrum of bone disease known as renal osteodystrophy.

Chronic renal failure will cause death if untreated and these patients are maintained on long-term dialysis, which may be via the bloodstream (haemodialysis) or through the peritoneal cavity (peritoneal dialysis), until renal transplantation can be performed. This is usually from a recently deceased compatible donor (cadaveric transplant) or may be from a related live donor. It is important that the donor and recipient are well matched in immunological terms to avoid problems of transplant rejection. This may be hyperacute (where pre-existing antibodies exist), acute (where there is a cell-mediated reaction causing damage to the tubules and interstitium) or chronic (where long-term vascular damage occurs, inevitably resulting in failure of the grafted kidney).

SUMMARY BOX
CHRONIC RENAL FAILURE

- Chronic renal failure is caused by a heterogeneous group of disorders including glomerular disease, diabetes, vascular diseases, chronic infection and polycystic disease.

- Patients present with progressive failure of renal function with systemic effects on electrolytes, calcium and bone metabolism and anaemia.

- Unless treated, patients will eventually die of disease; treatment is by dialysis or renal transplantation.

Vascular disease

Hypertension itself may damage the kidney, or hypertension may be caused when the kidney is damaged in the long term by atheromatous disease. This can be caused by narrowing of the renal artery leading to renal ischaemia, which causes a reduction in the glomerular filtration rate, stimulating the juxtaglomerular apparatus to release renin which converts angiotensinogen to angiotensin and raises the systemic blood pressure. The extent of kidney damage in atheromatous disease is greater in the elderly, when there is atheroma elsewhere, in cigarette smokers, in systemic hypertension and in coexisting diabetes. The degree of renal damage in hypertension is decreasing because the likelihood of chronic renal failure is much reduced as a result of better antihypertensive drugs and improved patient compliance.

Polycystic kidney disease

This disease may arise in the neonatal period as an autosomal recessive condition when it is almost inevitably fatal. However, the adult form of the condition is inherited as an autosomal dominant disease and affects 1 person in 1000. It is nearly always bilateral and may present with haematuria, hypertension, chronic renal failure, or an asymptomatic mass, possible picked up on abdominal ultrasound. It may be associated with liver disease including congenital hepatic fibrosis and cysts or with intracranial berry aneurysms, possibly leading to subarachnoid haemorrhage. The kidneys are completely replaced by cysts of varying sizes containing clear and sometimes haemorrhagic fluid. The intervening stroma may contain some functioning renal parenchyma but as the disease progresses this is replaced by cysts, ultimately causing renal failure requiring dialysis or transplantation.

Neoplasms
Urothelial tumours

Most tumours of the urothelium are transitional cell in type. They are relatively common tumours accounting for 1–2% of all malignancies and the vast majority occur in the bladder, although identical tumours can occur in the renal pelvis, ureters and urethra. They are more likely to occur in males rather than females and are a disease of middle age and later in urban and industrialized societies. Urothelial neoplasms are good examples of the effect of chemical carcinogenesis. β-Naphthylamine is a chemical used in the synthesis of azo and aniline dyes and pigments, whose metabolites are released in the bladder urine by the effect of β-glucuronidase usually associated with acidity. There is a long latent period, 20 years or more, from the time of exposure to the development of neoplasia but the relative risk of bladder tumours is in the order of 50 times in this group. It is also seen in those who use similar chemicals in the textile, printing, plastics, rubber and cable industries and in fishermen who use maggots. Cigarette smoking increases the risk by some two to four times and rarer associations are with analgesic abuse, tryptophan metabolites and cyclophosphamide. Infection with the *Schistosoma* parasites are associated with an increased incidence of squamous carcinoma. It is likely that there is a 'field effect' as a result of exposure to carcinogenic agents, and urothelial tumours are often multiple and recurrent, arising in a background of an unstable epithelium. Most tumours arise de novo but a minority occur in the setting of carcinoma in situ, which is difficult to detect cystoscopically and is associated with a worse prognosis.

Pathologically, most tumours are low grade and have a papillary, fern-like growth pattern projecting above the epithelial surface. Grading is based on the epithelial appearances, particularly how closely the cells resemble the cell of origin (urothelial), the extent of nuclear pleomorphism and the number and type of mitoses. As tumours enlarge and become less differentiated, they tend to become less papillary and more solid. The stage of tumour relates to the extent of spread of the tumour, initially within the bladder. Most low-grade papillary tumours do not invade below the basement membrane into the submucosa, whereas as tumours become more high grade and more solid, they are more likely to invade submucosa and deep muscle. The stage of the tumour is an important determinant in prognosis.

Kidney

Renal cell carcinoma is the commonest primary tumour of the kidney. It accounts for 1–3% of all solid cancers and for 85–90% of all renal tumours (most of the remainder are of urothelial origin, see above). It is more common in men than in women and is a disease of the middle-aged and elderly (50–80 years). Again smokers are at increased risk and some unusual genetic associations are known including von Hippel–Lindau syndrome. Patients may present with a palpable mass or a lesion found incidentally on investigation of other abdominal conditions. Rarely, it may present with haematuria or with paraneoplastic syndromes including hypercalcaemia, polycythaemia or Cushing's syndrome.

Pathology. Grossly, the tumours tend to occur at the poles of the kidney (upper more than lower) and usually are solitary masses between 3 and 15 cm in diameter. They have a predominantly yellow cut surface with areas of haemorrhage and cystic degeneration. Tumour may

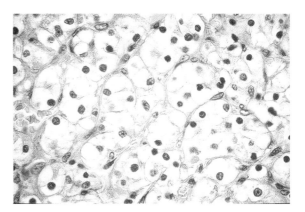

Fig. 11.10 Kidney: clear cell carcinoma. Histological section of a typical renal cell carcinoma showing clear cell features.

extend into the renal capsule or perinephric fat, into the renal pelvis and calyces, into the kidney elsewhere as satellite nodules and into the renal vein, often at the hilum and extending into the inferior vena cava. Histologically, the commonest pattern is as sheets of clear cells (Fig. 11.10), which are rich in glycogen and fat, the latter giving the tumour its characteristic yellow appearance. Other cell types include granular eosinophilic cells and spindle cells, while solid and papillary patterns may also be seen. The tumours have a very vascular stroma giving rise to the often haemorrhagic gross appearance. Behaviour of these tumours is unpredictable. Many have an indolent slow-growing course while others (up to 25%) have metastasized at the time of diagnosis. The renal vein involvement described above may give rise to haematogenous metastases in lungs and bones, while there may also be regional lymph node involvement, spread to the adrenal glands, brain and the opposite kidney. 5-Year survival is approximately 45%, which is reduced to 15–20% if there is renal vein or perinephric spread. Small tumours (less than 2–3 cm in diameter) may be found whose biological behaviour is uncertain. While they are unlikely to metastasize, it is probably best to treat them aggressively with surgery.

Wilms' tumour

One of the commonest intra-abdominal tumours of childhood is Wilms' tumour (nephroblastoma), most presenting between the ages of 1 and 4 years. These are very aggressive tumours which have often spread to the lungs at the time of diagnosis. They are composed of a mixture of epithelial and mesenchymal (blastemal) elements, often embryonal in appearance and may contain heterologous components such as muscle, bone or cartilage.

Despite the aggressive clinical behaviour, current treatment modalities combining surgery, chemotherapy and radiotherapy provide excellent long-term survival figures.

Prostate

This is the commonest form of cancer affecting men and is a leading cause of cancer deaths. It is a disease of increasing age particularly involving the elderly between 65 and 80 years. It is rare in Orientals but is common in Caucasians and those of Afro-Caribbean origin. It is probably related to hormonal influences, with androgens such as testosterone and its metabolites playing a role in its growth and because of the known effect of anti-androgens in its treatment.

It must be distinguished from the other more common disease of benign nodular enlargement of the prostate (Fig. 11.11). In this condition, there is a combination of glandular hyperplasia and stromal fibromuscular hypertrophy, occurring most often in the central zones of the prostate gland, particularly the median lobe. This leads to urinary retention and infections.

Pathology. Grossly, most prostatic carcinomas arise in the peripheral zones of the prostate gland, especially posteriorly where the tumour can be palpated by digital rectal examination. It has a gritty firm texture, is of yellow-grey colour and tends not to be nodular (unlike benign nodular enlargement/hyperplasia). The vast majority of tumours are adenocarcinomas and the degree of glandular differentiation forms the basis of one of the most frequently used grading systems (the Gleason grade); perineural infiltration is a characteristic histological feature. Staging of these tumours is important because many men as they get older will develop symptoms of

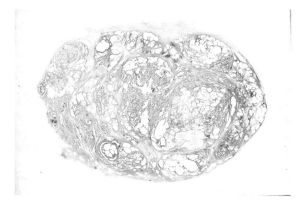

Fig. 11.11 Prostate: benign nodular enlargement. Whole mount histological section of prostate gland showing well-marked glandular hyperplasia typical of benign nodular enlargement.

urinary outflow obstruction requiring surgery. Approximately one-third of men over 50 years will harbour a stage A tumour (early incidental tumour confined to the gland) and over two-thirds of men over 80 years will do so. The long-term significance of such a finding is uncertain and is reflected in the different managements on either side of the Atlantic, the approach being much more aggressive in the USA. The tumour may spread into surrounding tissues such as the base of the bladder, seminal vesicles and perirectal tissues, via lymphatics into para-aortic lymph nodes and via the bloodstream to bone, where characteristic osteosclerotic/osteoblastic metastases develop, or to liver and lungs. A marker of spread of prostatic carcinoma is serum prostate-specific antigen (PSA) which is elevated in metastatic disease. However, there is considerable overlap between the 'normal' range and that associated with disseminated disease, so that PSA cannot yet be used as a screening test for prostate cancer. The prognosis depends on the grade (Gleason) and stage of the tumour with Stage A and B disease (incidental/localized to the gland) having a 50–80% 10-year survival and Stage C and D disease (local extension/metastatic) having a 10–40% 10-year survival.

Testis

These are rare tumours but they have a tendency to occur in young adults and, before the development of chemotherapy, had a very high mortality rate. Nowadays, the availability of combination chemotherapy has increased the survival rates. Most testicular tumours (90–95%) are of germ cell origin while the remainder are of interstitial cell or lymphoid origin. They have been increasing in incidence recently and tend to occur in higher socio-economic classes. Risk factors for the development of testicular tumours include cryptorchidism (undescended testis) in up to 10% of cases, gonadal dysgenesis and a history of previous germ cell tumours. It is now generally accepted that all germ cell tumours arise from a precursor lesion in the testis known as intratubular gem cell neoplasia (ITGCN) where there is a proliferation of atypical cells resembling undifferentiated germ cells. Seminomas are composed of undifferentiated germ cells, accounting for 50% of germ cell tumours, while teratomas are derived from multipotent cells which may show endodermal, mesodermal and ectodermal differentiation.

Seminomas. These are the commonest form of germ cell tumours and have a peak incidence in the fourth and fifth decades. Grossly, they are well-circumscribed masses between 3 and 5 cm in diameter, of uniform texture, white or tan in colour, and rarely show haemorrhage or necrosis. Histologically, they are composed of a single large cell type with pale cytoplasm and single prominent nucleolus. They lie in sheets with interspersed lymphoid aggregates with occasional granulomas.

Teratomas. These occur at a slightly younger age, in the late 20s, and occasionally may occur in children. The tumours tend to be larger than seminomas, may be multicystic and often show areas of haemorrhage and necrosis. Histologically, the tumour is composed of tissues from all three germ layers, most commonly containing skin, glial (neural), bronchial and gastrointestinal tissues, smooth muscle, cartilage and fat, and occasionally extra-embryonic tissues. The classification is related to the degree of differentiation: containing mature ('normal' tissues), undifferentiated, anaplastic, yolk sac (α-fetoprotein positive), and choriocarcinomatous (human chorionic gonadotrophin positive) elements. In general, seminomas do not show similar areas. The tumours spread locally to the surrounding tissues, especially epididymis, at a late stage; via lymphatics to iliac, lumbar and para-aortic lymph nodes; and by blood-borne spread to liver, lungs, brain and bones, earlier in teratomas than in seminomas. Prognosis generally is very good in response to radiotherapy for seminomas and to chemotherapy for teratomas.

SUMMARY BOX
URINARY TRACT NEOPLASMS

- In the kidney, tumours may be derived from the tubules (renal cell carcinoma), or from the urothelium in the pelvis (transitional cell carcinoma).
- In the bladder, most tumours are of urothelial origin (transitional cell carcinoma) which may be associated with exposure to dyes and cigarette smoking.
- Prostatic carcinoma is a disease of elderly men which presents with bladder outflow problems, UTIs or distant metastases to bone; it must be distinguished from the more common benign nodular enlargement of prostate.
- Testicular tumours are usually of germ cell origin and include seminomas which have a peak incidence between 30 and 50 years and teratomas which present between 20 and 30 years.

ASPECTS OF RENAL DISEASE OF PARTICULAR RELEVANCE TO DENTISTRY

- Metabolism of prescribed drugs may be impaired in patients with renal failure.
- Drug-induced gingival overgrowth may be seen in renal transplant recipients.

FEMALE GENITAL TRACT

Vulva

This is lined by squamous epithelium and thus many of the same conditions which affect the skin may also occur in the vulva. The common infections of the vulva are with *Candida albicans* and herpes simplex, type 2. Human papillomavirus (HPV) infection causes genital warts and is associated strongly with neoplasia (see below). A number of cysts, e.g. of Bartholin's glands, and benign tumours, e.g. papillary hidradenoma, also occur at this site.

Non-neoplastic epithelial disorders affecting the vulva include squamous hyperplasia and lichen sclerosus, which may present as leukoplakia due to hyperkeratosis in both conditions. In squamous hyperplasia, as its name implies, there is epidermal hyperplasia but in lichen sclerosus there is thinning of the epidermis with flattening of the rete ridges. There is an increased risk of neoplasia in both conditions, which is greater in squamous hyperplasia.

Vulval intraepithelial neoplasia (VIN) is the spectrum of pre-invasive neoplasia in the vulva, analogous to that in the cervix, and is associated with HPV infection. There may be synchronous involvement in other sites such as vagina and cervix. Squamous carcinoma is more common in elderly women and gives rise to local lymph node involvement. Paget's disease of vulva, unlike that of the breast, is associated with underlying carcinoma in only about 25% of cases. Other malignant tumours at this site include melanoma and basal cell carcinoma.

Vagina

Infections of the vagina are usually venereally transmitted including *Gardnerella vaginalis*, *Neisseria gonorrhoeae*, *Candida albicans* and *Trichomonas vaginalis*. Subepithelial glands occur in the vagina in the rare condition of vaginal adenosis, associated with in utero exposure to diethylstilboestrol; very rarely, clear cell carcinoma may arise from this condition. Vaginal intraepithelial neoplasia (VaIN) is analogous to the situation in the cervix. Squamous carcinoma of vagina is a rare tumour mainly of elderly women, which often gives rise to local invasion.

Cervix

Non-specific inflammation of the cervix occurs with the use of intrauterine contraceptive devices (IUCDs), prolapse of the cervix and ectopy. *Chlamydia trachomatis* is an intracellular organism often transmitted venereally which causes cervicitis often associated with lymphoid follicle formation ('follicular cervicitis').

Cervical intraepithelial neoplasia (CIN) is strongly associated with HPV infection. Some HPV subtypes including 6 and 11 tend to cause simple warts (condyloma acuminatum) (Fig. 11.12) whereas subtypes 16, 18, 31 and 33 are associated with CIN and carcinoma. Risk factors for squamous neoplasia include an early age of first intercourse, frequency of intercourse and multiplicity of sexual partners. Cigarette smoking has also been implicated. The severity of CIN is graded according to the level of the epithelium at which maturation occurs: thus

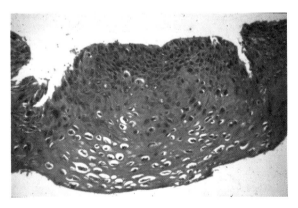

Fig. 11.12 Cervix: human papillomavirus. Full-thickness biopsy of cervical squamous epithelium in which enlarged cells with clear cytoplasm and crumpled nuclei, characteristic of koilocytes, are present, indicating HPV infection.

CIN1 shows maturation about one-third of the way up the epithelium while CIN3 shows maturation between two-thirds and full thickness. The higher the grade of CIN the more likely is the risk of invasive neoplasia. This is the basis of cervical cytology screening where smears of cells derived from the cervix are examined for the characteristic nuclear abnormalities (dyskaryosis) which correspond to the histological appearances. If recognized early, these lesions may be treated locally with laser ablation or diathermy.

Squamous carcinoma may be microinvasive, which has a negligible risk of lymph node metastasis, or frankly invasive where metastases are more likely. The prognosis of cervical carcinoma depends on the stage of disease, which relates to the extent of local spread within the pelvis and to the presence and extent of lymph node metastases. Treatment of extensive disease is by radical surgery.

Uterus

Endometrium

This is lined by glandular epithelium which changes with the menstrual cycle in response to oestrogen and progesterone levels, affected by FSH and LH levels. Non-neoplastic conditions affecting the endometrium include luteal phase insufficiency, endometritis due to chlamydial infection and tuberculosis, and iatrogenic conditions secondary to hormones such as the oral contraceptive pill and hormone replacement therapy and the presence of an IUCD.

Endometrial polyps are common in peri- and post-menopausal women and have little potential for malignant change. Endometrial hyperplasias occur in response to unopposed oestrogen stimulation and are classified as simple, complex and atypical, the last of which has a high risk of malignant change.

Endometrial adenocarcinoma may arise from atypical hyperplasia or develop in atrophic postmenopausal endometrium. Tumour may spread locally into cervix and vagina, via lymphatics to local and regional lymph nodes or via the bloodstream. Tumours may also arise from endometrial stroma, giving rise to endometrial stromal sarcomas. Combined tumours including glandular and stromal elements may occur and are referred to as mixed Müllerian tumours. They may contain so-called heterologous elements such as cartilage and bone.

Myometrium

Foci of glandular tissue may be found within the myometrium, referred to as adenomyosis, which is a form of endometriosis. The most common pathology affecting the myometrium is benign smooth muscle tumours or leiomyomas, more commonly referred to as 'fibroids' (Fig. 11.13). These can become very large and tend to be multiple. They present clinically as an abdominal mass, excessive bleeding from the endometrium and urinary problems due to pressure effects on the bladder.

Ovary

The normal functions of the ovary are to provide ova on a cyclical basis for potential fertilization and to produce female sex hormones.

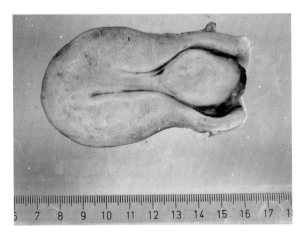

Fig. 11.13 Uterus: leiomyoma. An opened uterus demonstrating a typical pedunculated submucosal leiomyoma ('fibroid').

SUMMARY BOX
UTERUS

- The normal endometrium is responsive to the cyclical secretions of oestrogen and progesterone.
- Non-neoplastic conditions of the endometrium include infections and conditions related to hormones or IUCDs.
- Endometrial hyperplasia arises as a result of unopposed oestrogen activity and may be simple, complex or atypical.
- Adenocarcinoma may arise from atypical hyperplasia or from atrophic postmenopausal endometrium.
- Stromal tumours may also occur either alone or as part of mixed Müllerian neoplasia.
- Myometrial tumours (fibroids) are very common, presenting with excessive uterine bleeding, abdominal masses or pressure effects on the bladder.

Non-neoplastic cysts of the ovary may arise from various inclusions and structures within the ovary including mesothelial lined, epithelial inclusion, follicular, luteinized follicular, corpus luteum, corpus albicans and endometriotic forms.

Endometriosis

This is the presence of endometrial glands and stroma outside the uterus including ovary, pelvic peritoneum, pouch of Douglas, cervix, vagina, vulva, bladder, small and large intestines. In the ovary they are a cause of severe pain with the accumulation of large amounts of blood, producing so-called chocolate cysts.

Neoplasms

These may arise from a number of elements within the ovary, including epithelium, germ cells, sex-cord stroma and connective tissue.

- Epithelial tumours may give rise to a range of types including serous, mucinous, endometrioid and Brenner neoplasms. All types may be benign or malignant and an intermediate form of borderline malignancy exists which is of low malignant potential. Mucinous tumours may give rise to spread within the peritoneal cavity known as *pseudomyxoma peritonei*. There may be a family history of ovarian and other neoplasms, sometimes associated with the BRCA1 gene. Most of these tumours present at an advanced stage and are a significant cause of death, spreading predominantly within the abdominal cavity.

- Germ cell tumours include dysgerminomas, which are the female counterpart of seminomas in males, and teratomas which are tumours capable of differentiating along all three germ cell lines: ectoderm, mesoderm and endoderm. Mature cystic teratomas may contain a mixture of germ cell constituents including teeth, hair and sebaceous material. Yolk sac tumours and chorio-carcinomas are germ cell tumours differentiating along extraembryonic lines.
- Sex-cord stromal tumours arise from the component of the ovary which normally produces hormones and include thecomas, granulosa cell tumours, Sertoli–Leydig cell tumours, gonadoblastomas and steroid cell tumours.
- The ovary may be the site of metastatic tumours from elsewhere in the genital tract including the endometrium and from extragenital sites such as stomach, colon and rectum, and breast. These may be confused with primary ovarian neoplasms.

SUMMARY BOX
OVARY

- Non-neoplastic ovarian cysts include mesothelial, follicular, corpus luteum, corpus albicans, epithelial inclusion and endometriotic forms.
- Endometriosis (endometrial glands and stroma outside the uterus) occurs commonly in the ovary, causing chocolate cysts and pain.
- Neoplasms:
  - may be of epithelial, germ cell and sex-cord stromal origin
  - may be solid or cystic and can be benign, borderline or malignant
  - are common malignancies which cause significant mortality because they present late in the disease.

Fallopian tubes

The commonest pathology affecting the tubes are infections secondary to infection in the endometrium or related to an IUCD. Organisms involved include *Chlamydia*, *Bacteroides* and less commonly gonococcus. Such infections may be a significant cause of infertility by causing obstruction of the tubal lumen. Tumours of the tube are rare. Ectopic pregnancy may develop within the Fallopian tube and can cause severe pain and life-threatening haemorrhage.

BREAST DISEASES

The breasts are part of the female reproductive system primarily designed for the purpose of lactation after pregnancy. They consist of epithelial structures organized as acinar tissue in lobules, in which lactation occurs, leading via ductal structures to the nipples on the skin surface of the anterior chest wall. Breast development is part of puberty and adolescence and is mediated by cyclical hormone production of oestrogen and progesterone, in response to the pituitary hormones: follicle stimulating hormone (FSH) and luteinizing hormone (LH). During pregnancy, the breasts enlarge in preparation for lactation, in response to the pituitary hormone prolactin, with increased secretions within the lobules and epithelial hyperplasia. If the mother chooses to breast-feed, lactational secretion continues. After the menopause the breasts involute through a process of atrophy.

Inflammatory conditions of the breast

Acute bacterial mastitis is a complication of lactation with infection of the breast tissue, particularly by *Staphylococcus aureus* and less commonly by *Streptococcus pyogenes*. Duct ectasia is a non-infective inflammatory process in response to release of duct contents. Fat necrosis occurs after trauma, particularly in obese women.

Proliferative conditions

Fibrocystic disease is a range of responses by breast tissue to disturbances of normal hormonal stimulation. There may be a palpable breast lump requiring excision biopsy. Histological changes include adenosis, sclerosing adenosis, epithelial hyperplasia, papillomatosis, cyst formation, apocrine metaplasia and fibrosis. In general, these conditions do not predispose to malignancy, although atypical hyperplasia may increase the risk slightly. In men, development of breast tissue may occur (gynaecomastia) associated with some drugs and chronic liver disease.

Neoplasms
Benign tumours

These include fibroadenoma which is a very common lesion in younger women. It presents as a palpable mobile mass, sometimes referred to as a 'breast mouse' and consists of a mixture of glandular and stromal elements. Treatment is usually by surgical excision and there is little or no risk of malignancy. Duct papillomas are less common tumours which occur in middle-aged women and present with a blood-stained nipple discharge. They arise in larger ducts and consist of papillary growths of epithelium over fibrovascular cores. Solitary lesions carry no risk of malignancy but rare individuals with multiple papillomas have an increased risk of carcinoma. Pure adenomas are rare but tubular and lactating adenomas occur in younger women and nipple adenomas present with a bloody nipple discharge and skin ulceration.

Carcinomas

These are very common carcinomas in western populations, and breast carcinoma is the commonest malignant tumour in women in the UK. Risk factors include increasing age, a long interval between first menstruation (menarche) and the menopause, an older age at first pregnancy, obesity and a high fat diet, previous atypical hyperplasia on biopsy, and a positive family history. Recently, the BRCA1 and BRCA2 genes have been identified, which increase the risk of developing carcinoma in susceptible individuals. Aetiologically, tumours are responsive to high oestrogenic stimulation with relatively lower progesterone levels. However, there is no relationship with use of the oral contraceptive pill.

Non-invasive carcinomas include ductal carcinoma in situ (DCIS) and lobular carcinoma in situ (LCIS). DCIS may present as a palpable mass and is being recognized more frequently with the use of breast-screening programmes (Fig. 11.14). They can be of solid or comedo types and are treated by surgical excision. The ultimate

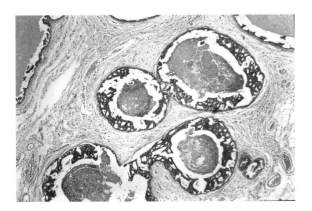

Fig. 11.14   Breast: intraduct carcinoma. Histological section of a ductal carcinoma in situ of breast showing central necrosis within the expanded ducts.

outcome of DCIS is uncertain but it is likely that they progress to invasive malignancy in 20–30% of cases. LCIS rarely presents as a palpable mass but in premenopausal women, has a 25–33% risk of developing invasive lobular carcinoma. In postmenopausal women, LCIS is usually seen in breasts adjacent to infiltrating lobular carcinoma.

Invasive carcinomas of the breast are most commonly of ductal type (85%) with infiltrating lobular carcinoma accounting for 10% of the total. Less commonly seen variants include mucinous, tubular, papillary and medullary carcinomas. Invasive ductal carcinoma (IDC) is the characteristic form of breast carcinoma presenting as a palpable mass. On sectioning it has a typical scirrhous (fibrous) reaction, cutting with the consistency of an unripe pear. Histological differentiation is related to the extent of gland formation, mitotic activity and nuclear pleomorphism.

Breast carcinomas can spread in different ways. Paget's disease of the nipple often presents with an eczema-like erosion of the nipple skin which on histological examination consists of pale-staining malignant tumour cells growing along the epidermis. It is associated with underlying DCIS or invasive ductal carcinoma, although direct connection between Paget's disease and the underlying neoplasm may not be seen. Tumours may directly infiltrate the overlying skin or underlying muscle. Spread via lymphatics causes axillary node involvement and may also cause node involvement elsewhere. Haematogenous spread is common to organs such as lungs, bone, liver and brain.

The prognosis in breast carcinoma is related to a number of factors. In general, the wider the tumour has spread the worse the prognosis. Staging systems exist, particularly the TNM classification, which help to determine prognosis and help to plan appropriate treatment. Some types of carcinoma have a better prognosis than the usual IDC type, including medullary, mucinous, tubular and invasive lobular carcinomas. Low-grade tumours as identified by the degree of differentiation (nuclear pleomorphism, mitotic activity, gland formation) have a better prognosis compared with high-grade tumours. Tumours which are oestrogen and progesterone receptor-positive have a better prognosis and are more responsive to hormonal treatment. Rapidly growing tumours as determined by growth kinetic methods have a poor prognosis.

Less common malignant tumours involving the breast include phyllodes tumour, angiosarcomas, lymphomas and tumours of mesenchymal origin.

SUMMARY BOX
BREAST

- Inflammatory conditions include bacterial mastitis, duct ectasia and fat necrosis.
- Fibrocystic disease is a form of proliferative disease with a variety of features.
- Benign tumours are common and include fibroadenomas, duct papillomas and pure adenomas.
- Non-invasive malignant tumours may be of ductal or lobular origin.
- Malignant tumours are usually of ductal origin although lobular carcinoma and other variants may occur; this is the commonest form of malignancy in women in the UK.
- Paget's disease is associated with underlying ductal neoplasia.
- Prognosis is related to the stage of disease, histological type, oestrogen receptor status and rate of growth of the tumour.

CASE STUDY 11.1
LOIN PAIN

A 72-year-old male presented to his general practitioner with an episode of severe loin pain. On examination, he was noted to have a temperature of 39.7°C and was tender in the right loin. Investigations were performed including urine and blood tests.

After appropriate treatment, his pain, tenderness and temperature improved, although haematuria which was present previously was noted to have persisted. He was referred to the Urology Unit at his local hospital where a number of investigations were performed, after which he was offered surgery.

1. What was the most likely cause of his presenting symptoms in this case?
2. What underlying conditions might have predisposed this man to these problems?
3. What treatment is likely to be offered in this case?

Suggested responses

1. This man had signs and symptoms of a urinary tract infection (UTI), probably an ascending pyelonephritis from pre-existing cystitis. Urine tests would have shown the presence of protein, red blood cells and white cells as a result of the infection, while culture of the urine would probably have demonstrated the presence of significant numbers of microorganisms (greater than 100 000 per cubic millimetre). Possible organisms include *E. coli*, *Proteus* and enteric streptococci. Blood tests should be done to determine if there is any evidence of renal damage such as raised blood urea and creatinine levels or evidence of coexistent diabetes.

2. In a man of this age the most likely underlying cause of UTI is prostatic disease, either benign nodular enlargement or prostatic carcinoma. This leads to retention of urine and, after micturition, there is often residual urine in the bladder which acts as a culture medium for bacterial infection. Diabetes mellitus, especially of maturity-onset type (type II), is common in this age group and should be excluded, as diabetics are prone to infections at many sites. Prostatic carcinoma is associated with raised levels of prostate-specific antigen (PSA) in the serum. Very high levels are seen where there is extensive extraprostatic disease, particularly in the presence of bone metastases which may be of osteoblastic/osteosclerotic type.

3. If prostatic carcinoma has been excluded (or at least considered unlikely) on PSA measurements, then transurethral resection of prostate (TURP) is the usual procedure to allow free passage of urine and complete emptying of the bladder, thus reducing the risk of infection. If prostatic carcinoma is suspected, TURP may provide histological confirmation, after which treatment such as hormonal manipulation may be offered since prostatic carcinoma is a hormonally responsive lesion. Haematuria may be the presenting feature also of bladder carcinomas of transitional type; this condition can be excluded at the time of TURP by undertaking cystoscopy before resection of prostate.

12 Bone and joint diseases

Normal bone metabolism

Bone is a specialized connective tissue, which despite its apparently rigid structure is a dynamic organ that undergoes change throughout life, although this is greater at some periods, e.g. in childhood, than others, e.g. middle life. Its main function is to provide structural support to the skeleton and in some areas it provides a protective covering for vital underlying organs, such as the rib cage for the heart and lungs and the skull for the brain. It is also an important store of minerals, especially calcium and phosphate, which are important for cellular metabolism throughout the body and are released from bone under hormonal influences as required. Structurally, it is composed of large amounts of parallel arrays of cross-linked type I collagen fibres, a matrix rich in proteins, hydroxyapatite crystals and bone cells (osteocytes) which interconnect with each other and the extracellular matrix. A number of different bone types exist, including:

- lamellar bone where the collagen fibres are arranged in parallel arrays; this is the normal pattern for most bones
- woven bone where the collagen fibres are deposited in a haphazard arrangement, where the cells are large and the bone is variably calcified and weak; this is the form seen in many skeletal disorders (see below) and may also occur in soft tissues
- cortical bone which is found on the outside of long bones and is more dense than lamellar bone, contains little marrow and is composed of lamellae arranged concentrically around a central Haversian canal.

Bone is a dynamic tissue and is constantly being remodelled. Multinucleated giant cells within bone which are capable of eroding bony surfaces are called osteoclasts. They act in response to a number of stimuli including parathyroid hormone (PTH), 1,25-dihydroxycholecalciferol (the active form of vitamin D) and prostaglandin E2, and may be inhibited by calcitonin, prostacyclin and some drugs. Following the action of osteoclasts, they disperse and are replaced by mononuclear cells which lay down reversal or cement lines; these allow the movement of bone, which has the effect of dissipating energy. Osteoblasts are cells which lay down an organic matrix known as osteoid and, under correct conditions, osteoid is mineralized adjacent to already mineralized bone. This proceeds for a variable length of time, after which the residual matrix is calcified and a resting line is deposited. Bone is remodelled in response to mechanical stress according to changes in electrical charge (piezoelectric forces) so that bone is deposited in areas under compression and resorbed in areas under tension.

Fracture healing

The principles of fracture healing are the same as those for wound healing generally (as previously described) but a number of specific features relate to fracture repair. An example of bone fracture healing is the response to tooth extraction within alveolar bone (Fig. 12.1). At the site of extraction there is disruption of soft tissues and blood vessels with the formation of a haematoma along with damage to the periodontal ligament and the surrounding alveolar bone. There is an influx of macrophages to the site with an ingrowth of new blood vessels from the adjacent alveolar region. Osteoclasts resorb dead bone and osteoblasts lay down osteoid in the form of fracture callus. This is later calcified and remodelled

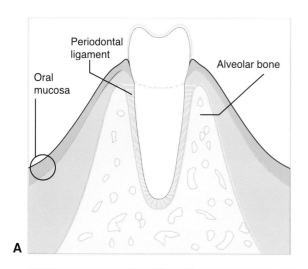

A

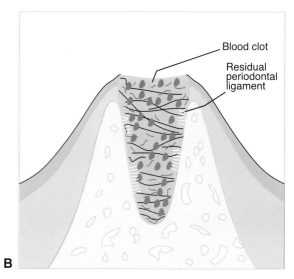

B

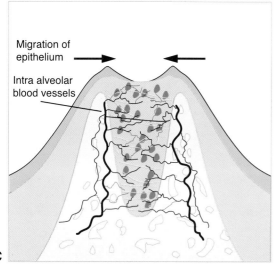

C

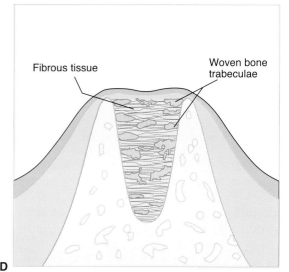

D

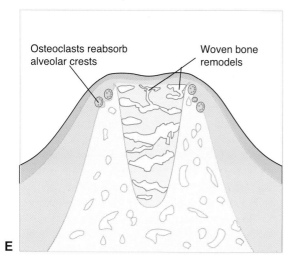

E

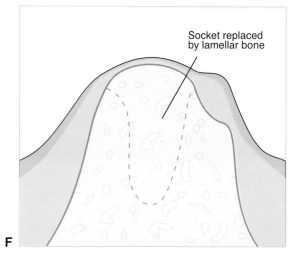

F

Fig. 12.1 Pattern of wound healing after dental extraction. A. Normal tooth socket with tooth within alveolar bone surrounded by periodontal ligament. **B.** 2–3 Hours after extraction, the socket is filled with blood clot and residual periodontal ligament. **C.** After 2–3 days, the socket has undergone an inflammatory process with polymorph infiltration followed by macrophage infiltration; early granulation tissue has developed with ingrowth of new blood vessels. In addition, osteoclasts will have commenced the removal of dead bone fragments. **D.** 2–3 Weeks after extraction, the cellular infiltrate has reduced but there is continuing vascularity with development of new fibrous tissue from fibroblasts and woven bone from osteoblasts. **E.** At 2–3 months, the woven bone is still undergoing remodelling while the overlying oral mucosa is fully developed; the alveolar crests are being reabsorbed by osteoclasts. **F.** At 2–3 years post-extraction, the tooth socket is completely replaced by lamellar bone.

into lamellar bone over a period of 2–3 months. In addition to the factors described previously which may affect general wound healing, bone fracture healing may also be impaired by poor apposition of the fractured ends because of wide displacement, entrapped viable soft tissue or excessive mobility, the presence of foreign bodies or large amounts of necrotic bone, the presence of infection, e.g. owing to severe gingivitis/periodontitis in tooth sockets, and corticosteroid therapy. Fractures may occur as a result of minimal trauma and repair may be delayed if the underlying bone is abnormal, so-called pathological fracture. Possible causes include metabolic diseases of bone such as osteoporosis, osteomalacia and Paget's disease and primary or secondary bone tumours.

Infections of bone

The commonest organism that causes osteomyelitis is *Staphylococcus aureus*, which is carried haematogenously to the metaphysis of long bones in children and the vertebral bodies in adults. Less commonly, the infection may spread through the epiphyseal plate to cause arthritis. If untreated, abscesses may form either within the medullary cavity or in the periosteal tissues. Reaction to this inflammation leads to infiltration by granulation tissue which erodes the bone to form a sequestrum and when the periosteal bone surrounds this area an involucrum is formed. Less severe infection causes small abscesses within densely sclerotic bone (Brodie's abscess). Diagnosis is made on the clinical and radiological presentation and is confirmed by bacterial culture. Treatment is usually the use of antistaphylococcal antibiotics, often given intravenously, but may require surgery to remove the sequestrum and involucrum with packing by bone chips.

The bones may become infected with *Mycobacterium tuberculosis* (see Chs 3 and 9) usually secondary to

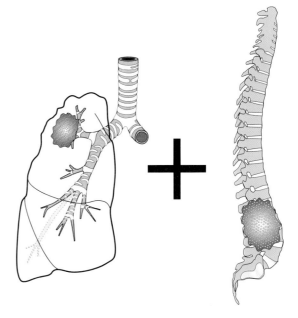

Fig. 12.2 Spread from secondary tuberculosis in lung apex, causing single organ involvement in the vertebrae leading to deformity (gibbus, Pott's caries).

pulmonary tuberculosis (Fig. 12.2) but infection may also spread from the intestines or the kidneys. The vertebral bodies are the most commonly involved bones. Infection begins in the medullary cavity close to the intervertebral disc and then destroys the adjacent bone with little reactive bone formation (so-called Pott's caries). This causes deformity of the vertebrae with spinal compression (gibbus), and infection can sometimes track along the iliopsoas muscle, pointing in the inguinal region. Diagnosis is made on the clinical and radiological features and is confirmed on biopsy (showing characteristic caseating epithelioid granulomatous inflammation in which acid-fast bacilli may be seen) and on microbiological culture.

Metabolic bone diseases (Fig. 12.3)

Osteoporosis (Fig. 12.3B)

This is a reduction in bone density due to an imbalance between deposition and resorption rates, in which the bone is normally mineralized and the bone shape is maintained. It is most commonly seen with increasing age as all people lose bone mass from the fifth decade onwards at the rate of 10% per decade in cancellous bone. This can be detected on dental radiography but is more usually screened by radiography of forearm bone.

The exact mechanism is uncertain but hormonal influences, especially a lack of oestrogen, are thought to be important since osteoporosis is seen particularly in women around and after the menopause and can be prevented by the use of hormone replacement therapy (HRT). It may also be observed in patients with disuse atrophy of bones, either in the short term related to immobilization after fractures or in the long term related to paralysis due to neurological disorders. Patients with hyperthyroidism and hyperparathyroidism may also develop osteoporosis and it is a frequent accompaniment of corticosteroid therapy for a variety of conditions and of Cushing's syndrome. Patients with liver disease, especially of alcoholic aetiology, may also suffer from osteoporosis.

Grossly, the bones affected most commonly are the long bones of the limbs and the vertebral bodies. Histologically, the main feature is a reduction in bone trabeculae within cancellous bone, with preservation of cortical bone and bone marrow. Clinically, there is an increased tendency to fracture, particularly in elderly women, affecting the hips (neck of femur) and wrists (Colles' fracture) and there may be compression fractures of

thoracic vertebrae causing back pain and anteroposterior bending of the spine (kyphosis). Management is aimed at prevention, and treatment is by symptomatic repair of fractures.

Osteomalacia (Fig. 12.3C)

This is a condition of adults in which there is normal bone structure and normal deposition of osteoid but there is a failure of mineralization because of a lack of calcium. This occurs in vitamin D deficiency, caused by dietary lack or intestinal malabsorption, chronic renal failure, renal tubular acidosis, and various genetically determined disorders especially of phosphate metabolism. Within bones, there are often central, normally mineralized trabeculae but unmineralized peripheral trabeculae and cortical bone. This results in bone pain with microfractures in the cortex (Looser's zones), especially in the lower limbs. In long-standing disease, there may be bowing of the legs. In children, where the condition is known as rickets, the changes occur in a skeleton which is still developing so that there is an increase in unmineralized osteoid around epiphyseal plates. This occurs especially at the osteochondral junctions of the ribs producing a 'rickety rosary' appearance, and also in the skull bones producing marked bossing of the skull, and in the lower limbs, causing bone deformities leading to severe bowing.

Parathyroid bone disease

Parathyroid hormone (PTH) causes the resorption of calcium from bone by increasing osteoclastic activity and its control is closely maintained by a feedback mechanism related to plasma calcium levels and PTH release from the parathyroid glands. PTH also increases renal calcium resorption and phosphate excretion. Primary hyperparathyroidism may be due to diffuse hyperplasia of all four glands or, more commonly, to a single autonomous adenoma, where the level of PTH is outside normal feedback mechanisms. Skeletal changes vary considerably in severity and are radiologically visible in only 35% of cases. The most common form of presentation is with renal stone disease. All bones are affected to some extent but cancellous bones show the most marked effects. Histologically, there are increased osteoclast numbers, as well as increased numbers of osteoblasts. There is osteoclastic erosion of periosteal surfaces, especially of phalanges, with tunnelling resorption of bone trabeculae. Initially the eroded bone is replaced

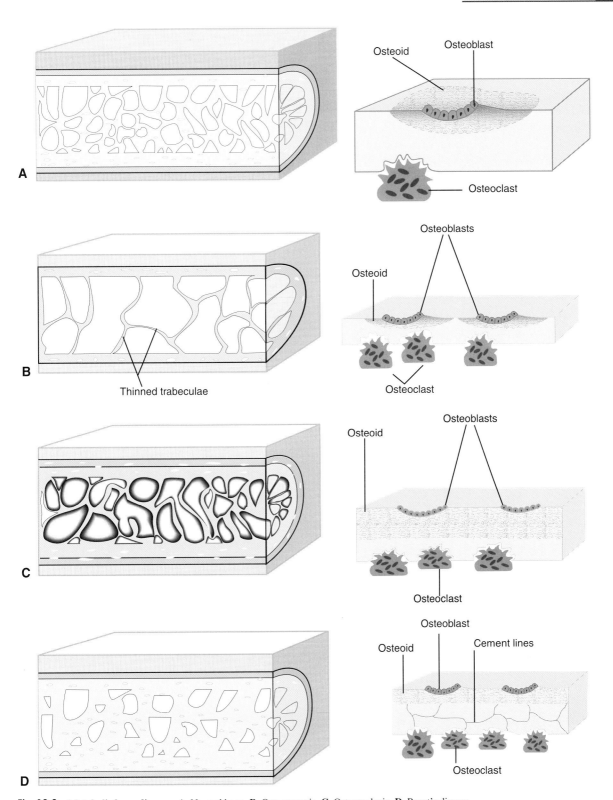

Fig. 12.3 **Metabolic bone diseases. A.** Normal bone. **B.** Osteoporosis. **C.** Osteomalacia. **D.** Paget's disease.

by fibrous tissue and the clusters of osteoclasts may resemble a giant cell tumour. Giant cell granulomas of the jaw have similar histological features and hyperparathyroidism must be excluded by serum calcium estimation. Secondary hyperparathyroidism is most commonly due to prolonged stimulation of the parathyroids in response to low plasma calcium levels in chronic renal failure, caused by excess calcium loss in the urine. This leads to diffuse hyperplasia of all parathyroid glands with constant excessive secretion of PTH. Similar features to those of primary hyperparathyroidism may also be seen on radiology and histopathology.

Renal osteodystrophy

This is the combination of features seen in bone that are related to chronic renal failure. Bone changes are of two main types:

- those due to a failure of conversion of 25-hydroxycholecalciferol (vitamin D_3) to the active form of the vitamin, 1,25-dihydroxycholecalciferol
- those due to secondary hyperparathyroidism because of vitamin D deficiency, excess calcium loss in the urine and retention of phosphate.

There may be a combination of lesions in bone including excessive bone erosion and failure of mineralization of osteoid. The osteoid in renal osteodystrophy may be further damaged by the accumulation of aluminium at potential sites of mineralization, which occurs as a result of the use of aluminium salts as phosphate-binding agents designed to prevent excessive accumulation of phosphate in patients on haemodialysis.

Paget's disease (Fig. 12.3D)

This is a condition characterized by excessive resorption of bone by abnormal large osteoclasts, which is of unknown aetiology but may be related to viral infection of these cells, possibly by canine distemper virus. The disease progresses in waves at various sites throughout the skeleton and each burst of bone resorption is accompanied by uncoordinated osteoblastic activity resulting in deposition of large amounts of woven bone having a 'mosaic' pattern. As time passes, the involved bone becomes sclerotic and structurally unsound and is prone to fracture. The intervening marrow becomes fibrotic and vascularity is increased, occasionally to the extent of precipitating high output cardiac failure. Complications

include fractures, bone pain, overgrowth of jaw, hypercementosis, spacing of teeth, osteomyelitis following dental extraction, nerve compression syndromes and, rarely, in long-standing disease, osteosarcoma. Calvarial thickening is almost universally present producing a leonine facial appearance.

SUMMARY BOX
METABOLIC BONE DISEASE

- Osteoporosis is usually a generalized reduction in bone density leading to an increased risk of fractures.
- Osteomalacia is due to inadequate mineralization of bone matrix in adults usually because of a lack of calcium or vitamin D metabolites.
- Parathyroid bone disease is associated with increased levels of parathyroid hormone which mobilizes calcium from bone, where cystic and haemorrhagic lesions may be seen ('brown tumours').
- Renal osteodystrophy is of two main types, related to vitamin D abnormalities or secondary hyperparathyroidism; there may be excessive bone erosion or failure of mineralization of osteoid.
- Paget's disease is a condition of unknown aetiology characterized by increased bone turnover; complications include pain, fractures, jaw overgrowth, spacing of teeth, nerve compression syndromes and increased tendency to osteosarcoma.

Tumour-like conditions of bone

Fibrous dysplasia can result in solitary, craniofacial or multiple bone swellings, which typically present in childhood or early adult life. Early lesions are fibrous and these mature into radiodense fibro-osseous tissue which merges into the surrounding bone. Growth arrest occurs at skeletal maturity. Ossifying fibroma, by contrast, has a similar microscopic appearance but is sharply delimited from the surrounding bone and has unlimited growth potential. Cherubism is an uncommon genetic disorder which can also result in fibro-osseous lesions in the jaws. Solitary and aneurysmal bone cysts may also occur in the jaws and elsewhere in the skeleton. Enostoses of the jaw may be a presenting feature of Gardner's syndrome. Exostoses are developmental defects, and so-called 'brown tumours' are the tissue manifestation of hyperparathyroidism.

Neoplasms of bone

The commonest neoplasm affecting bone is metastatic disease. Any extraskeletal malignant tumour may metastasize to bone and the majority of bone metastases, including those from breast, lung, kidney and thyroid primaries, are lytic and thus capable of causing hypercalcaemia. Less commonly they may be osteoblastic (osteosclerotic) producing new bone, especially if they have arisen in the prostate gland or breast. Clinically, patients with metastatic carcinoma of bone often have severe pain, nerve and spinal compression, replacement of bone marrow leading to a leukoerythroblastic anaemia, and hypercalcaemia. They occasionally respond to radiotherapy but this is usually a palliative measure and indicates advanced disease.

Primary tumours of bone are relatively rare and may be either benign or malignant. They are classified on the basis of their histological appearances and degree of differentiation rather than their presumed cell of origin, which in many cases is unclear.

- Bone-forming tumours include osteoid osteoma, which is a disease of adolescents affecting the lower limbs and is often extremely painful. Giant cell tumours are thought to be of stromal cell origin, which attract osteoclasts to the tumour, and are usually benign tumours occurring around the knee joint in people between the ages of 20 and 40 years. They may recur locally.
- Osteosarcoma is the commonest primary malignant tumour of bone (Fig. 12.4) and has a bimodal pattern of age distribution, being seen mainly in the teens and early 20s around the knee joint, but it can also develop in the elderly at the sites of Paget's disease. It is a highly malignant tumour and has often spread via the bloodstream to the lungs at the time of presentation,

although it metastasizes only rarely to lymph nodes. It is now treated very successfully with aggressive chemotherapy combined with early surgery and radiotherapy.

- Chondroma is a benign tumour of cartilage and consists of lobulated mature cartilaginous tissue found in the centre of the bones of hands and feet of young adults.
- Chondrosarcoma is a malignant tumour of cartilage in patients between 30 and 60 years of age, mainly in the pelvic bones, proximal long bones and shoulder girdle region. It may spread locally and may also metastasize distally.
- Tumours of fibrous tissue may also arise in bone, including non-ossifying fibroma, which affects the metaphyses of long bones in the lower limbs of adolescents and young adults, chondromyxoid fibroma which affects the tibias of a similar age group, and fibrosarcoma, which affects patients between 20 and 60 years and has characteristic lytic lesions which are rich in collagenous fibres but do not produce either cartilage or bone.
- Vasoformative tumours may arise in bone, including solitary angiomas (multiple angiomas occurring as part of an inherited syndrome), and rarely the malignant form, angiosarcoma.
- Ewing's sarcoma is a highly malignant tumour of bone which arises in children and adolescents; it is composed of small round hyperchromatic cells, and metastasizes extensively. This is probably a tumour of primitive neuroectodermal origin and is associated with characteristic cytogenetic abnormalities.
- Chordoma is a malignant tumour of primitive notochord origin which usually arises in the sacral region of patients over the age of 40 and causes local bone destruction and invasion.

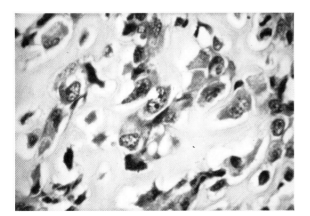

Fig. 12.4 Histological section of bone tumour showing pleomorphic malignant tumour cells with intervening stroma consisting of tumour osteoid, characteristic of osteosarcoma (osteogenic sarcoma).

SUMMARY BOX
BONE NEOPLASMS

- The commonest tumour involving bone is metastatic carcinoma, especially from breast, lung, prostate, kidney and thyroid primaries.
- Primary neoplasms may be benign or malignant, and may arise from bone, cartilage or connective tissue elements.
- Malignant tumours include osteosarcoma, chondrosarcoma and Ewing's sarcoma; these commonly spread via the bloodstream to the lungs and generally have a poor prognosis.

Arthritis

Acute pyogenic arthritis may occur at any age and is usually monoarticular, except when complicating rheumatoid arthritis when it may be polyarticular. The commonest infecting organism is *Staphylococcus aureus*, although *Escherichia coli*, *Haemophilus influenzae*, streptococci and gonococcus may also cause infective arthritis. The main mode of spread is via the bloodstream but there can also be direct spread from nearby bone or soft tissue foci of infection, accidentally during intra-articular injections, e.g. of corticosteroids, and as a result of direct trauma. Clinically, the joint is painful and on examination is distended, hot and tender. Diagnosis is by bacterial culture of joint fluid and characteristic changes may be seen on synovial aspiration cytology. Histologically, the synovial surface is necrotic and the subsynovial tissues contain an infiltrate of polymorphs, plasma cells, lymphocytes and macrophages.

Tuberculous arthritis

This is usually a haematogenous complication of disease elsewhere, especially of the lung, but it may also arise from spread of adjacent bone involvement. Clinically, the involved joint becomes swollen and loses function but is not usually hot or tender. The diagnosis is made on culture of synovial fluid or tissue and the finding of typical caseating epithelioid granulomas on biopsy.

Crystal arthritis

There are two main types of crystal arthritis: gout and pseudogout. Gout occurs when microcrystals of sodium urate (in the presence of high serum levels of uric acid) precipitate into cartilage, synovium and periarticular tissues (Fig. 12.5). They are ingested by polymorphs in synovial fluid which degranulate in response and induce a severe acute arthritis, which is initially monoarticular, often the great toe, but later becomes polyarticular. Crystals outside synovium excite a foreign body type of inflammatory response, producing lesions in the soft tissues, e.g. the tip of the nose or the ear known, as gouty tophi. Pseudogout is caused by the precipitation of calcium pyrophosphate crystals in a similar manner to gout. This occurs especially in articular cartilage and is associated with the development of osteoarthrosis (see below).

Haemarthrosis refers to the presence of blood in the joint cavity. It is most commonly due to trauma and

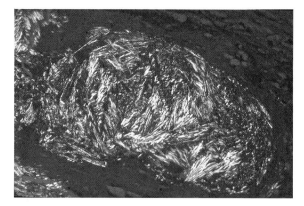

Fig. 12.5 Histological section of a gouty tophus viewed under polarized light, demonstrating characteristic urate crystals.

monoarticular but may also be seen with vascular lesions such as angiomas, villonodular synovitis and haemophilia. The presence of blood may mimic acute arthritis and it stimulates a macrophage response with changes in the synovium and subsynovial layers. In haemophiliacs who have repeated episodes, there is increased risk of degenerative joint disease.

Degenerative joint disease

This is the commonest form of joint disease affecting the general population. Most people develop some degree of joint disease with increasing age. When it affects synovial joints it is called osteoarthrosis (OA) for which the term osteoarthritis is a synonym, and when it affects intervertebral discs, it is called simply disc degeneration. OA may be of primary or secondary types. Primary OA is of unknown aetiology and affects multiple joints mainly in women over the age of 50 years. The joints particularly involved include the terminal interphalangeal joints and the first carpometacarpal joints of the hands, the knees and the spinal apophyseal joints. Secondary OA has a recognizable cause and may be seen in joints which have had previous trauma or surgery, especially in sportspersons; inflammatory joint disease such as rheumatoid disease; aseptic bone necrosis in conditions such as Perthes' disease in childhood and sickle cell disease; metabolic disorders such as ochronosis and haemochromatosis; and repeated episodes of haemarthrosis in haemophilia. Early in the disease there is fraying of the articular cartilage (fibrillation) followed by clefts in the underlying cartilage and progressive loss of the surface, leading to a smooth appearance (eburnation). The bone becomes thickened but may develop cysts and microfractures, and there is often gross deformity of the articular contour. This is accompanied by enchondral ossification with the formation of new bony outgrowths (osteophytes) at the margins of the articular surface. The deformed joint leads to ligamentous sprains and effusions in the joint which are the cause of severe pain in this condition. Histologically, there is hyperplasia of the lining epithelium with oedema and fibrosis but usually little or no inflammatory cell infiltration. Fragments of degenerate cartilage or bone may also be seen.

Temporomandibular joint (TMJ) dysfunction. This is a common pain syndrome particularly in young women. A distinctive pattern of TMJ arthropathy is seen, similar to the changes seen in OA but the joint shows considerable regenerative capacity with possible complete resolution.

Disc degeneration. This condition is also known as spondylosis and it may affect any intervertebral joint. The height of the affected disc is reduced and there is increased compressive stress on the annulus fibrosus with osteophyte formation at the vertebral rims. These bony outgrowths reduce the size of the intervertebral foramina with irritation and possibly compression of the nerve roots. Occasionally the nucleus pulposus of the disc or the annulus fibrosus may protrude through a tear and press on a nerve root causing leg pain possibly with a neurological deficit.

Rheumatoid arthritis

This is a condition of unknown aetiology which is possibly of autoimmune origin in which antirheumatoid factor antibodies may be found in the serum. It is a polyarthritis in which there is involvement of peripheral synovial joints of the fingers and wrists, but the knees and larger proximal joints may also be involved. Involvement of the cervical spine is common and may cause problems in dental practice. It affects women two to three times more often than it affects men and usually presents in the third or fourth decades. In involved joints there is thickening of synovium with a lymphoplasmacytic infiltrate and fibrin deposition. As the disease progresses, there is the formation of pannus with granulation tissue formation and destruction of cartilage at the periphery of joints (Fig. 12.6). Ultimately, there is erosion of the bone edges, increased soft tissue swelling and joint deformity and the affected joints are swollen, painful and warm, often with redness of the overlying skin. Joint dislocation is common and, with long-standing disease, the underlying bone shows secondary osteoarthritic changes and the associated muscle develops muscle wasting. Similar changes may be seen in extra-articular sites including

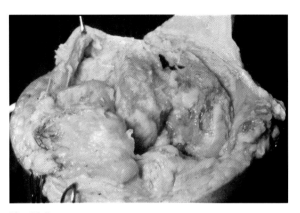

Fig. 12.6 The opened knee joint of a patient with severe rheumatoid arthritis in which there is marked proliferation of the surface synovial epithelium with destruction of the underlying cartilage.

mesothelial surfaces such as the pleura and pericardium. Nodules may be found in the subcutaneous tissues at pressure points, e.g. around the elbows, where there is central fibrinoid necrosis of collagen with surrounding palisaded histiocytic infiltration. Chronic disease is associated with the development of amyloidosis (of AA type), arteritis/vasculitis, pyoarthrosis, chronic peptic ulcer (possibly related to corticosteroid therapy), pyelonephritis and osteoporosis due to steroid therapy.

SUMMARY BOX
ARTHRITIS

- Infective arthritis is usually bacterial, usually arising from infections elsewhere.
- The two main forms of crystal arthritis are gout (uric acid) and pseudogout (pyrophosphate).
- Osteoarthritis is a common form of degenerative joint disease primarily affecting large weight-bearing joints.
- Rheumatoid arthritis is part of a systemic disease which involves symmetrically peripheral joints, and in which extra-articular features are common.

ASPECTS OF OSTEOARTICULAR DISEASE OF PARTICULAR RELEVANCE TO DENTISTRY

- Oral manifestations of metabolic bone diseases, especially osteoporosis and Paget's disease, may be detected on oral radiographs.
- Dentists may rarely detect primary bone neoplasms and genetic syndromes involving bone.
- Cervical rheumatoid disease may cause problems in dental practice.

CASE STUDY 12.1
BONE PAIN

A 37-year-old woman of Pakistani origin living in the UK presented to her GP complaining of low back pain and pain in the left hip region. The GP was familiar with her family background and knew that she had had four children. Her husband was unemployed and her GP suspected that there was a poor diet in the family.

The GP referred her to the local hospital for investigations. She was seen by doctors in the Metabolic Unit who ordered some blood tests. She was also referred for other investigations to look at her bone status.

Some weeks later when all the results of the investigations were available, she was seen again at the clinic and was recommended to have a bone biopsy. This was performed under local anaesthetic.

When the result of the biopsy was available she was seen again at the clinic and was advised about her diet and commenced on a specific drug treatment.

1. What are the likely clinical causes of this woman's problems?
2. What likely abnormalities in blood tests may be seen in this woman and what investigations may elucidate the cause of her problems?
3. What are the likely appearances in the bone biopsy in this woman's case?
4. What are the possible complications of this disease if untreated?

Suggested responses

1. This woman may have problems of osteoarthritis affecting the lower back and hips, which may be a complication of problem pregnancies and prolonged labour. She may have some form of metabolic bone disease causing her bone pains. At her age, osteoporosis is unlikely, especially before the menopause. Thus, the most likely cause of her problems is osteomalacia, because of her probable poor diet and possible lack of vitamin D as a result of impaired absorption from the gut, compounded by the presence of phytates in chapatti flour, and failure to convert vitamin D into its active form by the skin.

2. There may be anaemia as a general manifestation of poor nutrition. Specifically related to her bone status, the calcium levels will be at the lower end of the normal range or reduced, as will the phosphate levels. Alkaline phosphatase (of bony origin) will be elevated, indicating increased bone turnover. Vitamin D levels will also be reduced. The parathyroid hormone (PTH) levels will be increased as an attempt to increase calcium levels. Radiological investigations of the whole skeleton will show reduced mineralized bone mass. This will lead to deformities of weight-bearing bones, especially in the pelvis and hip regions. This can be confirmed on more detailed investigations such as bone densitometry. Small fractures, so-called 'Looser's zones', may also be detected and these may be identified on radioisotope bone scans.

3. The trabecular bone will have increased osteoid deposition on the surface, in which calcification will be deficient, and cortical bone may also be thinned.

4. There may be secondary osteoarthritis with more severe pain, and there is an increased tendency to bone fractures. These may lead to further deformities and sometimes to nerve compression injuries or paralysis.

13 Central nervous system diseases

Dentists may encounter diseases of the central nervous system (CNS) in a variety of forms including the after-effects of strokes, intracranial haemorrhages, tumours and degenerative conditions. Patients with sensory loss and facial pain often present to dentists and these conditions may be a manifestation of primary nervous system pathology.

CEREBROVASCULAR DISEASE

This is the cause of the condition known as a cerebrovascular accident (CVA) or 'stroke', which has a high mortality rate and, in the survivors, leads to significant morbidity. There are three main groups, the largest being infarction (more than 80%) with intracerebral haemorrhage (more than 10%) and subarachnoid haemorrhage (5%) being less common causes. A condition that causes a significant neurological deficit which lasts less than 24 hours is termed a transient ischaemic attack (TIA).

Cerebral infarction

Aetiology

Cerebral infarcts may arise from embolization from a major vessel such as the aorta or carotid artery, from embolization from the chambers of the heart in patients with atrial fibrillation or recent myocardial infarction, or from direct vessel occlusion within the brain or its major arteries. Risk factors for the development of cerebrovascular disease are as for general vascular disease and include hypertension, cigarette smoking, hyperlipidaemia, diabetes and a positive family history of vascular

disease. Less common conditions associated with cerebral ischaemia are vasculitides, fat or air emboli, vasospasm in migraine, hypercoagulable states and cerebral venous thrombosis.

Clinical picture

This depends on the vessel involved (Fig. 13.1). The commonest vessel to be occluded in cerebrovascular disease is the middle cerebral artery, which results in the loss of use and feeling in the contralateral arm, face and lower limb with dysphasia and spasticity and increased

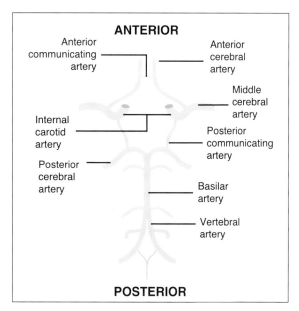

Fig. 13.1 Schematic representation of the arterial blood supply of the brain via the circle of Willis.

197

reflexes. The vertebrobasilar artery territory is the next most commonly involved vessel and causes damage to the cranial nerves, resulting in double vision, facial weakness, vertigo, dysphagia, dysarthria, ataxia and motor and sensory loss in both arms or legs. Less commonly, clinical signs include loss of vision (ophthalmic artery), loss of use and feeling in the contralateral leg (anterior cerebral artery) and dementia (multiple small infarcts).

Gross appearances

The size of the infarct depends on which vessel is occluded, whether hypertension is present or not, and the state and patency of the other vessels in the circle of Willis. In the first 2 days after infarction, the brain shows an oedematous area with loss of the distinction between grey and white matter, necrosis and possible haemorrhage into the infarcted area. Over the next 2 weeks, because of the high lipid content of cerebral tissue, the infarcted tissue undergoes liquefactive necrosis. From 2 weeks onwards, the necrotic area is cleared and is marked by the appearance of a cystic cavity, often with a surrounding zone of brown tissue owing to the accumulation of haemosiderin in macrophages (Fig. 13.2). This inevitably results in disruption of the tracts running through the damaged area.

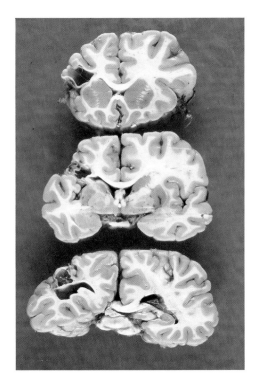

Fig. 13.2 Brain: cerebral infarct. Series of slices of brain in which there is well-developed cystic infarct of the right cerebral hemisphere in the territory of the middle cerebral artery.

Histological appearances

In the first 2 days, there is pallor of tissue with neuronal degeneration and minimal polymorph infiltration. Later, there is loss of neurons and cell processes, of glial cells and of vessels in the area, with replacement by macrophages and fluid. Because cerebral neurons are permanent cells, they are not capable of regeneration and the

brain replaces the damaged tissue with scar tissue (gliosis) produced by glial cells. As time goes on, the damaged area becomes a cystic cavity. Smaller infarcts show less cystic change, while microinfarcts show gliosis with spaces around vessels.

Intracerebral haemorrhage (Fig. 13.3)

This is seen particularly in patients with long-standing essential hypertension that is untreated or inadequately treated. In hypertension, there is intimal thickening of arterioles, with hyalinization of the walls and microaneurysm formation. Major intracerebral haemorrhages occur in basal ganglia, cerebellum and the pons region of the brain stem. This leads to a sudden rapid rise in intracranial pressure that causes rapid distortion of the brain and death within a few days. A less common cause is rupture of an arteriovenous malformation.

Subarachnoid haemorrhage (Fig. 13.3)

Most cases (65%) of subarachnoid haemorrhage occur as a result of rupture of a saccular 'berry' aneurysm in the

---

SUMMARY BOX
CEREBROVASCULAR DISEASE

- Cerebrovascular accidents or 'strokes' are a major cause of mortality; significant neurological impairment lasting for less than 24 hours is a transient ischaemic attack.

- The commonest cause is cerebral infarction, with associated atheroma and emboli in the heart or major vessels; other risk factors include hypertension and diabetes mellitus.

- Grossly, the infarcted area appears soft and necrotic in the early stages, then undergoes liquefactive necrosis and ultimately becomes cystic.

- Less common causes of strokes are intracerebral and subarachnoid haemorrhage.

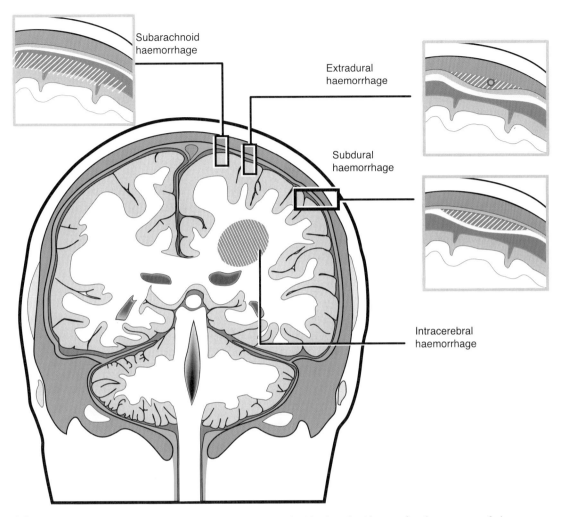

Subarachnoid haemorrhage

Extradural haemorrhage

Subdural haemorrhage

Intracerebral haemorrhage

Fig. 13.3   Intracranial haemorrhage. Intracranial haemorrhages may be (a) subarachnoid, most often due to rupture of a berry aneurysm; (b) extradural, due to tearing of a meningeal artery; (c) subdural, due to trauma to veins; or (d) intracerebral, commonly due to hypertension.

circle of Willis, with rupture of an arteriovenous malformation contributing 5% of the total; in approximately 25% of cases, no cause can be identified. The common sites of aneurysms are at the bifurcation of the internal carotid artery with the posterior communicating artery, followed by the bifurcation of the anterior communicating with the anterior cerebral artery and then at branches of the middle cerebral artery in the sylvian fissure. The aetiology of these aneurysms is unknown but is probably multifactorial. Aneurysms may be found in 1–2% of adults but rupture tends to occur in the sixth decade and is more common in women than in men (female to male ratio 3:2). Approximately 10% of patients die during the first bleed, which presents with a severe posterior headache with signs of raised intracranial pressure.

Without surgical intervention, another 30% will die over the next few days. The presence of blood in the subarachnoid space acts to cause spasm of the vessels in the circle of Willis, especially around the brain stem, which may cause infarction. The haemorrhage in the subarachnoid region may also extend into the brain substance itself causing intracranial haemorrhage. If the patient survives, there may be residual neurological deficits or hydrocephalus.

Head injury

Head injuries are a major cause of admissions to hospital every year and a significant cause of death, especially in a young age group. They cause a range of pathological features, depending on the site and type of injury.

- *Extradural haemorrhage.* This occurs when there is a fracture of the temporal bone with tearing of the underlying middle meningeal artery. Characteristically, patients regain consciousness after the initial injury but later deteriorate; the time of apparent normality is referred to as the 'lucid interval'. If untreated, death occurs rapidly.

- *Subdural haemorrhage.* This often occurs as a consequence of relatively minor trauma and is a result of tearing of veins. Gradual accumulation of blood leads to chronic subdural haematomas, possibly bilateral, which may cause minor neurological abnormalities, but if a large haematoma develops, the prognosis is worse.

- *Subarachnoid haemorrhage.* Traumatic haemorrhage in this region is often thin and patchy and rarely causes significant clinical abnormalities.

- *Brain contusions and lacerations.* There may be brain damage at the site of impact ('coup') with damage to the opposite pole of the brain owing to contact with the bony skull ('contrecoup').

- *Intracerebral haemorrhage.* When this is seen as a result of trauma, it is associated with a poor outcome.

- *Diffuse axonal injury.* Shearing stresses acting on the brain cause stretching of nerve tracts and tearing of axons, which leads to a variety of neurological symptoms.

SUMMARY BOX
INTRACRANIAL HAEMORRHAGES AND TRAUMA

- Intracerebral haemorrhage is most commonly caused by hypertensive vascular disease.

- Subarachnoid haemorrhage usually occurs as a result of rupture of a berry aneurysm at the branch points of the circle of Willis; many patients die from the initial haemorrhage, subsequent rebleeding or arterial spasm.

- Subdural haemorrhage is caused by relatively minor trauma which causes tearing of veins, leading to gradual accumulation of blood in the subdural space.

- Extradural haemorrhage occurs as a consequence of temporal bone fractures with tearing of the underlying middle meningeal artery; accumulation of blood causes brain compression, brain shift and raised intracranial pressure.

- Non-missile injuries may cause cerebral contusions, diffuse axonal injury and secondary brain damage.

Raised intracranial pressure (Fig. 13.4)

This may be caused by the presence of blood within the cranial cavity, as in the various forms of intracranial haemorrhage described above, diffuse cerebral oedema, abscess formation, neoplasms and hydrocephalus. Because the skull is a bony box, once the sutures have closed in infancy, there is only a limited space for the brain to expand in the situation of raised intracranial pressure. In addition, within the skull, there are fibrous bands which separate the right and left sides of the cerebral cortex (falx cerebri) and which separate the cerebrum above from the cerebellum below (tentorium cerebri); these fibrous septa may also complicate the consequences of raised pressure, particularly as the cranial nerves traverse the tentorium.

Grossly, in intracranial pressure, there is brain shift which may be lateral, especially in the cerebral hemispheres, causing herniation of the cingulate gyrus below the falx, or downward with tentorial herniation where part of the temporal lobe, mainly the hippocampus, is pushed down over the tentorium to compress the upper brain stem. Lesions in the posterior fossa or the cerebrum lead to herniation of the cerebellar tonsils, which are pushed downwards into the foramen magnum; this process is called coning and leads to damage to the vital centres in the medulla and brain stem and to death. Rarely, the brain will herniate outwards through sites of skull fracture.

Clinically, patients with raised intracranial pressure have a reduced level of consciousness, as assessed by the Glasgow Coma Scale, and may have a slow pulse rate and high systemic blood pressure. An important clinical sign is identifying a unilateral lack of reactivity in the pupillary reflex owing to compression of the oculomotor (third cranial) nerve as it crosses the tentorium. Similarly, it is important to examine the optic fundus for signs of papilloedema, which indicates raised intracranial pressure and is a contraindication to the performance of a lumbar puncture.

SUMMARY BOX
RAISED INTRACRANIAL PRESSURE

- Space-occupying lesions in the brain such as tumours, blood clots and abscesses, along with associated oedema, cause raised intracranial pressure.

- Initially there is a reduction in CSF, then pressure atrophy and a reduction in blood volume.

- Ultimately there is no longer a possibility of compensation and the brain shows features of lateral shift and herniation at characteristic sites.

- Coning leads to compression of vital centres and death if untreated.

- Clinically, patients have bradycardia, hypertension and pulmonary oedema; papilloedema may be found with other cranial nerve compression syndromes.

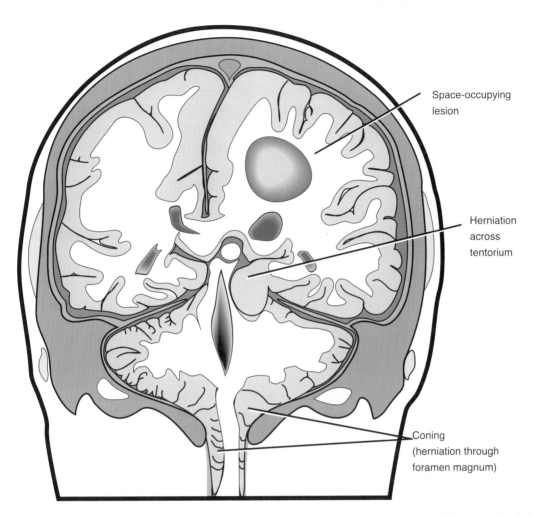

Space-occupying lesion

Herniation across tentorium

Coning (herniation through foramen magnum)

Fig. 13.4 The consequences of raised intracranial pressure, e.g. due to a space-occupying lesion, include shift across the midline away from the site of the lesion with compression of the lateral ventricles, herniation across the tentorium cerebri in the hippocampal region, and coning (downward shift of the cerebellum, brain stem and cord into the foramen magnum).

Intracranial neoplasms

In children under the age of 15 years, tumours of the central nervous system are the second commonest group of neoplasms after leukaemias. In adults, primary CNS neoplasms are very rare, approximately 4 per 100 000 population.

More frequently, brain tumours in adults are secondaries from a variety of sources, particularly lung, breast, colon and rectum, kidney, malignant melanoma and thyroid. Metastatic tumours are usually multiple, though occasionally single, and are well-defined, sometimes haemorrhagic, lesions. The surrounding brain tissue is often oedematous. The effects of secondary tumours depend on their site within the brain. They may cause epilepsy, hemiparesis, personality change, headaches and decreasing levels of consciousness.

Childhood tumours

In children, approximately 60% of primary tumours occur infratentorially and in order of frequency, the commonest tumours are astrocytomas, medulloblastomas and ependymomas. Other forms are rare.

- Astrocytomas which occur in the cerebellum are slow growing and have a typical pilocytic appearance. They are amenable to surgical treatment and if completely excised are associated with a normal life expectancy. They do not require radiotherapy.

- Medulloblastomas arise from primitive cells in the cerebellum. These are rapidly growing tumours which are poorly differentiated and can spread quickly within the brain via the cerebrospinal fluid (CSF). They respond to both chemotherapy and radiotherapy and have an approximately 50% 5-year survival rate.
- Ependymomas arise from the ependymal lining, mainly from the fourth ventricle, and fill the ventricle, possibly infiltrating the surrounding brain tissue. They respond poorly to radiotherapy and are difficult to resect surgically, which leads to a 5-year survival of only 33%.

Tumours in adulthood

In contrast to the situation in childhood tumours, approximately 60% of primary tumours in adults occur supratentorially. They are classified according to their presumed cell of origin: from glial cells leading to astrocytomas, oligodendrogliomas and ependymomas; from neuronal cells leading to neurocytomas (rare); from both neuronal and glial cells leading to gangliogliomas (rare); from lymphoid cells leading to primary CNS lymphomas; from meninges leading to meningiomas; and from Schwann cells of cranial nerves leading to schwannomas.

- Anaplastic astrocytomas are the commonest primary tumours in adults. They are ill-defined grey-white masses with poor definition from surrounding brain tissue and may be haemorrhagic. Microscopically, they are cellular tumours with nuclear pleomorphism and mitotic activity. Some of the tumour cells stain positively for glial fibrillar acidic protein (GFAP), a marker of glial differentiation. The majority of patients with this tumour die approximately 18 months after presentation.
- Glioblastoma multiforme presents as a large poorly defined mass with irregular borders which may extend into the opposite cerebral hemisphere, producing brain shift, and shows extensive haemorrhage and necrosis (Fig. 13.5). Microscopically, they are very cellular tumours with marked nuclear pleomorphism, including multiple giant cell forms, abundant mitotic activity, a characteristic pattern of ribbon necrosis and vascular proliferation. Despite treatment, most patients are dead 9 months after presentation.
- Fibrillary astrocytomas usually present in a younger age group (15–40 years) and are often difficult to see grossly. The tumour cells have GFAP-positive fibrillary processes and may show cystic degeneration,

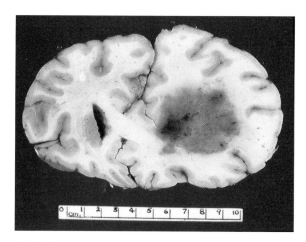

Fig. 13.5 Brain: glioblastoma multiforme. Slice of brain showing prominent right-to-left brain shift and compression of the right lateral ventricle by an expanding tumour mass within the left cerebral hemisphere, typical of a high-grade astrocytoma (glioblastoma multiforme).

although mitotic activity is absent. The overall survival rate is 24–48 months with most tumours transforming into anaplastic astrocytomas.
- Oligodendrogliomas are uncommon tumours which are slow-growing gelatinous masses in the frontal or temporal lobes. The tumour cells are characteristically 'box-shaped' and have a fine capillary network with frequent calcification. Survival is generally good from 3 to 20 years or more.
- Meningiomas account for 15–20% of all primary intracranial tumours. They arise from arachnoidal cells and are slow-growing tumours which form solid well-defined masses that indent the underlying brain. They are more common in women than in men and usually occur after the age of 60. The commonest location is parasagittally. Histologically, the tumour is composed of sheets and whorls of cells which look like arachnoidal endothelial cells; there are very few mitoses and occasionally calcified psammoma bodies may be found. Treatment is by surgical removal, but if untreated, these tumours may be fatal as a result of raised intracranial pressure.
- Schwannomas (neurilemmomas) are tumours of Schwann cell origin which commonly arise from the vestibular portion of the eighth cranial nerve. They are more common in women than in men and present with tinnitus and deafness. They are slow-growing tumours in the cerebellopontine angle, microscopically composed of spindle cells set in vascular stroma, sometimes with hyalinized vessels. Treatment is by surgical

resection and complete cure is the rule. Occasionally, these tumours can be bilateral and, in this case, are indicative of an inherited neurofibromatosis (von Recklinghausen's syndrome, central type 2). Tumours may arise from other cranial nerves including the trigeminal (V) and the facial (VII) nerves causing problems such as sensory loss or facial pain, although such problems may also develop after viral infections and, in many cases, no specific cause can be found.

SUMMARY BOX
INTRACRANIAL NEOPLASMS

- The commonest tumours involving the brain are secondary carcinomas from sites such as lung, breast, colorectum, kidney and thyroid, and metastases from melanoma.
- Primary brain tumours are the second commonest type of neoplasm in children (after leukaemia) but are relatively less common in adults.
- In children, tumours usually arise below the tentorium in the posterior fossa and include astrocytomas, medulloblastomas and ependymomas.
- In adults, most tumours arise above the tentorium; the commonest type arises from glial cells.
- Tumours may also originate from the meninges or from cranial nerves.
- Intracranial tumours present as space-occupying lesions, usually with the features of raised intracranial pressure.

Epilepsy. This is a condition characterized by seizures which may be generalized or focal and are associated with abnormalities on electroencephalographic (EEG) examination. In many cases no specific cause is ever found and the condition is presumed to be due to an abnormal focus of electrical activity within the cerebral cortex. Less commonly, epilepsy may be the presenting feature of an intracranial neoplasm or other mass lesion, or may be a complication of previous head injury, meningitis or neurosurgery. Specific anticonvulsant drugs may be of benefit but may have side-effects, including phenytoin which causes drug-induced gingival overgrowth.

Degenerative brain disease

Cerebral neurons are the largest cells in the body and have vast surface areas, with axons up to 1 metre in length containing neurofilaments, intermediate filaments and microtubules. They require oxygen and glucose for nutrition and are very susceptible to damage by toxins such as alcohol. When these cells undergo lethal damage,

they cannot be replaced. Neurons are also important in the metabolism of the adjacent Schwann cells and endothelial cells.

Dementia is characterized clinically by disorders of higher brain function, leading to loss of intellect, disorientation in time and place, memory loss especially for recent events, change in personality and speech disturbance. When it occurs before the age of 60, it is termed pre-senile. Causes of dementia include Alzheimer's disease, Lewy body disease, Huntington's chorea, Pick's disease, Creutzfeld–Jacob disease and multi-infarct states.

Alzheimer's disease

This is a degenerative disease of unknown aetiology, which affects women more than men over the age of 50. It is one of the commonest causes of dementia, which occurs in up to 15% of the population over the age of 80. The brain is atrophied, weighing less than 1000 g, and shows compensatory dilatation of the lateral ventricles. Microscopically there are characteristic neurofibrillary tangles, which are intraparenchymal thickenings of paired helical filaments, and neurofibrillary plaques, which are masses of granules and filaments, often with a core of amyloid, in the neuropil. The vessels may also show amyloid angiopathy and there is a loss of cholinergic neurons. A similar condition occurs in middle-aged people with Down syndrome (trisomy 21). It has been shown that there is a genetic abnormality on chromosome 21 in Alzheimer's disease, in the amyloid precursor protein P gene region. Some cases of Alzheimer's disease may be familial, associated with mutations of this gene.

Parkinson's disease

This is a relatively common disease in the general population, which in the idiopathic form is of unknown aetiology. Secondary causes include some psychotropic drugs, trauma and a post-encephalitic form. Clinically, patients may have rigidity of facial expression and movement, so-called 'cogwheel' rigidity, or abnormal movements such as a resting tremor and 'pill-rolling' of the hands. It is characterized by degeneration and loss of neurons from the substantia nigra and loci cerulei, with a reduction in neuromelanin. It may be possible to identify Lewy bodies, which are granular eosinophilic intracytoplasmic inclusions in neurons. Some patients may go on to develop dementia as part of their Parkinson's disease, while others may develop diffuse Lewy body disease, which is another cause of dementia, with Lewy bodies being found in parietal, temporal and frontal cortex.

Multiple sclerosis

Myelin is the material produced by oligodendrocytes in the brain and by Schwann cells in the peripheral nervous system and which surrounds neurons in peripheral nerves, spinal cord and the white matter in the brain. Multiple sclerosis (MS) is the commonest cause of demyelinating disease. The cause of MS is unknown, although it is thought to involve a combination of genetic and environmental factors resulting in an inflammatory response in the CNS, targeted at one or more of the components of the oligodendrocyte–myelin unit. Clinically, patients present in a variety of ways, particularly related to visual disturbances due to retrobulbar neuritis or optic atrophy and to limb weakness. There is a tendency to relapses and remissions, but the disease generally is a chronic one with gradual progression to invalidity. The immobility which accompanies this disease leads to an increased tendency to lower respiratory infections, and where bladder innervation is impaired, urinary infections and progressive renal impairment may also occur. Grossly, the demyelinated foci appear as well-defined firm grey areas around the horns of the lateral ventricles, particularly in the occipital lobes but also in the optic nerves and the brain stem. Histologically, there is loss of myelin and oligodendrocytes, with collections of macrophages and lymphocytes around vessels and demyelinated areas, and as the disease progresses gliosis is noted. In the cerebrospinal fluid, protein levels are raised, often with oligoclonal IgG bands.

Guillain–Barré syndrome. Demyelination may also occur in the peripheral nervous system as a primary phenomenon, when the Schwann cells are damaged by pressure, ischaemia or inflammation. Here there is segmental loss of the myelin sheath, with subsequent remyelination. In Guillain–Barré syndrome, the damage to the myelin sheath is caused by inflammation, probably as a result of an immune reaction. It causes loss of motor function which starts peripherally and ascends, ultimately causing respiratory failure requiring assisted ventilation. Treatment is with corticosteroids and general supportive measures, until recovery occurs.

Motor neuron disease

This is a disease of unknown aetiology involving the middle aged and elderly, which is more common in men than in women. It affects the motor neurons in the cerebral cortex, cranial nerve nuclei and the anterior horn cells of the spinal cord, causing degeneration and later disappearance. It also causes degeneration of the nerve processes, leading to lack of innervation of muscle and consequent atrophy. Patients have progressive loss of muscle power and finally develop respiratory insufficiency through respiratory muscle involvement.

SUMMARY BOX
DEGENERATIVE/DEMYELINATING BRAIN DISEASES

- Dementia is a disease of the elderly associated with disorders of higher brain function; the commonest type is Alzheimer's disease.

- Parkinson's disease is a disorder of nuclei of the basal ganglia; clinically, patients have abnormalities of movement and facial expression; secondary causes include drugs and trauma.

- Multiple sclerosis is characterized by demyelination of white matter in the brain; the cause is unknown but associations with autoimmunity and viral infections have been shown.

- Motor neuron disease is a disease of unknown cause of the middle aged and elderly, affecting the motor neurons in the cortex and anterior horn cells in the spinal cord.

INFECTIONS OF THE CENTRAL NERVOUS SYSTEM

Meningitis

Meningitis is infection of the meningeal lining of the brain and spinal cord and may be caused by a variety of organisms including bacteria (Fig. 13.6), mycobacteria, viruses and fungi. The clinical pattern of disease depends to a great extent on the age of the patient and the microorganism involved. Diagnosis is on clinical suspicion of the condition, confirmed by examination of the cerebrospinal fluid (CSF). In bacterial meningitis, there is an increased white cell count, especially polymorphs, raised proteins and reduced glucose. Gram staining may reveal the presence of the causative organism, and culture on appropriate media allows specific identification of the cause and the antibiotic sensitivity of the organism.

Neonatal meningitis

Neonates in the first 4 weeks of life are at particular risk of meningitis, especially if they are of low birth weight

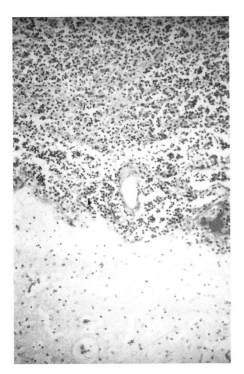

Fig. 13.6 Purulent meningitis. Histological section of brain (below) with meninges (above) in which there is a dense polymorph infiltrate typical of acute bacterial meningitis.

and premature. The risk is greater if there are congenital anomalies, traumatic birth and maternal genitourinary infection, as the organism is often transmitted just before or during delivery. The usual agents involved are Group B streptococci, *Escherichia coli* and *Listeria monocytogenes*, and presentation is often non-specific with respiratory distress or features of septicaemia. *E. coli* infections are associated with high mortality (up to 30%). Streptococcal infections are seen particularly in children of infected mothers, while listeriosis is caused by eating soft cheeses, pâtés, cook–chilled meals and ready to eat poultry, all of which should be avoided by pregnant women. *Listeria* may also cause miscarriages, stillbirths and other severe illness in the neonate.

Meningitis of childhood and adolescence

The commonest causes of meningitis in this period and of meningitis overall are *Neisseria meningitidis* and *Haemophilus influenzae*, although the latter organism is seen less frequently now as a result of the introduction of the Hib vaccine as part of the standard vaccinations in the first 6 months of life. The meningococcus (*Neisseria meningitidis*) is a small Gram-negative diplococcus which spreads from its natural habitat in 5–30% of the population in the oro- or nasopharynx. Cases may be sporadic or part of a fast-spreading epidemic. *Haemophilus influenzae* infection also usually arises from the upper respiratory tract, especially in children before the age of 4. In both instances, invasion of the organism into the bloodstream is the first stage in infection, which depends on the virulence of the organism and the host response. Bacteraemia (the presence of organisms in the bloodstream) allows adherence of the organism to the endothelium and crossing of the blood–brain barrier. This leads to an acute inflammatory response in the meninges, with a dense neutrophilic infiltrate, which can rapidly lead to increased intracranial pressure, cerebral ischaemia, obstructed CSF flow, coma and death, unless treated as a matter of urgency. Patients present with headaches, neck stiffness and photophobia, and in meningococcal infection, may have a skin rash as a result of septicaemia. It is important to take blood cultures before commencing antibiotics but examination of CSF can be delayed. Prophylactic treatment of relatives or contacts of affected patients may be necessary, depending on clinical circumstances.

Meningitis of adulthood and old age

The commonest cause of meningitis in patients over the age of 30 years is pneumococcus. This is often found as part of the normal flora in the pharynx and usually causes meningitis secondary to septicaemia from another site, such as pneumonia, ear infections and sinusitis. Occasionally, the CSF can be infected directly from skull fractures. Chronic alcoholics are at increased risk of meningitis of this type as are those who have had a splenectomy or are immunosuppressed for other reasons. The clinical presentation is as for meningitis in general without a skin rash but possibly with signs of infection elsewhere.

Tuberculous meningitis

This usually occurs as part of post-primary tuberculosis in children, and in the UK, is seen especially in children of Asian families. It may be seen in adults, particularly in those with relative immunosuppression, such as alcoholics and transplant recipients, often as a complication of secondary tuberculosis. It arises from rupture of a small caseous focus into the subarachnoid space. Clinically the presentation is often insidious with a long prodromal phase with low-grade fever and intermittent headaches. There is gradually developing meningism (signs of irritation of the meninges such as neck stiffness), cranial nerve palsies, drowsiness, coma and death. The CSF picture differs from bacterial infection, with clear fluid and raised white cells consisting predominantly of lymphocytes, which may cause confusion with viral meningitis, although in tuberculous infection, the CSF glucose is reduced (unlike viral infection where it is normal). Acid-fast bacilli may be difficult to identify and long-term culture may be required to confirm the diagnosis.

Viral infections

Viral meningitis. This is a less severe illness than either bacterial or tuberculous meningitis. Viruses usually reach the brain via the bloodstream or less commonly along neural routes, and common viruses include the echoviruses, coxsackieviruses, mumps and some other enteroviruses. Patients have mild clinical features of headache and mild pyrexia. The CSF shows greatly increased lymphocyte numbers, increased protein levels and normal glucose; it is usually clear and colourless. Most patients recover completely.

Viral encephalitis. This occurs less commonly than viral meningitis but is associated with a more severe clinical course, although many cases are mild and self-limiting. Herpes simplex type 1 is the commonest organism and causes perivascular mononuclear cell infiltration, cell lysis, viral inclusions and oedema. Some viruses cause subacute or latent infections, such as varicella zoster, which lies dormant in sensory ganglia and becomes activated occasionally, especially in periods of immunosuppression, and JC virus which causes progressive multifocal leukoencephalopathy. Subacute sclerosing panencephalitis is a poorly understood condition of children in which large numbers of viral inclusions may be found.

Other infections

Creutzfeld–Jakob disease (CJD) is caused by a prion, which has been transmitted via human growth hormone extracts. Recently a new variant CJD has been recognized but its exact mode of transmission is as yet unclear, similar to a transmissible spongiform encephalopathy called kuru in the East Indies.

Fungal infections of the CNS are rare except in immunocompromised patients such as leukaemics, transplant recipients and patients with HIV infection.

Organisms like *Candida* and *Aspergillus* usually have pre-existing pulmonary disease but cryptococcal infection and mucormycosis may arise without other manifestations.

In addition, patients with HIV infection and AIDS are prone to infection with these fungi as well as with atypical mycobacteria (e.g. *Mycobacteria avium-intracellulare*), viruses such as papovavirus and cytomegalovirus and parasites such as *Toxoplasma gondii* and *Entamoeba histolytica*. Particularly in AIDS, multiple infections are common.

SUMMARY BOX
INTRACRANIAL INFECTIONS

- Meningitis is infection of the lining of the brain often caused by bacteria:
  - in the neonatal period the common organisms are *Escherichia coli*, group B streptococci and *Listeria*
  - in early childhood *Haemophilus influenzae* type B is the most likely cause, although Hib vaccination is now available
  - in late childhood, adolescence and early adult life, the commonest organism is the meningococcus (*Neisseria meningitidis*)
  - in later adult life, *Streptococcus pneumoniae* is the commonest involved organism.

- Presenting symptoms vary with the age and the organism; a high index of suspicion is required and diagnosis is made by examination of the CSF.

- Complications include cerebral abscesses, hydrocephalus, cerebral infarction and epilepsy.

- Tuberculous meningitis may complicate primary or secondary pulmonary disease.

- Viral meningitis is usually relatively mild; viral encephalitis is a more severe condition often caused by herpes simplex.

- Immunocompromised patients have increased risks of CNS infections, especially with unusual organisms such as fungi, atypical mycobacteria, viruses and parasites.

ASPECTS OF CENTRAL NERVOUS SYSTEM DISEASE OF PARTICULAR RELEVANCE TO DENTISTRY

- Central nervous system lesions may present with pain, palsy or paraesthesiae in the oral region
- Dentists often encounter patients with neurodegenerative disorders including strokes and intracranial haemorrhages.

CASE STUDY 13.1
RIGHT-SIDED WEAKNESS

A 68-year-old woman was found collapsed at home by her daughter. When last seen the previous evening, she had been well. She was taking diuretics for mild heart failure but she was otherwise in good health. She had had a hysterectomy in the past. When her daughter found her, she was slumped in a chair and the right side of her mouth was drooped. Her daughter called the family GP.

The GP examined her and decided to send her to hospital. On admission there, her blood pressure was 170/105 mmHg, her pulse rate 130/min and irregular and her breathing rate 14/min. An electrocardiogram was performed, which showed atrial fibrillation but with possible ischaemic changes. Her speech was slurred and difficult to understand. Examination of her central nervous system revealed weakness of her right arm and leg with increased tone and tendon reflexes.

She was transferred to a geriatric ward where she was given intravenous fluids and feeding was instituted by naso-gastric tube. She was commenced on digoxin to control her heart rate and continued on diuretics at a lower dose than before. Over the next 2 weeks, her condition improved gradually. She regained some power in her arm, and with the help of physiotherapists, she sat out of bed and started to take some steps with a frame. Her pulse rate settled down to 80/min and was regular. Further ECGs did not show any evidence of recent myocardial infarction.

3 Weeks after admission, her condition deteriorated. She became short of breath and started to cough up thick green sputum. Her pulse rate increased to 120/min and was regular; her blood pressure was 150/95 mmHg; her respiratory rate was 28/min; and her temperature was 39.5°C.

A chest X-ray was performed which showed patchy areas of consolidation in both lower lobes. Sputum was sent for culture and she was commenced on intravenous antibiotics and fluids, and oxygen via nasal prongs, and given chest physiotherapy. Despite this intensive treatment, she did not improve and she died 2 days later.

The family gave permission for a postmortem examination.

1. What are the likely causes of this woman's collapse?
2. What condition did this woman have and what are the possible predisposing factors in her case?
3. What was happening to this woman's brain during her hospital stay?
4. What are the possible causes of the acute change in this woman?
5. What are the likely findings at autopsy in this woman's brain, heart and lungs?

Suggested responses

(see also Chs 7 and 9)

1. The usual causes for collapse in a woman of this age include myocardial infarction or cerebrovascular accident. Less likely, given that she was well a short time previously, are pneumonias, other overwhelming infections or pulmonary embolism, but the possibility of drug overdose (accidental or deliberate) should also be borne in mind.

2. The symptoms and signs described are those of a cerebrovascular accident (stroke) involving the left cerebral cortex. The causes of cerebrovascular accidents include thrombosis of cerebral vessels, cerebral embolism from sources such as atrial thrombosis associated with atrial fibrillation or mural thrombosis secondary to myocardial infarction, and intracerebral haemorrhage, possibly hypertensive in nature. In this woman's case, she has atrial fibrillation; possible ischaemic changes on ECG might suggest a recent myocardial infarct; her blood pressure is high although this may be associated with some degree of raised intracranial pressure rather than a primary cause of her problems.

3. After the initial event of cerebral infarction, there is inevitably some degree of cerebral oedema around the site of damage. As time passes, this oedema settles down and the area of liquefactive necrosis is resorbed by macrophages (microglial cells) and gliotic scar tissue is laid down in the brain. This minimizes the degree of damage and there is often an improvement in clinical symptoms and signs.

4. These are the signs of infection (tachycardia, pyrexia) and with the history of a productive cough and tachypnoea, this is likely to be pneumonia. Patients with strokes are at risk of developing pneumonia, typically bronchopneumonia by infection with organisms such as *Haemophilus influenzae* or *Streptococcus pneumoniae*.

5. Autopsy findings:
    a. *Brain.* This will probably show an area of softening in the left cerebral cortex, typically in the area of distribution of the middle cerebral artery, often involving the internal capsule. This will have undergone liquefactive degeneration, but cyst formation is unlikely at this stage. There may also be some degree of cerebral artery atheroma.
    b. *Heart.* This woman had atrial fibrillation so there may be residual atrial thrombosis, although the treatment with digoxin should reduce the likelihood of this. The causes of atrial fibrillation include ischaemic heart disease (coronary artery atheroma ± signs of old myocardial ischaemia, i.e. fibrosis), hypertensive heart disease (left ventricular hyper-

trophy) and valvular heart disease, especially post-rheumatic (mitral ± aortic fibrosis). There was also a history of cardiac failure, so that the heart is likely to show dilatation of all four chambers, particularly the ventricles.

c. *Lungs.* There should be evidence of bronchopneumonia, patchy areas of consolidation centred on bronchi and bronchioles in both lower lobes. There may also be evidence of cardiac failure, with oedema and congestion of the lungs.

CASE STUDY 13.2
FACIAL PAIN

A 22-year-old woman began to experience attacks of facial pain. The pain was intense and caused her to contort her face for several seconds during attacks. It was triggered by touching parts of the face, moving her lip or by eating. She attended her dentist who examined her face and teeth and also radiographed her jaws. No local cause for the pain was found and she was referred to a Dental Hospital.

In the clinic, the patient was reluctant to let staff touch certain areas of the face during the examination. Touching these areas triggered an electric shock sensation. Both sides of the face were involved. The patient was referred urgently to a neurologist who noted a unilateral lack of pupillary reflex and signs of papilloedema. Her blood pressure was 160/95 mmHg and pulse rate was 42/min. A computerized tomography (CT) scan showed bilateral lesions in the cerebello-pontine angles. These were removed by a neurosurgeon.

The pathologist reported the lesions as consisting of tumours composed of palisaded spindle cells in a vascular stoma. Hyalinized vessels were present and the spindle cells stained with S100 antibody.

The patient's recovery was uneventful. She was referred to the Medical Genetics Department for further advice.

1. Facial pain of a similar character to that described may be caused by trigeminal neuralgia. Which features in the patient's clinical history suggest the possibility of a CNS lesion as an alternative diagnosis?
2. Explain the loss of pupillary reflex and signs of papilloedema. What is their significance?
3. Suggest a diagnosis on the basis of the CT scans and histopathological findings.
4. Why was the patient referred to the Medical Genetics Department?

Suggested responses

1. Trigeminal neuralgia causes an electric shock-like facial pain, possibly related to vascular pathology in the trigeminal ganglion. This patient was not typical in that she was under 50 years of age at presentation, and suffered bilateral facial pain. In such a case CNS lesions, for example multiple sclerosis or a space-occupying lesion in the cerebello-pontine angle, should be suspected.

2. Lack of reactivity of pupillary reflex is due to compression of the oculomotor (third cranial) nerve as it traverses the tentorium. Papilloedema is due to an accumulation of axoplasm in the optic papilla when axonal flow is impeded. These are important signs of raised intracranial pressure. Further indications are the raised blood pressure and reduced pulse rate, resulting from autonomic imbalance and hypothalamic compression.

3. The histopathological features are those of schwannoma. Two main patterns are seen: densely packed spindle cells with frequent nuclear palisading (Antoni A areas) and more loosely structured tissue, which may show cystic degeneration (Antoni B areas). The most common site is the vestibular branch of the 8th cranial nerve in the cerebello-pontine area, and the tumour is often referred to as 'acoustic neuroma'. Cells in schwannomas can be identified by using the tumour marker, S100.

4. Bilateral 8th nerve schwannomas and meningiomas are often a feature of central neurofibromatosis (neurofibromatosis, NF2), which is an hereditary disorder.

14 Endocrine diseases

Endocrinology is the study of hormones, which are chemical agents secreted into the bloodstream by specialized glands throughout the body to influence the activity of cells at distant sites. Similar effects are possible on a localized basis where cells are influenced by the secretions of adjacent cells (paracrine) and on an even more local basis where the secretory products of a cell influence the action of that particular cell (autocrine). All these regulators of cellular activity act via receptors which are proteins either on cell membranes or within target cells. The interaction of hormones with their receptors then triggers a series of diverse intracellular mechanisms culminating in a specific action of the target cell.

HORMONES

There are three main classes of hormones:

- peptides or proteins: these form the majority of hormones and range from short 3-amino acid sequences (thyrotrophin-releasing factor) to large glycoproteins with subunits (pituitary gonadotrophins)
- amino acid derivatives: only a few hormones fit into this category, e.g. adrenaline and thyroxine
- steroid hormones, which are all derivatives of cholesterol.

Although many of these hormones have diverse structures and biological effects, they have evolved from a common source and many act in a similar way through a superfamily of receptors which share structural and functional features.

A number of factors may affect hormone secretion (Fig. 14.1), including:

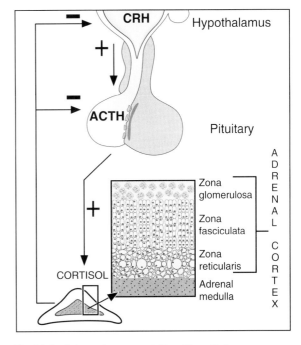

Fig. 14.1 Schematic representation of hypothalamo–pituitary–end-organ axis, using the adrenal cortex as the model. ACTH = adrenocorticotrophic hormone; CRH = corticotrophin-releasing hormone.

- Hypothalamic factors may stimulate or inhibit hormone synthesis and release.
- There may be a pulsatile or episodic pattern of release, such as of gonadotrophin-releasing hormone (GnRH).
- There may be a circadian pattern of secretion producing peak levels of hormone at different times of the day and night, as is seen particularly with adrenocorticotrophic hormone (ACTH) and its end-organ

hormone, cortisol, but similar patterns may also be observed with prolactin, thyroid-stimulating hormone (TSH), growth hormone (GH) and parathyroid hormone (PTH).

- Stress may precipitate the increased synthesis and release of hormones such as ACTH, GH and prolactin.
- Feedback mechanisms from the end-organ-secreted hormones or changes in metabolic products as a result of hormonal action may alter the rate of secretion from the controlling gland.
- Other hormones, not related to feedback mechanisms directly, and drugs, prescribed or taken for other effects, may also have an impact on normal endocrine responses.

PITUITARY GLAND

The pituitary gland lies in a bony cavity at the base of the skull and is connected to the hypothalamus by a stalk containing a series of portal capillaries and nerve fibres (Fig. 14.2). The gland, which weighs approximately 0.5 g, is divided into (a) the anterior pituitary (adenophypophysis) which comprises 75% of the gland and is regulated by a variety of stimulatory and inhibitory hormones from the hypothalamus, and (b) the posterior pituitary (neurohypophysis) which is a collection of specialized nerve endings derived from the hypothalamus.

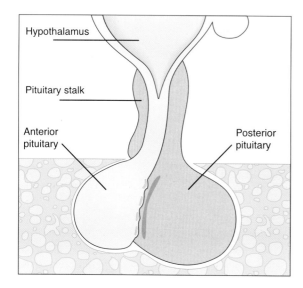

Fig. 14.2 Schematic representation of normal pituitary, demonstrating relationship of pituitary to hypothalamus and between anterior (adenohypophysis) and posterior (neurophypophysis) aspects of the gland.

There are six hormones secreted by the anterior pituitary under the influence of the hypothalamus:

- Thyroid-stimulating hormone (TSH) is secreted in response to thyrotrophin-releasing hormone (TRH) and acts on the thyroid gland to cause secretion of the thyroid hormones, thyroxine (T_4) and tri-iodothyronine (T_3).
- Adrenocorticotrophic hormone (ACTH) is secreted in response to corticotrophin-releasing hormone (CRH) and acts on the adrenal cortex to elicit secretion of cortisol.
- The gonadotrophins, luteinizing hormone (LH) and follicle-stimulating hormone (FSH), are secreted in response to gonadotrophin-releasing hormone (GnRH) and act cooperatively on the ovaries in women, leading to oestrogen and progesterone production, and on the testes in men, leading to testosterone production.
- Growth hormone (GH) is secreted in response to growth hormone-releasing hormone (GHRH) and acts on a variety of tissues to modulate metabolic activity; its secretion may be modified by circulating levels of, for example, glucose and free fatty acids.
- Prolactin secretion is inhibited by dopamine. Prolactin acts on the breasts to produce lactation and also has effects on gonadal function.

The posterior pituitary gland secretes two hormones which are produced in the hypothalamus and are passed along nerve fibres to be stored in granules in the terminal bulbs of nerves close to veins:

- vasopressin, also known as antidiuretic hormone (ADH), which is important in the regulation of plasma osmolality, and
- oxytocin which is released in response to breast-feeding and at the onset of labour.

Hypopituitarism

This is a clinical syndrome which varies in presentation depending on the age of the patient. In infancy or childhood, there may be short stature or impaired development; in the reproductive period, women may present with amenorrhoea or infertility while men may have reduced libido or an absence of secondary sexual characteristics; and in the elderly, symptoms such as hypoglycaemia or hypothermia may be related to ACTH or TSH deficiency. This is an uncommon condition in which there may be a failure of one or more pituitary functions. Possible causes include tumours of the pituitary, either primary or secondary; infarction, particularly associated with pregnancy (Sheehan's syndrome); trauma; congenital malformation; infections, especially tuberculosis; and diseases of the hypothalamus.

Overactivity of the pituitary

This is usually due to the presence of a tumour. Adenomas (benign tumours of glandular tissue) have been described for all the pituitary hormones but TSH- and gonadotrophin-secreting tumours are rare. GH- and ACTH-secreting tumours occur more frequently, while the commonest tumour of the pituitary gland is a prolactinoma.

Hyperprolactinaemia causes amenorrhoea and galactorrhoea (milk production in the absence of pregnancy) in women, while in men the usual presenting feature is due to pressure effects of the enlarging pituitary on the optic nerves. Other causes of increased prolactin levels must be excluded before a diagnosis of prolactinoma can be made. These include stress, drugs, hypothyroidism and idiopathic hypersecretion. Treatment is by suppression of prolactin secretion with bromocriptine or by surgery (hypophysectomy).

Growth hormone excess is usually due to a pituitary adenoma (Fig. 14.3) and in childhood causes rapid linear growth ('gigantism') and in adults causes acromegaly. After fusion of the bony epiphyses, excess GH leads to a protruding jaw, 'spade-like' hands, coarse facial features, soft tissue thickening, sweating and impaired glucose tolerance or even diabetes mellitus. Diagnosis of GH-producing tumours is by biochemical means such as a lack of suppression of GH after a glucose load and the finding of raised levels of insulin-like growth factor-1 (IGF-1) in the serum. Radiological investigations such as

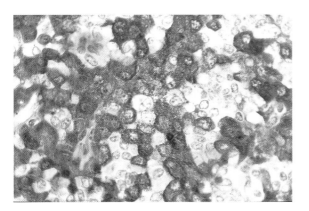

Fig. 14.3 Pituitary: GH adenoma. Immunohistochemical demonstration of growth hormone-producing cells in a pituitary adenoma from an adult patient with acromegaly.

computerized tomography (CT) and magnetic resonance (MR) scanning are useful to confirm the diagnosis. Treatment is by surgery, radiotherapy or drugs such as octreotide or bromocriptine, or possibly a combination of all three modalities.

SUMMARY BOX
PITUITARY GLAND

- The anterior pituitary produces ACTH, TSH, FSH/LH, GH and prolactin; secretion is controlled by feedback mechanisms through the hypothalamus.

- Hypopituitarism is commonly caused either by tumours or infarction; the effects are due to lack of stimulation of pituitary-dependent endocrine organs, especially the adrenal cortex, and lack of GH production.

- Tumours of the pituitary are benign neoplasms which cause their effects either by pressure on local structures, such as the optic nerve, or secretion of excess functionally active hormone.

- The posterior pituitary secretes antidiuretic hormone and oxytocin; damage to the hypothalamo–pituitary link can cause diabetes insipidus.

THYROID GLAND

This gland in the anterior aspect of the neck is essential for the normal maturation and metabolism of all the tissues in the body. It secretes T_4 and T_3 in response to TSH from the pituitary gland, which in turn is stimulated by TRH from the hypothalamus. The secretion of TRH and TSH is influenced by circulating levels of free (i.e. not bound to transport proteins) T_4 and T_3 in a negative feedback loop.

Hypothyroidism

This is caused by a deficiency of thyroid hormones which may be either primary (failure of the gland itself) or secondary (failure of TSH production by the pituitary). Clinically in adulthood, patients show characteristic features of weight gain, lethargy, cold intolerance, coarse dry skin and hair, hoarseness and slow relaxation of tendon reflexes. Most cases are due either to autoimmune destruction of the thyroid gland (Hashimoto's disease) or previous thyroid surgery or radiotherapy with radioactive iodine. The finding of autoimmune thyroid disease, in which there may be antibodies against thyroglobulin, thyroid microsomal antigen and TSH receptor, should lead to a search for other autoimmune phenomena such as Addison's disease, pernicious anaemia, insulin-dependent diabetes mellitus and vitiligo. Treatment of hypothyroidism is by lifelong replacement with T_4.

Congenital hypothyroidism occurs in 1 in 3500 births in the UK and is the subject of a well-established screening programme, where high levels of TSH indicate primary failure of the gland owing to dysgenesis. Many children appear normal at birth but if untreated they will go on to develop severe mental retardation and signs of cretinism such as a puffy face, protuberant tongue, umbilical hernia, muscle weakness and other neurological signs.

Hyperthyroidism (thyrotoxicosis)

This can be a very dramatic clinical disease. Patients may present with weight loss despite a normal appetite, heat intolerance, undue tiredness, diarrhoea, tremor, cardiac arrhythmias such as atrial fibrillation, angina and heart failure, muscle weakness especially proximal myopathy, subfertility in women, a goitre (enlargement of the thyroid gland) and in Graves' disease, eyelid lag and eyelid retraction. The commonest cause of hyperthyroidism is Graves' disease, which is an autoimmune disease where there are antibodies to the TSH receptor which appear to mimic the action of TSH, thus leading to a lack of the normal control mechanisms, and which causes a diffuse toxic goitre. Other causes include a toxic multinodular goitre, a solitary toxic adenoma, thyroiditis, iodine and iodine-containing drugs, and excessive ingestion of T_3 and T_4. Histologically in Graves' disease, there is evidence of hyperplasia of thyroid follicles which are lined by tall columnar cells and which contain little stored colloid. There is often a heavy lymphocytic infiltrate including lymphoid follicles with germinal centres. Treatment may be with antithyroid drugs, radioiodine and surgery, depending on the age and other clinical situation of the patient concerned.

Goitre

This simply means enlargement of the thyroid gland, which may be diffuse as in Graves' disease (see above), but is usually nodular. These nodules are composed of variably sized follicles, containing colloid to greater or lesser degrees, surrounded by fibrous tissue. As the nodules enlarge, they may cause pressure effects on adjacent structures such as the oesophagus and trachea (Fig. 14.4). Enlargement may occur suddenly as a result of haemorrhage into very vascular nodules and this results in

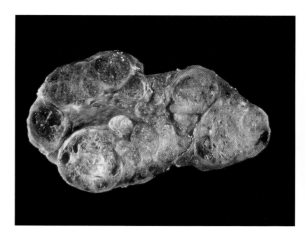

Fig. 14.4 Thyroid: nodular goitre. Slice of thyroid gland showing prominent nodularity with focal haemorrhage and calcification.

degenerative change with cyst formation and more fibrosis. Occasionally, these nodules may contain foci of papillary carcinoma (see below). In most cases, patients with multinodular goitres are euthyroid, but less commonly, they may be either hyper- or hypothyroid. Such goitres were seen more frequently in parts of the world where iodine deficiency had been a problem, such as the Derbyshire region of England and parts of Bavaria and Switzerland, but with the introduction of iodized salt, they are not seen much nowadays. Most cases are now due to inborn errors of iodine metabolism where incorporation of iodine into tyrosine in T_3/T_4 synthesis is impaired (dyshormonogenetic goitre) or as a result of exposure to iodine-containing drugs.

SUMMARY BOX
THYROID GLAND

- The thyroid gland secretes thyroxine (T_4) and tri-iodothyronine (T_3) whose secretion is controlled by a feedback mechanism through TSH.

- Hypofunction may be congenital or acquired in adult life; acquired causes include autoimmune destruction of the gland in Hashimoto's disease, and previous surgery or radiotherapy.

- Hyperfunction is usually due to excess T_4/T_3; patients present with features of increased metabolic activity and rarely with atrial fibrillation; the commonest cause is Graves' disease.

- Goitre means enlargement of the thyroid gland; common causes of nodular goitre are inherited abnormalities of iodine metabolism or lack of iodine.

Neoplasms

Papillary tumours of the thyroid gland tend to occur in young people who present with enlargement of the gland, which on radioisotope scanning is seen as a 'cold nodule'. The tumour is composed of papillary projections of thyroid epithelial cells with a characteristic nuclear morphology, where there is optical clearing, often with a single nucleolus, and overlapping or grooved nuclear membranes – so-called 'orphan Annie' cells named after the American cartoon character. Within the papillary cores, there may be laminated concretions of calcified material known as psammoma bodies. These tumours tend to be multifocal and metastasize early to regional cervical lymph nodes. Treatment is by local resection and long-term prognosis is usually quite good as distant metastases rarely occur.

Tumours of follicular origin may be benign or malignant. Benign follicular neoplasms (adenomas) may have a simple follicular structure but may have abundant colloid production (colloid adenoma), resemble fetal thyroid (fetal adenoma) or develop a marked oncocytic appearance (Hürthle cell adenoma). Malignant follicular tumours tend to occur in an older age group and spread via the bloodstream. The earliest form is seen as microinvasive follicular carcinoma where a predominantly encapsulated tumour shows vascular invasion in its capsule. Later, carcinomas metastasize widely, especially to lung.

Medullary carcinoma of the thyroid is a malignant tumour derived from calcitonin-producing cells (C cells) in the thyroid stroma and may be part of the multiple endocrine neoplasia (MEN) syndromes. The tumour cells are large and eosinophilic and are characteristically found in an amyloid stroma.

Lymphoma of the thyroid is rare and usually arises on the basis of pre-existing autoimmune disease where mucosa-associated lymphoid tissue develops. The usual tumour is a low-grade non-Hodgkin's lymphoma of B cell type (MALToma).

Other tumours are extremely rare and include sclerosing variants of papillary and follicular carcinomas, metaplastic (squamous) carcinoma and anaplastic carcinoma.

ADRENAL CORTEX

The adrenal cortex is divided into three zones:

1. zona glomerulosa – which secretes aldosterone and is regulated by the renin–angiotensin system in response to plasma sodium levels
2. zona fasciculata – which secretes cortisol and sex hormones and is regulated by ACTH secretion from the anterior pituitary, which in turn is regulated by CRH production by the hypothalamus, both of which are under feedback control by cortisol levels, and
3. zona reticularis – which is identical to zona fasciculata in the hormonal sense.

Hypofunction of the adrenal cortex

When lack of function occurs as a primary disease of the cortex itself, this is known as Addison's disease. It can be due to selective damage to the adrenal cortex, e.g. autoimmune attack of the cortex by antibodies reacting against steroid-producing cells, and may be associated with other autoimmune diseases affecting the thyroid, parathyroid, ovary and stomach. It may also be due to diffuse destruction of the adrenal cortex and medulla, e.g. by inflammatory conditions such as tuberculosis or other granulomatous disease, and fungal or viral infections, by metabolic disease such as amyloidosis, by neoplastic disease, especially metastatic carcinoma and lymphoma, and by vascular disease such as the Waterhouse–Friderichsen syndrome in acute meningococcal septicaemia. Adrenocortical hypofunction may also be caused by extra-adrenal factors such as iatrogenic glucocorticoid therapy, and ACTH deficiency due to pituitary or hypothalamic disease. Clinically, these patients may present with lethargy, anorexia, weight loss, excess pigmentation of oral mucosa and body creases and abdominal pain. The diagnosis may be suspected biochemically by the presence of low plasma sodium and raised plasma potas-

---

SUMMARY BOX
TUMOURS OF THE THYROID

- Tumours of the thyroid are of four main types with different clinical patterns.

- Papillary carcinomas occur in young people and have a high risk of lymph node spread.

- Follicular neoplasms may be benign or malignant, and are more common in elderly patients; in the most severe form, follicular carcinomas may cause widespread blood-borne metastases.

- Medullary carcinomas arise from calcitonin (C) cells and may be part of multiple endocrine neoplasia (MEN) syndromes; tumour-associated amyloid may be present.

- Primary lymphomas of thyroid are rare, often arise on a background of autoimmune disease and are usually of mucosa-associated lymphoid tissue (MALT) origin.

sium and urea and can be confirmed by dynamic tests of pituitary–adrenal function. Treatment is with life-long corticosteroid replacement.

Hyperfunction of the adrenal cortex

This may cause overproduction of (a) cortisol, (b) sex hormones and (c) aldosterone.

Cortisol excess causes Cushing's syndrome, in which patients develop characteristic physical features of moon face, buffalo hump, acne, baldness, increased abdominal fat, abdominal striae, thinning of the skin, easy bruising, muscle weakness, osteoporosis and systemic hypertension. The possible causes of cortisol excess include a pituitary adenoma secreting excess ACTH (so-called Cushing's disease), an ectopic source of ACTH, e.g. from a small cell carcinoma of bronchus, a benign adrenocortical adenoma, less commonly an adrenocortical carcinoma and iatrogenic Cushing's syndrome where patients are taking prescribed corticosteroids for other conditions. The condition can be mimicked in chronic alcoholics.

Histologically, the glands may be diffusely enlarged, either unilaterally or bilaterally, and may have a nodular appearance; they will weigh more than the normal 4–6 g. Adenomas are commonest in women between 30 and 50 years, and characteristically are solitary nodules more than 1 cm in diameter composed of large lipid-laden clear cells (Fig. 14.5). Carcinomas tend to be large lesions weighing in excess of 100 g and are more common in women; when Cushing's syndrome occurs in childhood as a result of a tumour, it is more likely to be a carcinoma than an adenoma. Grossly, carcinomas are large soft redbrown lesions with areas of haemorrhage and necrosis and microscopically there is abundant cellular pleomorphism. Adrenocortical carcinomas are associated with a poor prognosis with metastases to lymph nodes, liver, lungs, bone and the contralateral adrenal gland.

Sex hormone excess in early childhood may occur as a result of an inherited abnormality where one of the enzymes involved in steroid metabolism is reduced or absent (usually 21-hydroxylase), resulting in continuing ACTH stimulation of the gland because of a lack of feedback control (congenital adrenal hyperplasia). This leads to the production of intermediate metabolites which may be fatal and often lead to virilization in females and precocious puberty in boys. In later childhood and adulthood, sex hormone excess is more likely to develop as a result of neoplasia, particularly due to carcinoma.

Aldosterone excess is rare as a primary phenomenon (Conn's syndrome) and is most commonly due to a solitary adenoma of zona glomerulosa cells; less commonly it may be caused by adrenocortical hyperplasia or carcinoma. Patients present with polyuria and polydipsia, muscle weakness, paraesthesiae and hypertension. Biochemically, the plasma potassium is low, the sodium high and plasma renin levels are reduced. Secondary hyperaldosteronism where the plasma renin levels are elevated is much more common and is seen in cardiac, hepatic and renal disease.

ADRENAL MEDULLA

The adrenal medulla is composed of chromaffin cells similar to postganglionic neurons of the sympathetic nervous system and secretes either adrenaline or noradenaline. Similar groups of cells may be found in extraadrenal sites related to nerve ganglia and occasionally in the urinary bladder, gut and gonads. Uncommonly, there may be hypofunction of the adrenal medulla as a result of total destruction of the adrenal gland (see above). However, the commonest pathology of the adrenal medulla is the development of a tumour known as a phaeochromocytoma. This is a rare tumour but it is a recognized cause of systemic hypertension, which is usually sustained but may be episodic. Associated features include cardiac arrhythmias, cardiac failure, myocardial infarction and cerebral haemorrhage. Such tumours may occur as part of the MEN syndromes, in which case they are more likely

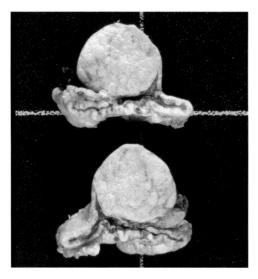

Fig. 14.5 Adrenal: cortical adenoma. Sections of an adrenal gland in which there is a solitary yellow nodule, typical of a benign adrenocortical adenoma.

to be bilateral. Sporadic cases tend to be unilateral. Phaeochromocytomas are tumours of 3–5 cm in diameter and weigh about 100 g, although occasionally they may achieve weights of 4 kg. They are well demarcated from surrounding tissues and have a brown cut surface with variable degrees of haemorrhage and necrosis; calcification may be present in the larger tumours. The tumour cells resemble those of the normal medulla, although larger with abundant granular cytoplasm. Pleomorphism is marked but mitoses are uncommon. A diagnosis of malignancy can only be made on the presence of metastases, usually to lymph nodes, lungs, liver and bone, since, like most endocrine neoplasms, morphological features alone are not a good predictor of behaviour.

SUMMARY BOX
ADRENAL GLAND

- The adrenal gland is composed of the adrenal medulla, which secretes the hormones adrenaline and noradrenaline, and the adrenal cortex which secretes glucocorticoids, mineralocorticoids and some of the sex hormones.

- The commonest pathology of the adrenal medulla is a tumour called phaeochromocytoma; the tumour may be part of the MEN syndromes.

- Hypofunction of the adrenal gland (Addison's disease) leads to problems with lack of mineralocorticoid and glucocorticoid secretion; it is commonly due to autoimmune destruction of the gland.

- Hyperfunction of the adrenal cortex with excess glucocorticoid production is called Cushing's syndrome, which may be caused by:
  – pituitary ACTH production (Cushing's disease)
  – hyperplasia or neoplasms of the adrenal gland
  – ectopic ACTH secretion
  – iatrogenic administration of corticosteroids or ACTH.

- Conn's syndrome is where there is excess mineralocorticoid production by the adrenal cortex, especially by an adenoma.

PARATHYROID GLANDS

These are a series of four glands intimately related to the thyroid gland in the anterior part of the neck. They secrete parathyroid hormone, which is involved in the maintenance of calcium homeostasis in the body. There are two main cell types: (a) chief cells which have a clear cell or eosinophilic appearance and (b) oxyphil cells which have a granular densely eosinophilic appearance. Parathyroid hormone (PTH, parathormone) raises blood calcium levels through several mechanisms including mobilization of calcium from bone, increased reabsorption of calcium from the kidney and by stimulating the production of 1,25-dihydroxycholecalciferol (vitamin D_3) in the kidney.

Hyperparathyroidism (see also Ch. 12)

This may be primary or secondary. Primary hyperparathyroidism occurs without any physiological stimulus and can be due to a solitary adenoma (80% of cases), diffuse hyperplasia of more than one gland (15–20%) and rarely carcinoma (2–3%). Excessive secretion of PTH leads to hypercalcaemia, hypophosphataemia and hypercalciuria. It usually occurs in middle age and is more common in women. Patients present with problems related to renal stone formation, bone disease such as osteitis fibrosa cystica and giant cell granulomas ('brown tumours'), peptic ulceration, pancreatitis, general tiredness and muscle weakness. Primary hyperparathyroidism may occur as part of the MEN syndromes, where hyperplasia is the most common pattern. Adenomas are usually tan-coloured and are composed predominantly of chief cells with variable components of clear cells and oxyphil cells. In hyperplasia, there is an admixture of all cell types with loss of the normal fat, but to make this diagnosis, all glands need to be examined. In common with other endocrine neoplasms, the diagnosis of malignancy is extremely difficult on histological grounds alone, but increased mitotic activity with capsular and vascular invasion are suggestive of a diagnosis of carcinoma.

Secondary hyperparathyroidism

This occurs in the presence of a physiological stimulus (hypocalcaemia) which is most commonly due to chronic renal failure but may also be seen in malabsorption syndromes and in vitamin D deficiency. The effect of secondary hyperparathyroidism is to raise the serum calcium to normal levels. Very occasionally, patients with secondary hyperparathyroidism may develop hypercalcaemia when cells within the hyperplastic glands become autonomous leading to inappropriately high levels of calcium, even to the extent of producing an adenomatous nodule (so-called 'tertiary hyperparathyroidism').

Hypoparathyroidism

This is usually due to inadvertent surgical removal of the parathyroid glands in thyroid surgery and leads to hypocalcaemia, which causes increased muscular tone, spasms and tetany. There may be mental changes, epilepsy and cataract formation. Less commonly, hypoparathyroidism may be due to autoimmune disease or is associated with DiGeorge's syndrome which is due to a failure of development of the third and fourth branchial pouches, also causing T lymphocyte deficiency.

SUMMARY BOX
PARATHYROID GLANDS

- Four glands in the neck are involved in calcium metabolism through parathyroid hormone (PTH) and, indirectly, vitamin D metabolism.
- Hypofunction of the glands is usually due to inadvertent surgical removal of the glands during thyroid surgery but may be autoimmune in origin.
- Hyperfunction may be primary or secondary:
  - the usual secondary cause is renal failure causing calcium loss in the urine
  - primary overproduction may be due to an adenoma in 80% of cases, diffuse hyperplasia (15–20%) and, very rarely, carcinoma.

ENDOCRINE PANCREAS

Diseases of the exocrine pancreas have been dealt with in the section on the gastrointestinal tract (Ch. 10). The endocrine pancreas coexists with the exocrine pancreas with concentrations of hormone-producing cells in the islets of Langerhans. The four main hormones secreted are insulin, produced by the B or β-cells, glucagon, produced by the A2, A or α-cells, somatostatin, produced by A1, D or δ-cells, and pancreatic polypeptide, produced by the PP or F cells. The PP-rich area of the gland is in the tail region, suggesting that these cells derive from the ventral pancreas in embryonic development. The commonest disease of the endocrine pancreas is diabetes mellitus.

Diabetes mellitus

This is not a single disease but a metabolic state caused by inadequate insulin action, which may be due to an absolute or relative lack of insulin, characterized by glucose intolerance. Insulin promotes the uptake of glucose by cells and is important in the conversion of glucose to glycogen intracellularly. It also stimulates protein synthesis from amino acids and the uptake of free fatty acids

by adipose tissue. Lack of insulin leads to a generalized catabolic state where there is weight loss, hyperglycaemia, reduced protein synthesis, increased gluconeogenesis and hyperlipidaemia. The renal threshold for glucose, although raised, is exceeded, producing glycosuria and an osmotic diuresis which promotes severe thirst. The liver converts free fatty acids into ketone bodies (acetoacetic acid, β-hydroxybutyric acid and acetone) which generate hydrogen ions that in turn cause a metabolic acidosis. If untreated, this leads to disturbances of neuronal function and ketoacidotic coma. Another form of coma in severe untreated diabetics is hyperosmolar non-ketotic coma where there is severe dehydration and marked hyperglycaemia without ketoacidosis. These are both acute medical emergencies and if untreated may be fatal. Patients may present with recurrent infections and problems with wound healing including delayed healing of tooth sockets.

Diabetes mellitus fits into two main categories although rare secondary causes may also exist, including chronic pancreatitis, haemochromatosis, Cushing's syndrome, acromegaly, cystic fibrosis and glucagon-secreting islet cell tumours. Diabetes mellitus is thought to occur in up to 5% of the general population and is more common with increasing age, especially in obese patients.

Type I diabetes

Type I diabetes (insulin-dependent diabetes mellitus; IDDM) usually presents in childhood and there is a strong familial tendency. There is a marked selective reduction in the number of insulin-producing β-cells with an associated chronic inflammatory cell reaction (so-called 'insulitis'), possible due to an autoimmune response triggered by viral infections such as coxsackie B, mumps or rubella.

Type II diabetes

Type II diabetes (non-insulin-dependent diabetes mellitus; NIDDM) occurs in an older age group. Patients with this condition along with obese people and approximately 25% of the general population have evidence of resistance to the action of insulin, so that higher levels of insulin secretion are required for normal glucose metabolism. Eventually, the capacity of β-cells to cope with this increased demand is overwhelmed and the clinical picture of overt diabetes develops. Histologically, up to 70% of cases show the deposition of amyloid within islets.

Complications

Diabetic patients are at increased risk of the development of cardiovascular disease, which may affect either large (macroangiopathy) or small (microangiopathy) vessels.

Macroangiopathy.   Atheroma occurs earlier and to a more severe degree in diabetics and, coupled with the increased incidence of hypertension, it is not surprising that 80% of diabetics die from large vessel disease in the form of myocardial infarction, cerebrovascular disease and peripheral vascular disease.

Microangiopathy.   This leads to three main manifestations which are major causes of morbidity in diabetes:

- diabetic retinopathy where there are capillary microaneurysms, retinitis proliferans and cataracts leading to blindness
- diabetic nephropathy where there is hyaline thickening of the afferent and efferent arterioles of the glomerulus, thickening of the glomerular capillary basement membrane producing diffuse or nodular glomerulosclerosis (the latter the classical Kimmelstiel–Wilson lesions; Fig. 14.6), exudative glomerular capsular lesions and interstitial chronic inflammation, leading to the nephrotic syndrome and chronic renal failure
- peripheral neuropathy, which causes severe problems with foot care and secondary infection.

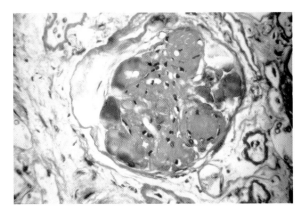

Fig. 14.6   Kidney: diabetic Kimmelstiel–Wilson lesion.
Histological section of a glomerulus from a patient with diabetic nephropathy, with prominent nodularity of the glomerular tufts. These have the appearances of nodular glomerulosclerosis, the Kimmelstiel–Wilson lesion.

SUMMARY BOX
DIABETES MELLITUS

- A common disease in which there is a relative or absolute lack of insulin, leading to glucose intolerance.
- Type I is characteristically juvenile-onset and insulin-dependent, associated with destruction of β-cells.
- Type II is usually maturity-onset and insulin-independent, and is a common cause of disease.
- Diabetes has effects on multiple organs, particularly blood vessels leading to increased atheroma, retinopathy, nephropathy and neuropathy.

Neoplasms

Tumours of the endocrine pancreas are relatively common. Like all endocrine neoplasms, it is difficult, if not impossible, to predict clinical behaviour on histological grounds alone. Most of these tumours cause problems through their secretory products, including insulin causing hypoglycaemia, glucagon producing diabetes and skin rashes, gastrin leading to severe peptic ulceration, vasoactive intestinal polypeptide causing watery diarrhoea and hypokalaemia, pancreatic polypeptide producing peptic ulcers and diarrhoea, and somatostatin causing mild diabetes. Occasionally, malignant tumours do occur with evidence of metastatic spread, usually to liver. It should also be remembered that similar clinical presentations and hormonal abnormalities may be produced by non-neoplastic islet cell hyperplasia.

Multiple endocrine neoplasia (MEN) syndromes

These are rare combinations of endocrine hyperplasias and neoplasia which are often familial.

- *MEN type I (Werner's syndrome).* This is a combination of a pituitary adenoma, an islet cell tumour of pancreas and hyperparathyroidism, commonly due to hyperplasia, occasionally with peptic ulceration and adrenocortical hyperplasia or adenoma.
- *MEN type IIa (Sipple's syndrome).* This comprises a phaeochromocytoma of adrenal medulla, medullary carcinoma of thyroid and parathyroid hyperplasia/ adenoma.
- *MEN type IIb.* This is similar to type IIa with the addition of mucosal neuromas, especially on the tongue, and ganglioneuromas of the bowel; hyperparathyroidism is less commonly seen.

SUMMARY BOX
ENDOCRINE PANCREAS

- The main hormones secreted by the endocrine pancreas are insulin (β-cells), glucagon (α-cells), somatostatin (δ-cells) and pancreatic polypeptide (PP cells).

- Tumours of the endocrine pancreas cause problems through their secretions:
  - glucagonomas cause diabetes and skin rashes
  - insulinomas present with hypoglycaemia
  - gastrinomas cause recurrent multiple peptic ulcers.

- It is difficult to predict clinical behaviour of endocrine tumours from histological appearances but malignant tumours with liver metastases may occur.

- Occasionally, pancreatic tumours may be part of the MEN syndromes.

ASPECTS OF ENDOCRINE DISEASE OF PARTICULAR RELEVANCE TO DENTISTRY

- Patients with acromegaly may present with overgrowth of the jaw and coarse facies.
- Addison's disease may be recognized through oral pigmentation.
- Dentists should recognize the characteristic features of Cushing's syndrome, especially when associated with corticosteroid therapy.
- Diabetic patients may present with dry mouth and oral candidiasis.

CASE STUDY 14.1
URINARY PROBLEMS IN DIABETES

A 55-year-old woman presented to her GP complaining of tiredness and feeling generally unwell. She suffers from diabetes mellitus and had been injecting herself with insulin twice a day for the last 15 years. On questioning, she described pain on micturition and occasionally noticed that her urine was frothy and smelly. Her GP asked her to provide a specimen of urine and sent part of this to the microbiology laboratory for culture and sensitivity. The GP tested part of the specimen herself and then prescribed a course of antibiotics.

A week later, she returned to her GP, having completed the course of antibiotics. The GP had received a report from the microbiology laboratory stating that *Escherichia coli* had been grown from the urine with greater than 10^6 organisms per mm^3. Although the pain on micturition had cleared up, the woman still commented that her urine was frothy. On examination, she was puffy around the eyes and her ankles

were very swollen; her blood pressure was measured at 170/110 mmHg, having been 140/95 mmHg at the previous visit. The GP again tested the urine. This time there was no blood present but the previous findings of glucosuria and proteinuria (++++) were still present. The GP took blood for further tests and referred the patient to the local nephrology unit.

The patient attended at the clinic where her history and examination were as before. In the meantime, her blood tests returned and showed a blood urea of 25 mmol/l (NR 2.8–6.8 mmol/l) and a blood creatinine of 340 μmol/l (NR < 88 μmol/l).

After explaining the position to her and outlining the risks, a percutaneous needle biopsy of kidney was undertaken, under ultrasound control.

1. What are the possible causes of the woman's symptoms?
2. What specific features might the GP identify by testing the urine herself?
3. What condition does this woman have?
4. What features are likely to be present in the biopsy from this diabetic woman?
5. What other conditions is this woman prone to?

Suggested responses (see also Ch. 11)

1. Diabetics are at increased risk of infection generally and in the urinary tract specifically, related to glycosuria (glucose in the urine). Thus, the symptoms of pain on micturition and 'smelly' urine are in keeping with a urinary tract infection (UTI). However, the frothy urine suggests the presence of protein and may indicate more serious underlying disease such as the nephrotic syndrome and chronic renal failure. The usual organisms involved in UTI are derived from the gastrointestinal tract and thus *Escherichia coli*, *Proteus*, *Streptococcus faecalis* and others.

2. The usual features tested for are the presence of (a) glucose, particularly important as a manifestation of diabetic control, (b) protein, which indicates the integrity of the glomeruli, and (c) blood, which might indicate infection or immunologically mediated disease.

3. This woman has evidence of chronic renal failure, probably of diabetic origin, confirmed on her renal function tests including blood urea and creatinine which are breakdown products of protein metabolism and are good markers of glomerular diseases. By combining quantitation of 24-hour excretion of creatinine with the blood level, an accurate assessment of glomerular filtration rate (normally greater than 120 ml/min) can be made.

4. The features of diabetic nephropathy are likely to be present including diffuse glomerulosclerosis, nodular glomerulosclerosis (Kimmelstiel–Wilson lesion), exudative lesions such as fibrin caps and capsular drops, accumulation of glycogen in renal tubules, hyaline changes in afferent and efferent arterioles, and increased atheroma in larger vessels.

5. Long-standing diabetics have an increased tendency to atheroma formation, and thus have increased risk of ischaemic heart disease and cerebrovascular disease, ocular lesions such as cataracts and proliferative changes in the retina, peripheral and autonomic neuropathy, and increased risk of infections in the lungs, skin and kidneys.

CASE STUDY 14.2
BITE PROBLEMS

A 45-year-old woman of Afro-Caribbean origin presented to her dentist with a recent history of difficulty with her bite. She noted that her back teeth were catching and that this was the first time she had noticed this. However, on questioning, she described loosening of her wrist after pregnancy over a 3-month period but this had cleared up spontaneously. On examination, her dentist identified an anterior open bite. Her dentist referred her to the Oral Medicine Clinic at the nearby dental school.

At the clinic, her history was confirmed and she also reported that her shoe size had increased and that she was having problems with sciatica. Prognathism was noted. A radiograph of her jaw showed reactivation of the growth condyle. A provisional diagnosis was made and she was referred onwards to the endocrinology clinic at the local hospital.

After her initial consultation, investigations were performed which confirmed the diagnosis. She was further referred to a neurosurgeon who removed her pituitary gland by the trans-sphenoidal route. Samples were sent to the histopathology laboratory.

1. What are the possible causes of this woman's presenting symptoms?
2. What investigations were required to confirm the provisional diagnosis and to identify the source of this woman's problems?
3. What is the likely underlying cause and what will the histopathologist see?

Suggested responses

1. A number of possible dental and oral causes should be considered for this woman's difficulty with her bite, including condylar hyperplasia, Paget's disease, brown tumours of hyperparathyroidism, cementoma, ameloblastoma and other intraosseous tumours. However, the combination of features suggest expansion of bone which may be related locally to a neoplasm or generally to acromegaly. General features include the change in occlusion, loose wrist, increased shoe size and sciatica.

2. The diagnosis of acromegaly is made on identification of elevated levels of growth hormone (GH) and of insulin-like growth factors (IGFs) which mediate the effect of GH on peripheral tissues, especially muscle, bone and soft tissues. If these levels are found to be elevated, then there is a need to identify the source of GH. This is usually due to a pituitary adenoma which may be recognized on radiological imaging such as computed tomography (CT) or magnetic resonance imaging (MRI) scans. If doubt exists, specific venous sampling of the pituitary region may be taken to confirm the pituitary origin.

3. The most likely diagnosis in this case is a functional (GH-secreting) pituitary adenoma. Histologically, these are benign tumours of glandular tissue composed of either acidophil or chromophobe cells. Immunohistochemistry will confirm GH production and there may be suppression of other pituitary activity with reduction or loss of ACTH, FSH/LH, TSH or prolactin production.

15 Diseases of the skin

The skin is a complex organ which is the body's first line of defence against a wide range of injurious stimuli, including irradiation, infection and trauma. It is involved in absorption and excretion of fluid, temperature regulation, immunological surveillance and sensory perception. For these reasons, the skin has evolved a vast array of responses to these situations which are beyond the scope of an undergraduate textbook. However, it is an area of particular interest to dentists since the squamous epithelium of the mouth develops many of the same conditions, and a basic knowledge of skin diseases is required to understand the pathogenesis of oral diseases at a later stage.

NORMAL SKIN (Fig. 15.1)

The skin consists of the superficial layer of epidermis overlying the dermis, in which the supporting connective tissue structures of collagen and elastic tissue are found. The epidermis (Fig. 15.1A) is composed of keratinocytes which mature upwards from the basal layer through the stratum spinosum and the stratum granulosum to the stratum corneum. These cells show complex interactions with each other and their underlying basement membrane. In the basal layer, melanocytes containing the pigment melanin are present, affording protection against the effects of ultraviolet radiation. Langerhans' cells are cells of the mononuclear-phagocyte system which act as antigen-presenting cells and are present in the suprabasal layers of the epidermis. The dermis is divided into the papillary (superficial) dermis around the rete ridges of the epidermis and the reticular (deep) dermis which extends to the subcutaneous fat (Fig. 15.1B). Depending on the part of the body, the dermis may contain specialized structures including hair follicles, and the sweat, sebaceous and apocrine glands. The dermis is richly supplied with blood vessels and nerves.

SUMMARY BOX
NORMAL SKIN

- The skin is the first line of defence against trauma, infection and irradiation.
- The epidermis consists of several layers including basal layer, stratum spinosum, stratum granulosum, stratum corneum and acellular keratin.
- The underlying dermis is divided into superficial papillary dermis and deeper reticular dermis; specialized dermal structures including sweat glands, sebaceous glands and hair follicles are present depending on the site.

INFECTIONS OF SKIN

Because of its position, the skin is prone to infection with a variety of microorganisms. Bacterial infections of the skin are usually caused by either staphylococci or streptococci. Impetigo is a highly contagious condition occurring in children, presenting as crusted blisters (vesicles) around the nose and mouth. In infancy, some staphylococci produce a toxin which causes disruption of the upper epidermis with widespread blistering, known as the staphylococcal scalded skin syndrome. Superficial infection of hair follicles caused by *Staph. aureus* leads to superficial folliculitis, which may lead to pus formation and the development of a boil, which is spreading infection in the dermis. Mycobacterial infection is less common nowadays but spread from a distant site of

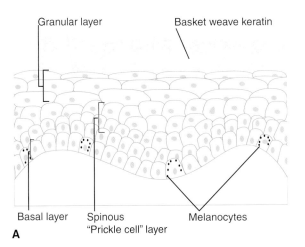

Granular layer   Basket weave keratin

Basal layer   Spinous   Melanocytes
A   "Prickle cell" layer

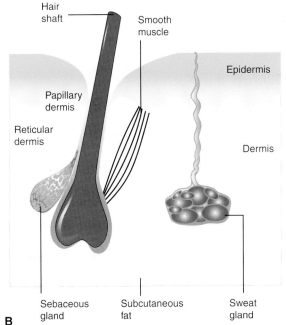

Hair shaft   Smooth muscle

Papillary dermis   Epidermis

Reticular dermis   Dermis

Sebaceous gland   Subcutaneous fat   Sweat gland
B

Fig. 15.1 Normal skin. A. Schematic representation of normal epidermis demonstrating maturation of cells from basal layers upwards, and including melanocytes in the basal layer.
B. Schematic representation of normal dermis showing relations of epidermis to papillary and reticular dermis and to subcutaneous fat, and including adnexal structures such as sebaceous and sweat glands.

tuberculosis may lead to lupus vulgaris, granulomatous inflammation of the dermis which destroys the skin appendages. Occasionally, atypical mycobacteria, e.g. *Mycobacterium marinum* from tropical fish tanks, may cause infections of the hands. On a world-wide basis, the commonest mycobacterial skin infection is leprosy which leads to raised nodules (papules) or plaques and there is often damage to nerves.

Fungal skin infections

These usually occur from spread of normal skin commensal organisms into the epidermis where they produce a variety of conditions depending on the site. These include athlete's foot caused by *Trichophyton* and *Epidermophyton* organisms, and ringworm caused by *Microsporum* and *Trichophyton rubrum*. In immunosuppressed patients, such as those with AIDS or on chemotherapy, fungal infection may be more deep-seated and lead to severe folliculitis spreading down hair follicles which is due to *Candida albicans*.

Viral infections

These are of three main groups: human papillomavirus, poxvirus and herpesviruses.

Human papillomavirus (HPV)

This is a DNA virus of more than 40 subtypes which lead to infections in a wide range of anatomical sites. In the skin, HPV types 2, 4 and 7 cause the common wart (verruca vulgaris) which occurs on the fingers and hands of children. The epidermis becomes thickened with prominent papillary folds and hyperkeratosis; typical infected cells with nuclear inclusions, irregular nuclei and keratohyaline granules may be seen. Plantar warts occur on the soles of the feet, are caused by HPV types 1, 2 and 4 and may be extremely painful. Genital warts (condylomata acuminata) are caused by HPV types 6 and 11. In the uterine cervix, HPV infection is associated with cervical intraepithelial neoplasia (CIN) and squamous carcinoma.

Poxvirus

Infection with a poxvirus leads to molluscum contagiosum, which is characterized by multiple raised pale papules on the face, trunk and limbs of children, although sexual transmission can also occur. These are well-circumscribed epithelial proliferations with a central keratotic core in which abundant large intracytoplasmic viral inclusions are present.

Herpesviruses

These cause blistering skin conditions. They include the common cold sore around the mouth which is due to herpes simplex virus (HSV) type 1, and the sexually transmitted genital herpes caused by HSV type 2. Infection with varicella zoster virus (VZV) causes the lesions of chickenpox (varicella) and shingles (herpes zoster). In childhood, chickenpox leads to widespread blisters. After recovery, the virus may survive in the posterior root ganglia and become reactivated within the dermatome involved as shingles. The lesions of HSV and VZV are similar histologically with oedema of keratinocytes leading to intraepidermal vesicle formation (see below), within which damaged epidermal cells with prominent intranuclear viral inclusions may be seen.

SUMMARY BOX
SKIN INFECTIONS

- Bacterial skin infections are common, especially with organisms such as streptococci and staphylococci; less commonly, mycobacteria may cause skin infections.
- Fungal skin infections usually arise from spread of skin commensals; in immunosuppressed individuals, more deep-seated infections may occur.
- Three main types of viral skin infections may occur: warts are caused by human papillomavirus (HPV); a poxvirus causes molluscum contagiosum; the herpesvirus group cause cold sores, genital herpes, chickenpox and shingles.

NON-INFECTIVE INFLAMMATORY SKIN DISEASES

Dermatitis refers to inflammation of the skin, which may involve either or both the epidermis and dermis. Some inflammatory skin conditions have characteristic features clinically and histologically but many are non-specific and may have many disparate causes. This is often called eczema.

Eczematous dermatitis

In acute eczematous dermatitis, the skin becomes itchy, red and tender. This leads to the formation of blisters (vesicles) in the epidermis, as a result of fluid accumulation between individual keratinocytes (spongiosis). Inflammatory cells from the dermis migrate into the epidermis causing these vesicles to rupture discharging clear fluid and then crusting over. The underlying dermis develops a chronic inflammatory infiltrate around blood vessels, and oedema fluid causes swelling. Secondary changes occur as a result of the intense itching experienced by the patient and, thus, repeated trauma leads to features of chronic dermatitis. This produces thickening of the epi-

dermis (acanthosis) and expansion of the surface keratin layer (hyperkeratosis). The rete ridges become elongated and the dermis becomes fibrotic with prominent thick-walled vessels. The term subacute dermatitis is used when there are chronic features along with evidence of acute damage such as spongiosis and vesicle formation.

Non-specific dermatitis

The causes of non-specific dermatitis are many and one of the commonest is atopic dermatitis. This is predominantly a disease of infancy and childhood and produces an intensely itchy rash that is scratched by the child causing secondary changes. It often improves with age but may persist into adolescence and adulthood. It is associated with excess IgE production in response to a range of stimuli, and affected patients often have a family history of atopic eczema or of hay fever and asthma.

Contact dermatitis

This may be of two types: irritant and allergic.

Irritant contact dermatitis

This is due to direct damage from exposure to substances such as detergents and alkalis (e.g. washing-up liquid or soaps) and is common in housewives or in other occupational exposure.

Allergic contact dermatitis (see Ch. 4)

This is a delayed type IV hypersensitivity reaction to substances such as rubber (which may be a particular problem for dentists), nickel (a common component of dental prostheses), dyes and cosmetics. In hypersensitivity to rubber, there is probably an inherited predisposition to develop hypersensitivity which is mediated by Langerhans' cells in the epidermis, leading to CD4-positive T lymphocyte cytokine activation. Gravitational dermatitis occurs in the lower limbs of people with varicose veins and often has a brown colour because of repeated leakage of blood with haemosiderin accumulation (varicose eczema).

Psoriasis

This is a common condition affecting 1–2% of the population and presents classically with oval red plaques with a silvery scale on extensor surfaces of elbows and knees and on the scalp. The underlying skin surface bleeds when the scale is lifted off. Some patients develop prominent nail changes and a few have a chronic arthropathy very similar to rheumatoid arthritis, although serological markers of rheumatoid disease are negative. There is a positive family history in about one-third of patients and associations with the major histocompatibility (HLA) system have been described. Histologically, there is evidence of hyperproliferation with acanthosis of the epidermis and thickening and elongation of rete ridges. On the surface there is parakeratosis with collections of neutrophil polymorphs (Munro microabscesses). The dermis is oedematous and the dermal capillaries are dilated and bleed easily.

Lichen planus

This is a common inflammatory condition of the skin which affects the flexor aspects of the forearms, wrists and ankles, as well as the genitalia and the oral mucosa where it produces white narrow streaks. On the skin, it causes small itchy papules, which are purple-red in colour often with delicate white lines on the surface. Histologically, the epidermis is acanthotic with a saw-tooth appearance and there is damage to the basal layer of epidermis, so-called liquefactive degeneration, with extensive lymphocytic infiltration of the dermo-epidermal junction. Damaged basal cells that have undergone apoptosis may be seen higher in the epidermis as Civatte bodies. The pattern of dense lymphocytic infiltration at the dermo-epidermal junction is referred to as 'lichenoid' and may be seen in other conditions that lack the clinical features of lichen planus and particularly in drug reactions.

Lupus erythematosus

This covers a range of conditions including chronic discoid lupus erythematosus (DLE) which affects only the skin and has no systemic involvement and systemic lupus erythematosus (SLE) where there is prominent vasculitic involvement of many organs, especially the kidneys, and where skin involvement may be minor. Serum autoantibodies against DNA and other nuclear factors are present in SLE and less commonly in DLE. In DLE, lesions occur on sun-exposed areas and consist of red scaly patches that heal with scarring. Histologically, the epidermis is atrophic and hyperkeratotic; there is degeneration of the basal layer similar to lichen planus and a patchy lymphocytic infiltrate around dermal vessels.

Direct immunofluorescence reveals IgG deposition at the dermo-epidermal junction (so-called lupus band), which is present only in affected skin in DLE but may be seen in apparently normal skin in SLE.

SUMMARY BOX
DERMATOSES

- These are inflammatory conditions which may affect either dermis or epidermis.
- Acute eczematous dermatitis may lead to blister formation.
- Atopic dermatitis is one of the causes of non-specific dermatitis.
- Contact dermatitis may be due either to direct damage or to a type IV hypersensitivity reaction.
- Psoriasis is a common condition associated with hyperproliferation of skin, and affected patients may have joint problems.
- Lichen planus may affect the oral mucosa as well as other skin sites.
- Lupus erythematosus may be either localized or systemic, and skin rashes are common.

BLISTERING SKIN CONDITIONS

These are classified according to the site of separation of the epidermis, whether intraepidermal or subepidermal or basal. Vesicles are less than 5 mm in diameter, whereas bullae are greater than 5 mm in diameter. Immunofluorescence (IF) studies for immunoglobulins, mainly IgG and IgA, and complement components, mainly C3, are useful in identifying the specific condition present (Fig. 15.2).

Intraepidermal blisters

These may occur (a) as a result of spongiosis due to fluid accumulation, as in atopic and contact dermatitis, (b) because of reticular degeneration following balloon degeneration and necrosis, as in herpesviral infections and some drug reactions including erythema multiforme, and (c) as a result of acantholysis, as in pemphigus vulgaris, where large flaccid bullae develop on reddened skin in middle-aged and elderly patients who have pemphigus antibodies in their serum and have positive IF for IgG and C3 in the epidermis or oral mucosa. Up to 50% of patients with pemphigus vulgaris present with severe oral blistering.

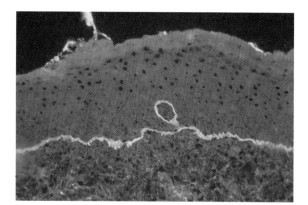

Fig. 15.2 Direct immunofluorescence for IgG from a biopsy of the oral mucosa showing benign mucous membrane pemphigoid.

Subepidermal or basal blisters

These develop from separation of the epidermis from the basement membrane or from separation of the epidermis and basement membrane from the underlying dermis. These conditions may be subclassified on the basis of the inflammatory cells within the vesicles.

Bullous pemphigoid

This is a disease of the elderly where large tense bullae occur especially on the lower limbs, and involvement of the oral mucosa is rare. Cicatricial pemphigoid (benign mucous membrane pemphigoid) involves the oral mucosa, eyes and genital regions. The characteristic inflammatory cell found is the eosinophil in the dermis and IF reveals IgG (and often IgA and IgM) and C3 along the basement membrane (Fig. 15.2). Eosinophils are also found in herpes gestationis, a rare blistering condition which develops in women in mid-to-late pregnancy.

Dermatitis herpetiformis

Neutrophil polymorphs are the predominant cell in dermatitis herpetiformis where there is subepidermal bulla formation with microabscess formation in the upper dermis. This condition affects young adults and is frequently seen in association with gluten-sensitive enteropathy (coeliac disease). IF demonstrates IgA in the dermal papillae.

Epidermolysis bullosa

In this condition, whether congenital or acquired, there is little or no inflammatory component. The site of separa-

tion varies in the congenital forms, which determines the prognosis: lethal in the early weeks of life in junctional epidermolysis bullosa; scarring in dystrophic epidermolysis bullosa; and good healing without scarring in epidermolysis bullosa simplex. The acquired form occurs in adult life with blistering on minor trauma affecting the hands or feet and may be associated with autoimmune diseases, malignancies or chronic inflammatory bowel diseases.

Erythema multiforme

This may follow preceding viral infections (particularly HSV) or exposure to drugs and is characterized by subepidermal bulla formation where the roof of the bulla is formed by necrotic keratinocytes.

SUMMARY BOX
BLISTERING SKIN CONDITIONS

- These are classified according to the site of separation of the skin; immunofluorescence may demonstrate immune-complex deposition.
- Intraepidermal blisters occur in atopic and contact dermatitis, viral skin infections and in pemphigus vulgaris.
- Subepidermal or basal blisters may be subclassified on the basis of the inflammatory cells present within the blisters:
  - eosinophils are common in bullous pemphigoid and herpes gestationis
  - neutrophils are common in dermatitis herpetiformis
  - few cells are seen in epidermolysis bullosa.

TUMOURS OF THE SKIN

Benign tumours
Basal cell papilloma

This lesion is also known as seborrhoeic keratosis and is a common benign warty growth, most often seen in the elderly on the face, chest and back. It has an exophytic growth pattern and is composed of cells resembling the basal layer of epidermis. Spherical masses of keratin in the form of horn cysts are present and melanin pigment is often prominent. This causes confusion with melanocytic lesions and leads to frequent excision biopsies. However, malignant change very rarely occurs in basal cell papillomas.

Squamous papilloma

This is most commonly a viral wart with koilocytes in the epidermis which is hyperkeratotic and acanthotic. Less frequently, squamous papillomas may be seen in the condition of linear epidermal naevi which are multiple hyperkeratotic warty lesions presenting at birth or in childhood, in a linear distribution on the trunk or the peripheries. Acanthosis nigricans is associated with internal malignancies such as carcinoma of the stomach or with endocrine diseases such as Cushing's syndrome or diabetes mellitus. The lesions are hyperkeratotic pigmented patches which are seen most often in the axillae, genitalia and neck regions.

Keratoacanthoma

This is a tumour-like lesion which causes confusion both clinically and histologically with squamous cell carcinoma. It occurs on sun-exposed skin, especially the face of adults, and presents as a rapidly growing nodule over an 8-week period, which involutes spontaneously over 6 months. Histologically, there is a well-defined shoulder of the lesion with a central crater filled with keratin, lined by proliferating squamous epithelium.

Malignant epithelial tumours

Basal cell carcinoma

This is the most frequently occurring malignant skin tumour which may develop on any part of the skin surface, especially in the elderly, and particularly on the face. They begin as a small nodule which undergoes central ulceration as the tumour grows, producing a characteristic raised rolled pearly edge. They are often multifocal producing a superficial pattern of spread; another pattern is the morphoea type where the tumour induces an intense desmoplastic stromal response. Histologically, they are composed of nests and downgrowths of basal cells from the overlying epidermis, showing typical peripheral palisading. They rarely if ever metastasize but have a propensity for deep local spread and require extensive surgery.

Squamous cell carcinoma

This is the next most common malignant skin tumour which arises on sun-exposed skin surfaces anywhere on the body, but especially on the face, ears, dorsum of the hands and lips. Apart from sun exposure, other risk factors include carcinogens such as tar and creosote and previously employed medicines such as arsenic. Long-term chronic irritation as seen at the edges of chronic venous ulcers and scars may also lead to the development of squamous cell carcinoma and there is an increased incidence of squamous carcinomas in immunosuppressed patients, especially renal transplant recipients. Histologically, most squamous carcinomas are well differentiated with abundant keratin production. They invade into surrounding tissues where they evoke a chronic inflammatory response and occasionally metastasize. The rate of metastasis, usually to lymph nodes, is higher in immunosuppressed individuals and from carcinomas arising in scars and ulcers and from the lower lip.

Premalignant conditions

There are two main premalignant lesions that may lead on to squamous carcinoma: actinic keratosis and Bowen's disease.

Actinic keratosis. This is also known as solar keratosis and occurs on the face, scalp and hands as irregular patches up to 1 cm in diameter with a hardened rough hyperkeratotic surface. Histologically there is atypia and dysplasia of cells in the lower half of the epidermis along with signs of solar damage of the collagen in the adjacent dermis.

Bowen's disease. This usually presents as a sharply defined red scaly patch which histologically shows full thickness dysplasia which may extend into adnexal structures. There is marked epithelial atypia with abnormal mitotic figures and multinucleated cells. In distinction to squamous carcinoma there is no invasion of the dermis and this rarely supervenes.

Adnexal tumours

These are much less common than tumours of the epidermis. They are most often seen in the head and neck regions and are usually benign, albeit with a tendency to recurrence. They may arise from sweat glands at various levels, from apocrine glands and from pilosebaceous follicles. Very rarely, malignant metastasizing tumours may occur, the two most common of which are eccrine sweat gland carcinoma and sebaceous gland carcinoma.

Melanocytic tumours (Fig. 15.3)

Melanocytes are a normal component of the basal layer of the epidermis (Fig. 15.3A and B) and are the cells of

SUMMARY BOX
NON-MELANOCYTIC SKIN TUMOURS

- Benign tumours include squamous papillomas (viral or non-viral), basal cell papillomas and keratoacanthomas.
- The commonest malignant tumour is basal cell carcinoma (BCC); it is associated with basal cell naevus (Gorlin's) syndrome.
- Squamous cell carcinoma (SCC) is associated with sun exposure.
- Adnexal tumours arising from hair follicles and sweat and sebaceous glands are rare but are most frequently seen in the head and neck regions.
- Cutaneous lymphomas are uncommon but are most often of T cell origin.
- Dermal tumours arise from normal dermal components; common lesions include fibrous lesions and vascular tumours.

origin of a number of important lesions including naevi, which are hamartomas or tumour-like conditions, and invasive malignant tumours.

Benign melanocytic tumours

Junctional naevus (Fig. 15.3C). This is composed of clumps of melanocytes situated at the dermo-epidermal junction. They are most common in childhood and adolescence and are seen as uniformly and deeply pigmented flat lesions (macules).

Compound naevus (Fig. 15.3D). This consists of a mixture of cells similar to those seen in junctional naevi along with clusters of cells in the upper dermis, which tend to become smaller the deeper they are situated in the dermis, probably indicating maturation. They are seen most commonly in adolescents and young adults and are typically raised nodular lesions with a slightly irregular surface but with uniform pigmentation.

Intradermal naevi (Fig. 15.3E). These are composed exclusively of naevus cells within the dermis and there is no epidermal or junctional component. They occur in adults and are raised lesions often with a smooth domed surface, in which pigmentation is less obvious than in the forms of naevi described above.

Blue naevi. These are variants of the usual naevi and are intradermal lesions consisting of very heavily pigmented melanocytes within irregular bands of coarse collagen. They appear blue-black through the epidermis, although on sectioning they are brown within the dermis. They are usually noticed first in childhood and grow slowly, achieving a large size in the buttocks, although

A. Normal

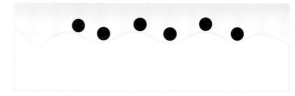

B. Lentigo

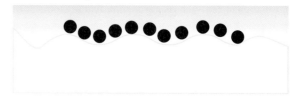

C. Junctional naevus

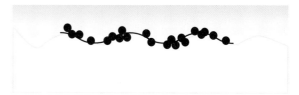

D. Compound naevus

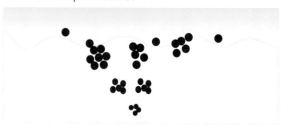

E. Intradermal naevus

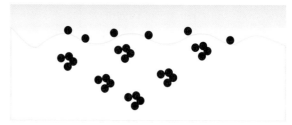

Fig. 15.3 Melanocytic lesions. A. Normal skin showing normal distribution of melanocytes in the basal layer. **B.** Lentigo (freckle) where there are increased numbers of melanocytes in the basal layer. **C.** Junctional naevus where there are clusters of naevus cells at the dermo-epidermal junction. **D.** Compound naevus where there are nests of naevus cells in the dermis with junctional activity of cells at the dermo-epidermal junction. **E.** Intradermal naevus where there are clusters of naevus cells only within the dermis.

smaller blue naevi arise on the arms and head. Very rarely, they may become malignant.

Spitz naevi. These are also known as juvenile naevi and, as this name implies, they occur in childhood. Histologically, they may show considerable pleomorphism and atypia, causing difficulty in differentiation from malignant melanoma. Clinically, they present as raised reddish-brown smooth-surfaced nodules.

Risk of malignant change. Most naevi are benign and have very little potential for malignant transformation. However, in a small minority, malignant change can occur. In these situations, it is the changes noted at the dermo-epidermal junction which predict progression. These include variation in size and shape of the melanocytes (cytological atypia) and loss of the normal rounded distribution of cell nests with flattening and extension along rete ridges (architectural atypia). Clinically, these changes manifest as an alteration in the size of an existing naevus, often with irregularity of its outline, colour or surface. Such changes are an indication of possible malignancy and should lead to an excision biopsy. In most cases, they are single lesions but occasionally, especially where there is a family history, may be multiple and form part of the dysplastic naevus syndrome.

Malignant melanoma (Fig. 15.4)

This malignant tumour of melanocytic origin is increasing in incidence and is seen particularly in white-skinned people. The main predisposing factor is exposure to ultraviolet (UV) light and is mainly due to increased sun exposure on holidays, possibly exacerbated by thinning of the ozone layer which reduces its filtering effect on sunlight. It is much less common in people of dark skins because of protection from UV irradiation by melanin pigment in the epidermis. It is slightly more common in women than men and occurs more frequently on the legs in women and on the trunk in men. It may also arise outside the skin from mucosal surfaces including the oral mucosa and the nose and from the pigmented choroidal epithelium in the eye.

A number of different patterns of malignant melanoma are recognized.

Lentigo maligna (Fig. 15.4A). This is a proliferation of junctional melanocytes occurring on the face of elderly men and women. Sometimes a raised solid nodule develops from these lesions representing the formation of an early nodular malignant melanoma (lentigo malignant melanoma).

A. Lentigo malignant melanoma

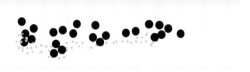

B. Superficial spreading malignant melanoma

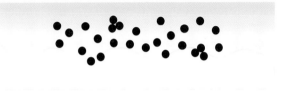

C. Nodular malignant melanoma

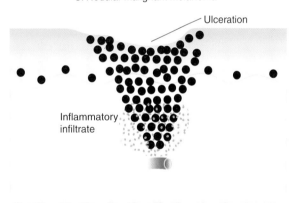

Fig. 15.4 Malignant melanoma. A. Lentigo maligna melanoma where there are malignant cells in the basal layers of epidermis and infiltrating the upper dermis. **B.** Superficial spreading malignant melanoma where there are malignant cells at the dermo-epidermal junction which spread upwards and laterally through the epidermis (horizontal growth phase). **C.** Nodular malignant melanoma where malignant cells migrate upwards into the epidermis (epidermotropism), possibly causing ulceration, and downwards into the dermis (vertical growth phase). The deeper the invasion into epidermis, measured in Clark's levels and Breslow thickness, the more likely that vascular invasion and distal metastasis will occur.

Superficial spreading malignant melanoma (Fig. 15.4B). This is the most common form of melanoma, presenting as a flat lesion with irregular edges and variable pigmentation. This can be either an in situ lesion, where the atypical melanocytes are confined to the epidermis, or invasive, where the atypical cells invade the upper dermis. This is the form of melanoma which is increasing in incidence, but if identified early, is also the form most amenable to curative resection.

Nodular malignant melanoma (Fig. 15.4C). This accounts for about 5% of the total of malignant melanomas and presents without a precursor lesion as a raised black-brown nodule.

Acral/mucosal lentiginous malignant melanomas. These are rare lesions occurring in the hands and feet, especially the soles of the feet, and occasionally beneath the nails (subungual) of the fingers and toes. Histologically, it is a form of superficial spreading melanoma and, although most common in white-skinned people, it is often seen in Orientals.

The histological diagnosis of malignant melanoma is made on the finding of atypical melanocytes arranged in clumps and nests in the upper and basal layers of the epidermis (in situ) and of similar clusters in the upper dermis (invasive). Tumours which spread along the epidermis, such as the superficial spreading type, are said to be in the horizontal growth phase, whereas those which invade into the dermis, such as nodular melanomas and later-stage superficial spreading malignant melanomas, are said to be in the vertical growth phase.

Spread of malignant melanoma. Malignant melanoma has the potential to metastasize via lymphatics to regional and distant lymph nodes and via the bloodstream to distant sites such as the lung, liver and brain but also to unusual sites such as the heart and gastrointestinal tract. These metastases may arise many years after the first presentation. In order for metastasis to occur, malignant cells must be able to enter lymphatic and blood vessels and, therefore, the deeper a tumour has invaded the dermis the more likely it is to spread as it encounters more vascular channels. This fact has led to the identification of prognostic factors in malignant melanoma. The Breslow thickness refers to the depth of invasion into the dermis measured from the granular layer of the epidermis: tumours less than 0.75 mm carry a low risk of spread; tumours between 0.76 and 1.5 mm have a moderate risk; while those greater than 1.5 mm in thickness carry a high risk of distant spread. This is mirrored by Clark's levels which describe the depth of invasion related to the skin structures: level 1 being confined to the epidermis, level 2 the papillary dermis and so on. This method is less reproducible than Breslow thickness measurement and is not as accurate in predicting outcome.

SUMMARY BOX
MELANOCYTIC SKIN TUMOURS

- Melanocytes are normal components of the basal layer of epidermis.
- Benign melanocytic lesions (naevi) may be intradermal, junctional or compound.
- Melanomas are malignant tumours of melanocytic origin; they may arise from pre-existing lesions or arise anew; they are associated with sun exposure.
- Features which may herald malignant transformation include changes in pigmentation, changes in size and shape, and itching.
- Malignant melanomas have a number of patterns; prognosis is related to the size and rate of growth of the tumour.

Cutaneous lymphomas

The skin may occasionally be involved by malignant lymphomas from elsewhere in the body. Less commonly, primary lymphomas may arise in the skin and these are usually of T cell origin. Mycosis fungoides is usually confined to the skin but may show lymph node and systemic spread. Sézary's syndrome refers to the presence of a generalized erythematous skin rash, enlarged lymph nodes and the finding of large atypical T lymphocytes in the peripheral blood.

Dermal tumours
Fibrohistiocytic lesions

These are relatively common tumours occurring in middle age and are composed of varying amounts of fibroblasts, producing collagen, and other mesenchymal cells including smooth muscle cells and blood vessels. In some, histiocytes are prominent and contain lipids giving a yellow appearance on a cut surface, while, in others, haemosiderin from leaking blood vessels gives a brown appearance on sectioning. Most present as raised nodules in which the overlying epidermis is acanthotic and hyperkeratotic. The vast majority of superficial dermal tumours are benign but two tumours with histological similarities may be encountered: dermatofibrosarcoma protuberans and malignant fibrous histiocytoma.

Vascular tumours

Most vascular lesions presenting in the skin are probably not true neoplasms but represent hamartomas (tumour-like malformations). These include capillary haemangiomas which present in childhood on the trunk, buttocks or face as strawberry naevi and grow, often alarmingly, before regressing spontaneously; cavernous haemangiomas which are similar though larger lesions which do not regress; and port-wine stains which present at birth on the face or neck as large flat red-purple areas which may continue to grow and do not regress. Pyogenic granulomas are common raised nodules with superficial ulceration composed of what appears to be granulation tissue with neutrophil polymorph infiltration. They occur commonly in the fingers and arms, and the head and neck region including the buccal and gingival mucosa. True vascular neoplasms include the glomus tumour, which often presents in the nail beds as exquisitely tender lesions, and angiosarcoma, a highly malignant tumour of vascular origin occurring in the elderly in the head and scalp. Kaposi's sarcoma is one of the defining lesions of AIDS. These lesions are often multiple and occur throughout the skin surface and especially in the oral mucosa. They are associated particularly with a specific type of human herpesvirus type 8 infection. They start as small reddish patches and expand into plaques and later nodules. Histologically, they consist of vascular channels within a spindle cell stroma showing variable degrees of pleomorphism.

ASPECTS OF SKIN DISEASE OF PARTICULAR RELEVANCE TO DENTISTRY

- Many immuno-inflammatory conditions occurring in the skin also involve the oral mucosa.
- Contact dermatitis is an occupational hazard for dentists especially using latex gloves.
- Dentists should be aware of the principles of patch testing since reactions to dental materials are increasingly being recognized.

CASE STUDY 15.1
MOUTH PROBLEMS AFTER HEPATITIS

A 48-year-old Italian woman attended her dentist because she had developed red sore gums and a rough sensation on the buccal mucosa over a 6-month period. Recently, the problem was becoming troublesome because painful ulcers appeared often after eating. Her medical history included gout and hepatitis many years previously. The hepatitis was detected when she presented for blood donation some years

earlier and was told that she had antihepatitis C virus (HCV) antibodies in her serum, later confirmed on a positive polymerase chain reaction (PCR) for HCV RNA. She took allopurinol for the gout but was otherwise fit and well.

On questioning, she recalled that she had experienced an itchy rash on the wrists, ankles and trunk 1 year ago but had not associated this with her oral condition. The rash had virtually resolved but a few raised and flat purple lesions with faint white surface striae remained on her wrists.

Intraoral examination revealed white plaques, striae and erythematous areas on the buccal mucosa and lateral tongue in a bilateral distribution. Superficial ulceration was present on the buccal mucosa and this was painful on examination.

An incisional biopsy was taken from the buccal mucosa and the pathologist reported this as 'consistent with lichen planus but that other forms of lichenoid mucositis should be excluded by clinical investigation'.

1. Several conditions can manifest as chronic, red, atrophic gingival lesions. What clinical term is used to describe this feature and which diseases may cause it?
2. Are there any possible links between the medical history and lichen planus?
3. Which histopathological features in the biopsy would lead the pathologist to the diagnosis?
4. Which other diseases may result in lichenoid mucositis?

Suggested responses (see also Ch. 10)

1. The clinical term 'desquamative gingivitis' is used to describe the clinical manifestation of several disorders. Lichen planus is the most common cause of desquamative gingivitis but cicatricial pemphigoid, bullous pemphigoid, pemphigus, plasma cell mucositis, allergic gingivitis and other chronic dermatoses can be indistinguishable clinically. Other lesions on the skin, mucosa or elsewhere may be helpful, but biopsy aided by immunofluorescence enables the distinction to be made.

2. An association between hepatitis C and lichen planus has been made from epidemiological evidence in Italy where the prevalence of hepatitis C is relatively high. Numerous drugs have been reported to trigger or amplify lichen planus, including allopurinols, antimalarials, gold, non-steroidal anti-inflammatory drugs and others.

3. In biopsies of oral lichen planus the epithelium may show parakeratosis or orthokeratosis and can be thickened or atrophic. A dense band of subepithelial lymphohistiocytic infiltrate consisting mostly of T lymphocytes is present and a key feature is liquefaction degeneration of the basal epithe-

lial cells. The degenerative process is due to apoptosis and it involves nuclear fragmentation, cytoplasmic shrinkage and ultimately swelling to form Civatte (colloid) bodies. Some T lymphocytes enter the lower layers of the epithelium and cytotoxic (CD8) cells are thought to mediate damage. Not all features are invariably present in oral biopsies, including the 'saw-tooth' rete processes which characterize the skin lesions of lichen planus. Immunofluorescence may show fibrin deposition at the basement membrane.

4. Lichenoid mucositis is a clinical term for an appearance which may be due to lichen planus, lupus erythematosus, lichenoid reaction to drugs and restorative dental materials, and graft-versus-host disease.

CASE STUDY 15.2
BLISTERS IN THE MOUTH

A 9-year-old girl complained of feeling unwell and was noted by her mother to have a slightly raised temperature. The next day her mouth became uncomfortable and numerous small blisters (vesicles) appeared on the gingivae, palate, buccal mucosa and tongue. These soon ulcerated and her tongue became progressively coated as she refused to eat. Cervical lymph nodes on both sides of the neck enlarged and became tender to touch. Fresh crops of vesicles developed over the next few days in the oral cavity and on the lips and circumoral skin. Painful blisters then appeared on the fingertips and her eyes also became inflamed. The gingivae became erythematous (reddened) and oedematous (swollen by fluid exudation). Her GP advised that she should stay away from school and should maintain an adequate fluid intake. After 10–14 days, the oral lesions had almost resolved, though the lesions on her fingers crusted and persisted for 6 weeks.

2 Years later she was taken on holiday to Spain and after a few days complained of itching and tingling of the lips. Within a few hours she developed small clusters of vesicles on the lips which quickly became crusted. These 'cold sores' healed within 10 days. Later she found that application of acyclovir cream to the sores at the itching stage prevented the eruption of the cold sores.

1. What is the most likely cause of the initial infection?
2. Which other viruses can cause infections in the oral cavity?
3. How was the virus transmitted to the fingers? What are these lesions called?
4. What mechanisms are involved in the development of the recurrent lesions manifesting 2 years after the primary infection?

5. Which factors may trigger recurrent cold sores?
6. What is the likely trigger factor in this case? How could it be avoided?

Suggested responses (see also Ch. 5)

1. The history strongly suggests infection with herpes simplex virus (HSV). There are two types of HSV, type 1 being most often associated with the oral region and type 2 with the genitalia, though overlap may occur. HSV is a DNA virus and the infection is transmitted by droplet spread or contact with the lesions. The clinical term 'primary herpetic gingivostomatitis' is used to describe the syndrome seen when a patient becomes infected for the first time by HSV and is usually seen in children and young adults. Intact vesicles are rarely seen; most often they break down into ulcers by the time the patient seeks advice. Primary infection by HSV may, however, be subclinical.

2. HSV is by far the most common virus to produce clinical oral infection. Various types of the coxsackievirus A produce two distinct clinical infections called 'herpangina' and 'hand, foot and mouth disease'. Measles virus produces small blue-white spots on the oral mucosa (Koplik's spots) in the early stages of infection. Chickenpox and shingles caused by the herpesvirus varicella zoster may involve the oral cavity. Glandular fever caused by the Epstein–Barr virus (EBV) can produce oral ulceration and petechial haemorrhages in the oral cavity but the appearances are rather non-specific. In immunocompromised patients, EBV may manifest as white papillary plaques on the lateral tongue, known as hairy leukoplakia. Cytomegalovirus (CMV) infection is also seen mainly in immunocompromised patients where it manifests as oral ulceration.

3. HSV is often transmitted from the oral cavity in primary herpetic gingivostomatitis to the hands as a result of finger-sucking. Infection of the nail bed is known as herpetic whitlow and is painful. Infection may be spread from the fingers to the eyes by rubbing.

4. Approximately one-third of those who have had primary herpes infection experience recurrent infection which manifests as local lesions without systemic illness. Most often these secondary lesions occur on the lips and circumoral skin, where they are known as cold sores or herpes labialis. HSV often remains latent in the trigeminal ganglion following primary infection and recurrences are due to reactivation. Viral particles migrate down the axoplasm and may be destroyed by cell-mediated immunity, shed asymptomatically or cause local infection. Recurrence is associated with transient or prolonged immunosuppression. In latency, HSV

DNA transcription is blocked. The sensory ganglion is an immunoprivileged site and antiviral drugs are ineffective in eliminating the virus from the ganglion.

5. Recurrent cold sores may be triggered by febrile illnesses such as the common cold, menstruation, trauma, ultraviolet light, stress and immunosuppression. In severe immunosuppressive states such as late-stage HIV infection, large and persistent herpetic lesions are a frequent feature.

6. Ultraviolet light is the most likely trigger factor in this case and the use of sun-block on the lips would prevent recurrences.

Further reading

It is not envisaged that this book alone will provide all the information required on pathology for students of dentistry, although it is designed to provide the essentials, to help in revision for assessements and to support PBL courses.

Other textbooks of pathology designed for undergraduate curricula, especially for medical curricula, provide another approach which may benefit some students. These include:

- General and Systematic Pathology, 3rd edition, ed. JCE Underwood, Churchill Livingstone, 2000
- Muir's Textbook and Pathology, 14th edition, eds. RNM MacSween & K Whaley, Hodder & Stoughton, 1992
- Pathologic Basis of Disease, eds. Robbins, Cotran & Kumar, Saunders
- Pathology, A Stevens & J Lowe, Mosby, 2000

while more detailed information is available in

- Oxford Textbook of Pathology, eds. JO'D McGee, PG Isaacson & NA Wright, Oxford University Press, 1992

There was no attempt in this book to supplant the excellent textbooks already available on oral pathology with which students will become familiar in their future careers. These include:

- Oral Pathology, 3rd edition, JV Soames & JC Southam, Oxford University Press, 1998
- Essentials of Oral Pathology and Medicine, 6th edition, RA Cawson & EW Odell, Churchill Livingstone, 1998

In immunopathology, students are referred to the excellent text

- Immunology, 5th edition, I Roitt, J Brostoff & D Male, Mosby-Wolfe, 1997

In genetics, a useful source of information is

- Human Molecular Genetics, T Strachan & AP Read, 2nd edition, Bios Scientific Publishers, 1996

No specific references to original articles have been given in this text. However, students familiar with the PBL approach will already have access to search engines for use on the internet which will allow them to retrieve up to the minute references on a range of topics, especially through systems such as Medline.

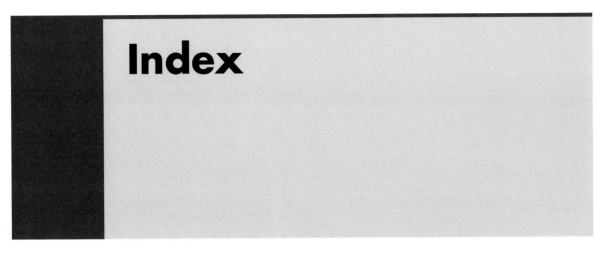

Index